# GENDER, STATE, AND MEDICINE IN HIGHLAND ECUADOR

PITT LATIN AMERICAN SERIES

John Charles Chasteen and Catherine M. Conaghan, Editors

# Gender, State, and Medicine in Highland Ecuador

## MODERNIZING WOMEN, MODERNIZING THE STATE, 1895–1950

### A. KIM CLARK

University of Pittsburgh Press

Published by the University of Pittsburgh Press, Pittsburgh, Pa., 15260

Copyright © 2012, University of Pittsburgh Press
Manufactured in the United States of America

Printed on acid-free paper

10 9 8 7 6 5 4 3 2 1


Library of Congress Cataloging-in-Publication Data

Clark, A. Kim, 1964–
    Gender, state, and medicine in Highland Ecuador : modernizing women, modernizing the
state, 1895–1950 / A. Kim Clark.
        p.      cm. — (Pitt Latin American series)
    Includes bibliographical references and index.
    ISBN 978-0-8229-6209-0 (pbk. : alk. paper)
    1. Women—Ecuador—Social conditions—20th century. 2. Women—Government policy—
Ecuador—History—20th century. 3. Women's rights—Ecuador—History—20th century.
4. Women—Medical care—Ecuador—History—20th century. 5. Medical education—
Ecuador—History—20th century. 6. Public welfare—Ecuador—History—20th century.
7. Ecuador—Social policy—20th century.    I. Title.
    HQ1557.C53 2012
    305.409866—dc23                                               2012006940

To my father-in-law, Eduardo Larrea Stacey

# CONTENTS

ACKNOWLEDGMENTS    ix

CHAPTER 1.   Gendered Experiences and State Formation in
             Highland Ecuador    1

CHAPTER 2.   Gender, Class, and State in Child Protection Programs
             in Quito    33

CHAPTER 3.   Governing Sexuality and Disease    78

CHAPTER 4.   Midwifery, Morality, and the State    112

CHAPTER 5.   The Transformation of Ecuadorian Nursing    143

Conclusion    184

NOTES    193
BIBLIOGRAPHY    235
INDEX    247

# ACKNOWLEDGMENTS

This book is more personal than any prior project. When I began to collect archival material for it almost two decades ago, I was working on a differently defined project; when I began to write this book, then too I thought I was writing a different book. Despite my initial intentions, I found myself pulled in by compelling historical situations and figures that I came across in the archival materials, the interpretation of which caught and held my imagination. If I had to identify a single starting point of that process, it would be my chance encounter in the archives in 1994 with a 1912 document referring to the teaching staff at the Escuela-Taller de Mujeres in Quito, where it became clear from the context that it was not public knowledge that one of the unmarried women teaching at the school, whose name I recognized, had given birth to a son two years previously.

I continued to turn that over in my mind as I discovered the conflict-ridden nature of women's work in paramedical fields, and even more so as the archives yielded up a clear social profile of some of Ecuador's first professional women: scientific midwives. I had a growing sense that there was a story to tell not only about restrictive gender ideologies and double morality—something that is self-evident in the historical record as well as in everyday life in highland Ecuador, including in the years since I began to visit and study the country in 1986—but also about the activities of particular kinds of women in the Ecuadorian public sphere *despite* those restrictions.

This is also a more personal project because of how much it depended ultimately on conversations with women (and men too) in Quito, both those belonging to my personal networks and those with whom I sought interviews because of their early professional activities. Given the still relatively few studies of gender history in early-twentieth-century highland Ecuador, conversations with women were particularly fruitful in helping me to understand the archival materials I was encountering, and many of those conversations included discussions of anecdotes from the archives that I was struggling to contextualize and interpret. I thank those friends and consultants for their patience not only in considering and responding to my questions but also in waiting for these research results, which seem to have been a long time in coming given the distinctly nonlinear research process involved.

I conducted thought-provoking (and highly enjoyable) interviews with Adrila Aguirre, Cecilia de Arellano, Iralda Benítez de Núñez, Ximena Cevallos, Clemencia Gía, Clemencia Larrea de Vela, María Clemencia (Morocha) Martínez de Larrea, María (Maruja) Martínez de Suárez, Piedad Mesías Mateo de Rubio, Georgina Morales de Carrillo, Fabiola Quevedo, Alcides Rubio, Elina Rubio, Rosa Santamaría, Aurelia Stacey, and Margarita Velasco. I also thank Dr. Eduardo Luna Yépez, fortuitously my neighbor in Quito, for his frankness and willingness to indulge my curiosity during a number of conversations about the history of the medical profession in Quito. My understanding of these materials has also been enhanced by conversations with many other friends in Quito over the years, including Alicia and Ximena Andrade, Rocío Bedón, Valeria Coronel, Antonio Crespo, Patricia de la Torre, Sonia Fernández, Ana María Goetschel, Mariana Landázuri, Raúl Mideros, Fabiola Montúfar, Martha Moscoso, Elena and Sandra Noboa, Mercedes Prieto, Catalina Rubio, Guadalupe Soasti, Luis Suárez, and Serena Van der Werff.

As I moved toward an interpretation of the processes explored in this book, feedback from colleagues and friends on conference presentations and chapter drafts has also been very helpful. My thanks to Michiel Baud, Marc Becker, John Clarke, Kendra Coulter, Juanita de Barros, Paulo Drinot, Lindsay Dubois, Nicola Foote, Margaret Kellow, Chris Krupa, Esben Leifsen, Shelley McKellar, David Nugent, Steve Palmer, Paul Potter, and Liz Roberts. Erin O'Connor deserves an extra measure of gratitude for reading through and commenting so helpfully on the entire manuscript. Colleagues and graduate students in the Anthropology Department at the University of Western Ontario engaged with various iterations of these materials during departmental research colloquia over a number of years. My thanks especially to a wonderful and supportive group of colleagues in the department who followed the evolution of this project with interest over a considerable period of time. Tracey Adams and Luz María Hernández Sáenz, colleagues in UWO's Faculty of Social Science with common interests in the social history of medicine and medical professionals, provided good company and constructive criticism of unwieldy chapter drafts over lunch. As the research and this analysis progressed, many conversations with Verónica Schild helped shape how I think about gender, social policy, and state formation.

Some of the most enthusiastic and evocative responses that I received to this work-in-progress, however, were from an audience of high-school history teachers gathered at the Congreso Ecuatoriano de Historia in July 2009, and in May 2010 from students and professionals at the Escuela Nacional de Enfermería and at the Escuela de Obstetricia of the Universidad Central. I greatly appreciate their interest in this research and their feedback on its principal findings. Of course, I alone am responsible for any errors of fact or interpretation.

Several research projects yielded archival materials and interviews relevant to this project, even though not all of those projects were initially oriented toward these problems. I am grateful for generous funding from Associated Medical Services, Toronto (for sustained support over three grants, despite delays in producing results as I took time away from research both for maternity leaves and to undertake nonresearch roles on campus); the Wenner-Gren Foundation for Anthropological Research, New York (for two grants); the Social Sciences and Humanities Research Council of Canada (SSHRC) (for a postdoctoral fellowship during which I first began to encounter these intriguing research materials); and the University of Western Ontario (for grants under the internal SSHRC and International Research Awards competitions as well as support from the Agnes Cole Dark Fund within the Faculty of Social Science).

The research that underlies this book spanned from postdoctoral work beginning in 1993, through my first sabbatical leave, culminating with the writing of the manuscript during my second such leave, interspersed with numerous shorter research trips to Quito. Too many people to name facilitated that research in Quito in a wide range of ways. Among them I would especially like to thank the friendly and helpful staff at the Museo Nacional de Medicina, housing the Archivo de la Asistencia Pública (AAP), the Archivo del Servicio de Sanidad (ASS), and the Archivo del Hospital Civil San Juan de Dios (AHCSJD), and the staff at the Archivo General de la Universidad Central (AGUC). Elena Noboa served intermittently and expertly as my research assistant, and her sister Sandra Noboa facilitated my access to the records of the Escuela Nacional de Enfermería. I am very grateful to them both for arranging a number of oral history interviews for me. Finally, I thank Fabiola Montúfar, who in a subsequent project facilitated a number of interviews relevant both to this book and another one in preparation, and Valeria Coronel for putting me in contact with Fabiola.

In the final stages of writing *Gender, State, and Medicine in Highland Ecuador*, I had a wonderful experience (again) with the University of Pittsburgh

Press. My thanks to Joshua Shanholtzer for his support for this project and to the whole Pitt team for their help in bringing it to completion. Two anonymous reviewers provided helpful and challenging comments that improved the text. I am grateful too for Ed Eastaugh's map-making skills, Amy Smith Bell's careful copyediting, and Bob Schwarz's expert indexing.

My family has facilitated this work in numerous ways: my children, Juliana, Marisol, and Alejandro, by their eagerness to visit Quito as often and for as long as possible; and my husband, Fernando Larrea, for his willingness to discuss Ecuadorian society in general and my data in particular over breakfast, lunch, and dinner for almost two decades now. I would understand much less, and no doubt have also conducted less research, if it weren't for him. More important, I can't imagine how I would juggle work and family, Canada and Ecuador, without him, nor would I want to imagine such a thing. I take this opportunity to thank my mother, Marilyn Clark, and my mother-in-law, Morocha Martínez, in general for providing such wonderful examples of strong and intelligent women and more concretely for their interest in this project and their willingness—in different ways and very different contexts—to discuss these ideas. My father, Phil Clark, has also taken an interest in this project, listening and responding avidly to stories of the female figures that populate it. Tía Aurelia Stacey lived part of this era and experienced some of the difficult processes discussed throughout this book; her death just as this project was reaching completion is deeply felt.

As I researched and wrote this work, however, no one has been more present in my mind than that infant born in 1910; although I knew he had been born out of wedlock, it was the discovery of that 1912 document that began to reveal to me the efforts made to hide that fact. Indeed, he lived the first years of his life apart from his mother, using a name that was not his own. Despite such difficult beginnings he grew up to be a man of extraordinary integrity—*construyendo patria* in Ecuador in ways perhaps more recognized than, but ultimately not essentially unlike, the women I discuss in the second half of this book. I dedicate *Gender, State, and Medicine in Highland Ecuador*, in loving memory, to my father-in-law, Eduardo Larrea Stacey.

GENDER, STATE, AND MEDICINE IN HIGHLAND ECUADOR

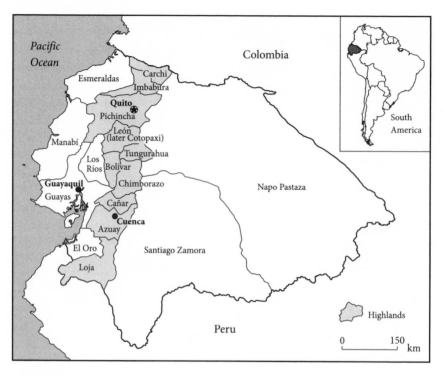

Political Divisions of Ecuador, c. 1920

# Gendered Experiences and
# State Formation in Highland Ecuador

This book explores the experiences of Ecuadorian women as both objects and agents of state formation, examining state practices, women's lives, and gender ideologies in the Ecuadorian highlands in the first half of the twentieth century. The subtitle *Modernizing Women, Modernizing the State* alludes on the one hand to state projects that attempted to modernize both women's behavior and the opportunities available to them, and on the other to the fact that some of the women involved were or became modernizers themselves. They seized on new opportunities and pressed the limits of those state projects in ways that perhaps were not anticipated. Thus they became active participants in the modernization of the Ecuadorian state, and in doing so they put their own imprint on processes that were also occurring elsewhere in a similar time period.

The analysis moves between two broad themes—state formation and patterns of women's experience and agency—bringing together a discussion of four general areas in which women's behavior was of interest to, and intervened by, state institutions. Child welfare and children's value (discussed in chapter 2) and prostitution and venereal disease (in chapter 3) were both arenas where women and girls became objects of state projects. New institutions, permeated by gender ideologies, were developed in these areas that increased the state's ability to act on gendered subjects and enlisted women's own participation in a range of ways. When we turn to examining midwifery and nursing (in chapters 4 and 5), however, we can see more clearly how women themselves became active agents in state projects.

Although child protection projects and control of venereal disease did turn Ecuadorian women into objects of state action, the operation of such programs also offered opportunities for women to exercise agency as they used state services to pursue their own goals. And while women who trained for new professional careers became state agents when they sought government employment, they were also the objects of state action via the provision of both new educational and employment opportunities and in the gendered ways they were objectified and their agency undermined (not always successfully) within state institutions. This book thus examines different permutations of how women were both objects and agents in the provision of social programs and state policy. What differs between chapters 2 and 3, and chapters 4 and 5, however, are some of the sources that allow a deeper reading of women's agency in the latter chapters. In their explorations of the functioning of specific state institutions and state programs, all of the chapters offer insight into processes of state formation, including attention to fissures within the state and specific ways that state and society were entwined, rather than constituting separate spheres of activity.

The period explored here is roughly the first half of the twentieth century, with significant changes initiated after the 1895 Liberal Revolution. The exact starting and end points in each chapter vary depending on the historical rhythms of the themes examined. For child protection policies, an early component of gendered social policy, we begin early in the liberal period and consider the decades up to passage of the 1938 Código de Menores, Ecuador's first Child Code. The history of antivenereal programs and prostitution control policies began later, with early projects from around 1910 but the Venereal Prophylaxis Service was only established in Quito in 1921. The heyday of antivenereal programs wound down after the 1943 discovery that penicillin was an effective treatment for syphilis, although the shift to new models was not immediate.

For midwifery, the first field of university study opened to women, stabilization of training began in the early 1890s, with a significant expansion of enrollments after the 1899 founding of the new Maternidad (lying-in hospital or maternity clinic) in Quito. For graduated midwives, state employment opportunities were expanded in 1935 with the establishment of a new maternal-infant health program within the Servicio de Sanidad (Public Health Service), so chapter 4 follows midwives up through the 1940s. Professional nursing came later, with the earliest classes begun in 1917, reorganization of nursing training in 1927, and a more profound transformation in models of nursing in 1942 with the founding of the National Nurses School as a collaborative effort of U.S. and Ecuadorian agencies. While chapter 5 begins with a consideration of early nursing projects, it focuses on the first decade of training at the Escuela Nacional de Enfermeras (1942–52), which allows a consideration of the challenges faced at midcentury by a new group of female professionals training and working in state institutions in highland Ecuador.

## Ecuadorian History Read through Women's Lives

Historical sociologist Philip Abrams has argued that "society must be understood as a process constructed historically by individuals who are constructed historically by society."[1]

In a suggestive discussion of the relation between individual and society, Abrams highlighted the ways that biological generations must be understood in conjunction with sociological generations. He argued that "the problem of generations . . . is a problem of the mutual phasing of two different calendars: the calendar of the life-cycle of the individual and the calendar of historical experiences. . . . New life-histories are constantly being lived in relation to new world-histories."[2] It was not so much that women gained new educational opportunities in Quito in the early twentieth century but that women of a specific age group did so. Moreover, "society" (including those women's social circumstances and positioning) made some of them particularly likely to be willing to grasp those new opportunities; their actions in doing so then propelled social change.

While we might think of the interplay of state projects and individual action in this context in terms of structure and agency, it is more useful to consider how state projects changed the terrain on which individuals could act, enabling certain possibilities and constraining others. Those state projects themselves were the contested results of conflict among dominant groups from the Ecuadorian coast and highlands, liberals and conservatives, and certainly church and state at the turn of the twentieth century. In other words, although they seem to form the structure within which women acted, those projects were themselves the result of human agency and struggle.[3] For those projects to then be realized—literally made real in life and not only confined to policy documents or official pronouncements—sometimes required substantial personal sacrifices, courage, and sheer stubbornness. One of my arguments is that social patterns can be discerned that suggest what kinds of women were more likely to display those characteristics, or rather, which social circumstances brought out those traits.

To illustrate these points, let us begin with accounts of some pioneering Ecuadorian women.[4] In 1921 Matilde Hidalgo became the first Ecuadorian woman to graduate as *doctora de medicina* (physician) from the Universidad Central in Quito. She had been born into what had been a middle-class family in the southern highland city of Loja in 1889. Because her mother was widowed just before Matilde's birth, she grew up in a fatherless household where her mother and older sister took in sewing to support the family and to allow her two brothers to continue their education. During her years as a primary student at a local Catholic school, Matilde had the opportunity to assist the nuns in their work at the small local hospital. She began to imagine pursuing a medical career. This would first require that she attend secondary school, but despite its status as a provincial capital, Loja did not have a secondary school for girls, although state schools open to young women had recently been established in the capital Quito and the main port of Guayaquil by the liberal governments that came to power in and after 1895.

Because there was only a secondary school for young men in Loja, Matilde petitioned in 1907 to be admitted to the Colegio Bernardo Valdivieso. Given that there was no explicit rule prohibiting women from attending, she was permitted to enroll. This created a scandal in Loja: female classmates from primary school were prohibited from speaking to her; she was mocked and insulted on her way to school; her mother was threatened with excommunication from the Catholic Church; and she had to manage difficult relationships with her male classmates. Following her graduation as *bachiller* in 1913 at the age of twenty-four, she applied to the medical program at Quito's Universidad Central. Despite her excellent grades, Matilde's application was rejected with the recommendation that she consider enrolling instead in the midwifery or pharmacy program—the only two areas of university study then open to women. She was more successful with an application to the undergraduate program in medicine at the Universidad de Azuay in the city of Cuenca (where she would be able to live with her brother and sister-in-law). Graduating as a licentiate in medicine in 1919, Matilde was finally accepted that year into the medical program at the Universidad Central to complete advanced studies. Unlike any of her male classmates, however, she was encouraged to enroll simultaneously in the third year of the midwifery program while she undertook her sixth year of medical studies, and the following year pursued the final year of courses in both programs.[5] She did her medical internship at the Maternidad, directed by Loja-born physician Isidro Ayora, where by definition Matilde would treat only female patients. In 1921 at the age of thirty-two she graduated as doctora de medicina from the Universidad Central.

Moving to Guayaquil—where her brother had by then settled with his family—Matilde took up positions in the Hospital General and then the Casa Cuna Juan Arzube Cordero (an orphanage). In 1923 she married lawyer Fernando Prócel, who had been her classmate in the *colegio* in Loja. The newlyweds settled in the southern coastal city of Machala, the capital of El Oro province, where Matilde established a medical practice and taught natural history at the state secondary school while Fernando practiced law and taught history there. In 1924 registration of voters began in preparation for the upcoming elections for Congress and Senate. At Matilde's request, her husband reviewed the 1906 constitution and offered his legal opinion that there was no explicit provision that women were ineligible to vote. On consultation, the minister of the interior agreed that the legislation referred only to "citizens" and did not specify that they must be male.[6] He therefore granted Matilde permission to vote in the May 1924 elections. In June a meeting of the Council of State determined that indeed Ecuadorian women who otherwise satisfied the requirements of citizenship—that is, who were at least twenty-one years of age and literate—were eligible both to vote and to be elected. Five years later, female citizens' right to vote was formally incorporated into Ecuador's 1929 constitution. Matilde Hidalgo de Prócel was thus not only the first Ecuadorian woman to vote in a national election but likely also the first Latin American woman to do so, since Ecuador was the first country in the region to approve female suffrage.[7]

In 1925 the Revolución Juliana (July Revolution) overthrew three decades of liberal rule in Ecuador, carrying physician Isidro Ayora to a cabinet post and then to the national presidency. With the reorganization of municipal councils by the revolutionary government, Matilde Hidalgo was appointed a municipal councilor for Machala by the central government. Soon thereafter, Matilde was appointed the provincial director of Asistencia Pública for El Oro, which placed under her supervision the province's curative health-care facilities. No other woman served in such a role in any Ecuadorian province during the first half of the twentieth century. Meanwhile, the expansion of women's formal political rights, initiated by Matilde Hidalgo, continued apace. In 1931 some fourteen thousand Ecuadorian women voted for the first time in national elections.[8] In 1936, Matilde herself was elected by popular vote to the Machala municipal council and was named vice president of the council. In 1941 she became the first woman elected to Congress, when she became supplemental representative for El Oro province. Matilde was not actually called on to serve in Congress in this capacity, but her election paved the way for the 1945 election to Congress of communist political activist Nela Martínez.

One of the women who joined Matilde Hidalgo in 1921 to celebrate her landmark graduation as a physician was teacher María Luisa Gómez de la Torre. Luisa had been born in Quito in 1887, the illegitimate daughter of Francisca Páez and Quito aristocrat Joaquín Gómez de la Torre. Although she attended the San Carlos Catholic primary school as a day student, Luisa was unable to register in any of Quito's three Catholic secondary schools for young women because of her illegitimate birth. However, in Quito in the first decade of the twentieth century there were two new secular educational options available to young women: matriculation in the Instituto Nacional Mejía, the state second-ary school established as a coeducational institution in 1897, or registration in the Colegio Normal Manuela Cañizares, a women's teacher-training facility founded in 1901 to staff the expanding network of state secular schools. In 1908, Luisa enrolled in the Colegio Normal. The requirements for admission were talent and dedication, rather than wealth and legitimate birth, and instead of learning embroidery and piano along with rudimentary lessons in arithmetic, grammar, and natural history, she would be able to prepare herself for a career there that would allow her to support herself financially.

Luisa began her studies at the Normal just three years after the first five *profesoras normalistas* graduated in Quito; she completed her studies in 1916. Thus her student era coincided with the presence at the Colegio Normal of the first of two German pedagogical missions.[9] The mission was contracted by the liberal government to reorganize the country's education system to base it on scientific, positivist thinking, moving from rote memorization to approaches that aimed to awaken students' interest and their analytical capacities through experiential and experimental study. Given the emphasis on developing a healthy body as well as an inquiring mind, physical education was promoted: students learned gymnastics and choreographed dance and went for hikes in the mountains surrounding Quito. This model of the active, healthy, mod-ern woman could not have been more different from the socially conservative norms promoted in the Catholic schools and within elite highland society.[10] Indeed, simply to enroll in the Colegio Normal was an inherently transgres-sive act, not least because the first teachers at the new secular state schools were Protestants.[11]

While an 1862 concordat between the Ecuadorian government and the Vat-ican required all Ecuadorian education from primary school to university to be in accordance with Catholic doctrine, this agreement lapsed following the Liberal Revolution. Luisa was not only publicly insulted on her way to classes but both she and her mother were excommunicated by the Catholic Church. Luisa spent much of her career teaching at Quito's Instituto Mejía; as physical education teacher there, she organized the first girls' basketball team in Quito. Later, when the Instituto Mejía became an exclusively men's school in 1935 and its remaining female students were sent to the Colegio 24 de Mayo—a women's secondary school that had been established in 1922 to provide a secular single-sex alternative in Quito to Catholic education—Luisa was the only female in-structor who remained at the Mejía.

While both the students and teachers at secular educational institutions challenged conservative social norms in Quito in the early twentieth century, by the mid-1920s Ecuadorian political life too was becoming more diverse and contested. When the socialist bookseller Leonardo Muñoz imported the first volumes of Marxist writings into the country, he found interested customers precisely among some of the teachers of the Mejía.[12] Similarly, among the participants in the 1926 founding meeting of the Partido Socialista Ecuatoriano in Quito were a number of Mejía staff members. The only woman who participated in that meeting was Luisa Gómez de la Torre. When a group of young conservatives disrupted the meeting, they saved their most damning insults for her, expressed in sexual terms. In her professional life she was also an activist, involved in defending working conditions by establishing such organizations as the Club de Profesores del Instituto Nacional Mejía and later the first Sindicato de Profesores (teachers' union) in 1937. She was also among the women who participated actively in the political events of 1944 in Quito, when a broad social coalition mobilized to bring down the government of Carlos Arroyo del Río and bring back to power for a second term José María Velasco Ibarra (a populist politician who would eventually serve five terms as national president), in what became known as the Revolución Gloriosa (Glorious Revolution).[13]

When Velasco Ibarra overthrew his own government's progressive 1945 constitution in a 1946 self-coup, Luisa Gómez de la Torre was among a group of women who publicly called for his resignation. After three decades as a teacher, Luisa was fired from her position at the Instituto Mejía. This led to a new stage in her life, as she turned increasing attention to working with indigenous activists who had founded the Federación Ecuatoriana de Indios in 1944. In association with illiterate peasant leader Dolores Cacuango, Luisa helped establish bilingual, bicultural schools for indigenous children within the grounds of state haciendas in the northern highlands.[14] In addition to the long list of her other transgressions, we can add Luisa's unusual cross-class and cross-ethnic friendship with Dolores Cacuango and their collaborative work in an indigenous literacy project. That project can rightly be seen as a precursor of the bilingual education programs that became central to the institutional history of the Confederación de Nacionalidades Indígenas del Ecuador (CONAIE) in the 1980s, facilitating CONAIE's emergence and development into the strongest indigenous rights confederation in Latin America at the end of the twentieth century.[15]

The lives of women like Matilde Hidalgo and María Luisa Gómez de la Torre provide revealing windows onto numerous dimensions of Ecuadorian society in the first half of the twentieth century. These were lives that were framed by important political processes—processes indeed in which these women participated—and that were equally marked both by new opportunities for education and employment and by admirable personal initiative that gave them the courage to seize such opportunities. Despite the many differences in the stories of these two women, there are also significant parallels. Both had a certain amount of cultural capital—certainly they were not among the illiterate poor—but they were also peripheral enough to elite Ecuadorian society that they were able to, or needed to, imagine a different life for themselves than contracting a good marriage and becoming adornments for and administrators of upper-class homes. They imagined lives in which they would become the subjects of their own histories, projects in which the ability to support themselves financially held a central place. They also faced some similar conflicts with respectable society, including with the Catholic Church. Finally, Matilde Hidalgo and María Luisa Gómez de la Torre were born just two years apart and into families lacking a father who could provide financial stability to the household.

These examples point to some of the ways that the options potentially available to young women in the early twentieth century were different from those available to their mothers and grandmothers. Those opportunities depended crucially on state projects established by the liberal governments that dominated Ecuadorian politics from 1895 to 1925. The existence of secular secondary schools—a cornerstone of liberal social policy—is an obvious example. Moreover, the liberal state tended to define rights in inclusive terms. Thus there was no explicit provision that women could not attend the men's *colegio* in Loja, nor was "citizen" defined in masculine terms. It was only social convention that determined that women were excluded from participation in secular secondary education, or for that matter from voting. Social convention was, however, very strong. This prompts a question: given both conservative social norms of appropriate female behavior, and new opportunities established in principle after the 1895 Liberal Revolution, just what kinds of women were most likely to have the nerve—or the lack of other options—to risk social disapproval by pursuing those new possibilities? The answer suggested by the lives of Matilde and Luisa is women who were neither entirely privileged nor fully marginal.

In 1903, Rosa Stacey was the first woman to begin study at the Instituto Nacional Mejía. Although the liberal state's flagship institution of secular education had been established as a coeducational institution six years earlier, she was the first woman who had dared to enroll. When she did, she was twenty-nine years old and apparently already a confirmed spinster. After completing her *bachillerato* at the Mejía she briefly directed and taught at Quito's Escuela-Taller de Mujeres, a trade school for working-class girls. Following her publication of a geography textbook, Rosa was awarded a scholarship to study at the Sorbonne in Paris, returning to Quito to direct the Colegio Normal Manuela Cañizares for many years. Her last name indicates her descent from Diego (James) Stacey, an Englishman who traveled to the Andes to fight for independence, widely believed in Ecuador to have been the nephew of Lord Byron (although it may be that Stacey was Byron's nephew in figurative rather than literal terms, perhaps via their Masonic relationship). Diego Stacey's son, Manuel Stacey Sanz, had various romantic liaisons, including a long-term relationship that produced four (illegitimate) children, the eldest of whom was Rosa.

Thus Rosa was born into a liberal family in Quito, whose father had a bohemian reputation. Clearly her family did not fulfill traditional Quito's ideals of conservative, Catholic, respectable society, despite the efforts of the women of the household to support themselves decently by taking in sewing, one of the few options available. Rosa herself is remembered as a very strong-willed woman.[16] She would have had to have been to take such a bold step as to enroll in the Instituto Mejía in 1903. Rosa's relatives (the grandchildren of one of Rosa's sisters) recount that her decision to do so came following an altercation with a client over the quality of a sewn item, after which Rosa swore to seek another way to support herself.[17] As the biographer of Rosa's nephew phrased it: "His ancestors were not people who were characterized by passivity and tranquility, but rather by courage, action, and participation in the important events of the time."[18] Rosa could certainly be included in this characterization.

Most of the female figures who populate this book did not have the public prominence of Matilde Hidalgo, María Luisa Gómez de la Torre, and Rosa Stacey, nor is it always possible to flesh out our understandings of their lives. The availability of archival documentation that offers information about the student days and working lives of midwives and nurses allows for a richer interpretation of some of those women in chapters 4 and 5. In contrast, it is rather more difficult to grasp the lives of poor girls and women who interacted with institutions of child protection and of women who used prostitution as one of their livelihood strategies. Although they had points of contact with various state institutions, relatively more dimensions of their lives were obscured from the view of the state.

The account offered here of women's experiences and agency in contexts not entirely, but sometimes in part, of their own making is undoubtedly partial. Nonetheless, I highlight the protagonism of particular kinds of urban women of the emerging middle sectors in building Ecuadorian modernity in the early twentieth century. This has been largely ignored in social histories of the country, with the notable exception of Ana María Goetschel's wonderful history of female education and female teachers (*profesoras normalistas*) in Quito in the same era. Consistent with the lives outlined earlier in this chapter, Goetschel also hints at the social conditions that might lead women to take advantage of new opportunities in a context of strong social disapproval. Consider, for instance, the following oral history anecdote from María Luisa Salazar (the director of the Colegio Normal Manuela Cañizares in the early 1980s) about how her mother had become one of the first normalistas:

> Before Eloy Alfaro became president [that is, during the battles of the Liberal Revolution], General Terán of the liberal army received help from my grandmother, a young widow with two daughters, when his troops stopped at her rural property in Patate. Eloy Alfaro heard of this and sent my grandmother a note to thank her and ask her to come to Quito. When she went, he told her: "A colegio is going to be opened and I want to give you the opportunity to educate your daughters. Women in the future will need to be educated; not just men, but women too." My grandmother looked frankly at her situation and decided to educate her daughters in the Normal, despite the recriminations of her conservative family: "You are going to lose everything, you are allying yourself with the liberals; if you are going to give your daughters a Godless education, then just say good-bye, we can no longer recognize you."[19]

This story points to a number of emerging patterns: the rejection by more conservative society of women's education in secular state institutions; a personalistic approach to recruitment of women for new roles, perhaps necessary given the social barriers at the time; and also the beginnings of what would become a more systematic emphasis on providing state protection to women without other male providers, a theme that runs through this book.

Salazar notes that her mother did not actually work as a teacher despite her training at the Normal, since after her marriage her husband wished her to stay at home. The acquisition of a male protector often led to new constraints as well as to new forms of security. A similar story is told in an oral history interview that María Cuvi Sánchez conducted with Rosario Mena de Barrera who, following her graduation from the Colegio 24 de Mayo with a diploma in commercial accounting, became the second woman hired to work in the new Caja del Seguro (social security office) soon after its 1937 founding. She withdrew with some regret from her professional life once she married lawyer Jaime Barrera.[20] As Mireya Salgado, the daughter of public health physician Eustorgio Salgado, recollected: "In my day we women did not work. There were girls who worked in stores selling fabrics, as vendors, that is all. Today girls become professionals and work in every field. But in my day women who had professional husbands did not work, our work was to stay at home raising our children."[21]

Salgado dreamed of becoming a physician like her father but did not pursue postsecondary education. This despite the fact that Salgado came from a family of strong liberal credentials: her father was one of five medical students sponsored by Eloy Alfaro's government to undertake advanced training abroad in the first decade of the twentieth century.[22] Moreover, at the time she was born, her maternal grandfather, Modesto Peñaherrera, was serving as minister of the interior during liberal general Leonidas Plaza's second term as president (1912–16). These anecdotes point toward social patterns that will be explored in later chapters: some of the contradictory experiences for women of having, or not having, male protectors; a changing terrain of opportunities structured by state programs and policies; and overlapping gender models that situated women in a variety of ways, both providing opportunities to maneuver among a range of options and riddling their lives with tensions. Without doubt, the contours of the pressures and limits on women changed, as new opportunities brought with them novel forms of social control.

### Women's Rights and Women's Opportunities in Political Context

This book is a study of state formation that conceives of those processes in terms of prosaic, everyday activities that entangle different social groups in a variety of ways. State formation does not start and end with broad political changes. Nonetheless, the larger political framework in Ecuador influenced the processes in important ways. Significant shifts in policy were clearly linked with broader political changes, both because policies toward disadvantaged groups (which were defined to include women in certain political moments) became symbolically important to represent changes in government, and because different political regimes brought new actors into the state, with different perspectives, interests, and lived experiences. Importantly, the historian Valeria Coronel has insisted on the weight of prior social struggles in the negotiations for social rights that occurred in different periods of Ecuadorian history. These were not just benevolent actions on the part of governments—although they were sometimes presented that way by government actors—but rather the result of alliances with and pressures from a variety of social groups.[23] We know more about the struggles of peasants and workers in this regard than of women.[24]

The 1895 Liberal Revolution constituted a fundamental political shift, bringing to power coastal agro-export and commercial elites who generally sought to modernize and open up the economy. They also promoted important social changes associated with the separation of church and state, asserting state control over areas that had previously been managed largely by the Catholic Church (such as education, marriage, civil registry, and social welfare institutions). While the three decades of liberal political domination (1895–1925) saw a number of internal shifts in political alliances and policy paradigms, another fundamental change came with the 1925 Revolución Juliana, when a nationalistic cohort of mid-ranking military officers joined with middle-class professionals to overthrow the liberals in a bloodless coup. The liberal project had wound down, with an economic crisis that led to government indebtedness to private banks in Guayaquil and thus increasing control of this "bancocracia" over government policies. A massacre of striking workers in Guayaquil in 1922 powerfully symbolized the displacement of the more radical aspects of the liberal project by repression and corruption. The Juliana governments between 1925 and 1931 engaged in an energetic process of reform, establishing Ecuador's Central Bank, nationalizing its railway, and passing a number of pieces of social legislation that, for instance, regulated working conditions and institutionalized female suffrage. Their administrative reforms involved coordination and harmonizing of state institutions, including a reorganization of the Servicio de Sanidad that moved its main office from Guayaquil to Quito and created provincial delegations to extend public health programs beyond Ecuador's main cities. Altogether, these reforms produced a more active, interventionist state, one effect of which was the considerable expansion of state employment, especially in Quito.[25] Indeed, by 1936 public employees constituted 16.6 percent of Quito's economically active population (5,893 people of a total workforce of 34,276 in the city's overall population of 101,668).[26]

The 1930s saw the advent of a new political environment, with a generalized economic crisis that was matched by an extraordinary degree of political instability: there were fifteen men who passed through the presidential offices in rapid succession in this decade alone. Although this was a "bust" period between Ecuador's earlier boom of cacao—undermined by the trade disruptions of the First World War and further threatened by crop diseases in the 1920s—and a later boom of banana production that took off in the late 1940s, scholars have proposed a more diverse set of experiences of this period.[27] In a context where global trade was reduced due to the global economic depression, there were efforts to expand industrial production of textiles and other consumer goods. There was also considerable migration to urban areas such as Quito. The decade was marked too by the emergence of populism, based on the social transformations associated with economic change, diversification, and urban growth. In a way, relative political stability emerged at the end of the decade under Carlos Arroyo del Río (1940–44), but the loss of half of Ecuador's territory to Peru in a 1941 war was one of the catalysts for another political revolution: the Revolución Gloriosa of 1944 that brought populist Jose María Velasco Ibarra back to the presidency. In 1948 the election of Galo Plaza Lasso, a modernizing landowner who was son of liberal president General Leonidas Plaza, initiated an extended phase of political stability, based in part on the consolidation of the banana boom in the 1950s.

While the latter part of the nineteenth century saw a number of shifts in political culture, it has been persuasively argued that in the decades immediately before the 1895 Liberal Revolution, Ecuadorian political discourse conceived of women's roles within the model of Catholic modernity forged by conservative president Gabriel García Moreno, who dominated Ecuadorian political life from 1859 until his assassination in 1875.[28] Unlike other Latin American countries where those decades saw processes of modernization pursued by liberals, García Moreno modernized the state, paradoxically, by tying it more closely to the Catholic Church.[29] In terms of women's contributions to the nation, the reference point of that model was primarily elite women, who were urged to influence the public sphere as "angels of the home," through their private moralizing influence over their sons and husbands.

Following the Liberal Revolution, a very different notion of women's potential contributions was presented by government leaders. President Eloy Alfaro, in an address to Congress on June 13, 1897, set out an ambitious plan to emancipate the female sex: "There is nothing as painful as the condition of the woman in our Patria, where relegated to domestic chores, the sphere of her intellectual activity is extremely limited, and even more narrow is the circle within which she can earn a living independently and honorably. To open new horizons, to include her in work that is compatible with her sex, to call on her to collaborate in the activities of science and art; to broaden, in a word, her field of action, improving her future, is a matter that we should not neglect."[30]

Eloy Alfaro went on to ask:

Why not open to woman the doors of the universities, so she can dedicate herself to the study of scientific professions? Why not provide, similarly, special institutes to train her in trades not incompatible with her sex? Why not give her a role in public employment, again as compatible with her sex? [ . . . ] And do not say, following the selfish pessimism of many, that all of these reforms in the education of the woman will deprive the home of her poetry and tranquility. To the contrary: the educated woman, the woman who knows a trade, the woman who works and acquires experience that gives her a more immediate contact with the real world, far from undermining domestic life, is a great support for the family, and a valuable treasure for the husband because, forging her soul in realism, her ideas about fidelity and honor—her greatest patrimony—become clearer and more perfect, and the moral education that the children of such women receive is therefore more solid.[31]

Eloy Alfaro thus called on the assembly to "perfect the protection that has been initiated by passing laws that emancipate the Ecuadorian woman from the narrow circle in which she lives, and giving her opportunities to raise herself up to a level that will offer her abundant resources for her honorable subsistence." Convinced of the importance of these issues, he explained that he had already initiated protective measures, hiring women to work in post offices and establishing a training course in telegraphy for señoritas. Indeed, some eighteen months earlier, he had decreed that effective January 1896, women would be hired to serve the public in postal offices in provincial capitals; the postal system would coordinate the sale of stamps, through a position that would be filled by a woman; and classes in telegraphy would be established in Quito and Guayaquil for women, providing them with credentials so that they could then be employed as telegraph operators. As the prologue to the decree explained: "It is the duty of government to improve the condition of the woman, providing her with honorable and decorous work."[32] This decree came only a few months after the Liberal Revolution and for the first time earmarked positions in the public administration for women.

Now, undoubtedly there is much here that suggests restricted definitions of appropriate forms of work for women. Nonetheless, that should not blind us to two other themes that were very significant in the context of the time. The importance and redemptive potential of *work* in this speech—and particularly the recognition that many women were seeking ways to support themselves honorably—is striking. The central position of women from nonelite sectors in this program of reform is also significant. In 1900 these sentiments were echoed and elaborated on when the minister of public education—key liberal intellectual José Peralta—presented his annual report to Congress. As he explained,

> The poor woman needs to create an independent situation for herself through
> her own work; she needs the workshop to elevate and ennoble herself, and
> thus to be able to fulfill her responsibilities; she needs an honorable wage
> which will become the best defense of her virtue and sentinel of her dignity.
> To redeem the woman by way of work is to moralize society, extirpating vices
> that are a fatal cancer for the people. To open up to the woman the professions
> and licit, lucrative industries is to double the nation's productive forces and to
> harness a new and enthusiastic factor of national prosperity. And these grand
> social and economic reforms will not be achieved except through the cre-
> ation and support of Industrial Schools, through the admission of women to
> university studies in fields of practical utility, in a word, through the decisive
> protection of women's work. Prostitution and pauperism cannot be detained
> through merely religious fears: women's virtue will not be preserved simply

through mystical practices. Experience dictates against the pretensions of Theology, and demonstrates the urgent need to place women under the protective shield of work, establishing institutions in which she can learn to earn a living honorably.[33]

The emphasis on work here was consistent with the liberals' emphasis elsewhere on labor issues. In that regard, they established a number of measures to loosen what they saw as traditional, backward, unproductive forms of labor control on highland agricultural estates, partly in an effort to generate flows of labor to coastal agro-export plantations.[34]

These also constituted attacks on the economic and political power of highland landowners, who as a group—although not always individually—were associated with the conservative rule of previous decades, a period that has been glossed by some scholars as characterized by the *estado terrateniente*, the large landowners' state.[35] With their social base in the more outward-oriented coast, the liberals represented their own program of reform as more secular, more modern, more liberating for productive working people of all kinds (implicitly including themselves in this category) and more open to external influence in general and the global economy in particular. Their emphasis in a wide range of areas on the importance of work and effort can be seen as part of the process of forging their own self-representation as economic entrepreneurs whose wealth, unlike traditional highland landowners, was based on effort and ingenuity rather than inheritance (regardless of whether those representations were accurate in individual cases). The liberals' general emphasis on labor issues was also consistent with the reconfiguration of the national population as human capital, which was particularly evident in relation to child health and welfare issues from the 1910s on.

For women the emphasis on the redemptive value of work had a distinctly moral tone, tied directly to preservation of their virtue and honor. In Peralta's comments it is clear how central women were, discursively, to the conflict between the Catholic Church and the liberal state. Key liberal reforms in the separation of church and state included the 1900 Law of Civil Registry in which the state seized control over information about births, marriages, and deaths from the Catholic Church, followed soon thereafter by the Civil Marriage and Divorce Law in 1902.[36] Civil marriage was characterized by the Catholic Church as state-sanctioned concubinage of women. Much worse, consistent with the reconfiguration of marriage as a contract rather than a sacrament, this law made it possible to dissolve the marriage contract. While in general the separation of church and state came later in Ecuador than in many other Latin American countries, Ecuador's divorce law was relatively early compared with most other countries in the region. The provisions for divorce in the 1902 law followed closely the reasons for which the Catholic Church itself allowed formal separations—infidelity, impotence, or a husband's attempt to prostitute his wife or children—which no doubt facilitated the law's passage in Congress. Much more controversial were the proposed 1910 amendments to the divorce law, which provided for divorce by mutual consent; despite heated debates in Congress, the law was ultimately passed.[37]

In 1911 a further law provided a concrete form of economic emancipation to married women: it allowed them to request partial separation of goods, which they could then independently administer. This law referred specifically to wealth brought into the marriage, not wealth gained during the marriage; and it required women to register their intention to separately administer those goods or property with a public notary. Of course, such a law really only applied to women who were in a position to bring some wealth into a marriage. It nonetheless was significant in undermining men's position as unilateral administrators of household property. Like other aspects of liberal reforms, many of these measures required action from the women involved to make them real and effective, action that surely was often difficult to take. Still, these legislative resources undoubtedly changed the terrain of gender relations in Ecuador. While these various processes were associated with a considerable secularization of social life in the early twentieth century, both the continuing weight of Catholic norms and the continuing participation of Catholic institutions in social policy areas are evident throughout this book.

The chapters explore the social effects of liberal projects and claims to expand women's opportunities, examining to what extent, and through which means, they became reality, especially in health-related areas. The expansion of state employment for women was based on the expansion of women's education—as is clear in the comments earlier of Alfaro and Peralta—since it depended on the acquisition of new skills. First it was necessary to establish the legal and institutional conditions for such study, however. In 1895 (just a month after the triumph of the Liberal Revolution) it had taken a presidential decree to recognize the secondary studies that a young Guayaquil woman, Aurelia Palmieri, had completed in 1893, since the Law of Education at the time did not recognize the possibility of women graduating with the high school diploma of *bachiller*.[38] The 1897 Congress formally recognized the right of women to opt for academic diplomas. This led some congressmen to respond to Alfaro's impassioned 1897 speech rather dismissively, saying they had already remedied the situation.

Indeed, in the 1897 constitution the state generally guaranteed the freedom of education (unlike the arrangements with the Vatican under the 1862 concordat), and made primary education both obligatory and free of charge. The 1897 founding of the Instituto Mejía as a coeducational secondary school was part of this process of establishing state-run secular education for both sexes. The founding of four Normal schools in 1901 (two women's schools in Quito and Guayaquil and two men's schools in Quito and Cuenca), with the purpose ultimately of staffing the expanding public education network, was another important step. For at least some Ecuadorian girls, the rapid growth of that network took education out of the two main venues where women's schooling had been provided until then: within the family and by Catholic religious orders. Secular education was one of the most important achievements of the Liberal Revolution, facilitating both a weakening of the influence of the Catholic Church over society and the dissemination of new skills needed for the modernization of the political and economic systems.[39]

Although this book explores the concrete effects of the expansion of healthcare training and careers for women, a quick look at a published source from the era indicates that in other fields, too, liberal claims to favor women's work were not empty words. A review of the information provided in Ecuador's 1909 *Guía comercial, agrícola e industrial* indicates that indeed women were appointed to positions in the postal system, as Eloy Alfaro claimed, particularly in the provinces of Guayas and Pichincha, the sites of Ecuador's two largest cities.[40] In coastal Guayas province, among the personnel of Guayaquil's administrative offices of the postal system, women made up 30 percent of the technical staff who merited being named in the guide, as well as the postal administrator in one of the province's four county post offices. Together these added up to fourteen women, ten of whom were single, two were widows, and only two were married. Although the numbers are small, that does not reduce the social significance of the emergence of these new areas of women's work, in which unattached women held a prominent place. In addition, in Guayaquil's port the entire statistical office of the Customs Service was staffed by "señoritas" (including one widow, who fit uncomfortably in the category of señorita except in the sense that she too lacked a husband), together amounting to another nine named female staff members in the guide.

In Quito, similarly, there were five women in each of the postal offices and mailbag sections of the postal system (in total, eight single women, one widow, and one married woman); another single woman served as one of four county post office administrators. Within the head offices of the institution in Quito, the interpreter in the office of the general director of the postal system was a single woman, and the sole bookkeeper within the accounts department was a married woman. In total, women made up some 45 percent (thirteen of twenty-nine) of the employees of the postal system in Pichincha province who were mentioned by name in the guide. The general director of the national postal system in 1909, Manuel Stacey, would have been well aware of women's abilities: he was the brother of Rosa Stacey. Unlike in Guayaquil, women had begun to make inroads in the telegraph system in Pichincha province; the telegraph operator in one of the local telegraph offices outside Quito was a single woman.

The guide indicates that women were also appointed in Quito to positions of responsibility within the National Library: they comprised the entire relatively small technical staff of the library, led by the library's director, Señora Zoila Ugarte de Landívar (perhaps best known as editor of Ecuador's first women's magazine, La mujer, and for her activities as a writer and a teacher). No doubt it was less controversial to appoint women to positions in institutions like the postal system and library, since these were relatively new forms of work in a process of expansion. They neither took positions away from men, nor had such work already been marked as masculine. Also noteworthy was the establishment of female workplaces, with women grouped together in specific offices within these institutions. In this and subsequent decades, there continued to be concern about women working alongside men, so it was more acceptable to have an entire office made up of women than to have a mixed workplace.

Despite the recollections of Mireya Salgado, there were increasing opportunities for white-collar employment for women, although as Rosa Mena de Barrera suggested obliquely, when women pursued careers they frequently remained single. While teaching was an area of rapid expansion of women's professional work for state institutions, in official references to the kinds of work and study appropriate for women, it is clear that health-care work also seemed particularly well matched to what were considered women's natural abilities. Women were thought to have special skills in areas that involved a combination of caring and technical work. It is striking that the Faculty of Medicine was the only faculty at the Universidad Central that admitted any female students at all until 1936, when a woman enrolled in the first-year program in the Faculty of Law.[41] Within the Faculty of Medicine, women were permitted first to study midwifery (beginning relatively early in the nineteenth century but significantly expanded and regularized in the liberal period), then were accepted into lower-level courses in pharmacy (beginning in 1904), and then began to study nursing (in 1917). Following Matilde Hidalgo's pioneering 1921 graduation as a physician, Lusitania Vivero became the first female doctor of dentistry in 1927.

What was it about medical, and especially paramedical, professions that seemed especially appropriate for women? In 1905, Luis A. Martínez, secretary of public education, phrased it like this in his annual report to Congress: "In the past year on an experimental basis we established a basic course [*curso in-*

*ferior*] in Pharmacy for señoritas. The initial results have surpassed all of the government's expectations, supporting yet again our conviction that the Ecuadorian woman has undeniable aptitudes for applied scientific study. . . . I think it is also necessary to establish in the universities of Quito and Guayaquil a special course for nurses, capable of forming adequate personnel for the service of hospitals and attention to patients, since the lack of knowledge for the appropriate application of the treatments prescribed by physicians can cause lamentable results."[42] While the first nursing classes were not established until 1917, what is evident from an earlier date is that women were considered well adapted to the careful application of knowledge created by others: that is, by men.

Some two decades later, Dr. Enrique Gallegos Anda, professor of clinical medicine at the Universidad Central, clarified some of these notions. In 1925 he was experiencing difficulties in running the Clinical Laboratory in Quito's Hospital Civil San Juan de Dios due to the inconveniences associated with employing male medical students as laboratory assistants. As he explained to the Junta de Beneficencia (the umbrella state organization that oversaw public health-care facilities), such students were not well suited to the work, because they had to leave the laboratory frequently to attend classes and they only took the position on a temporary basis while they completed their studies.[43] He elaborated:

> As a result, for some time I have thought that it would be more convenient to
> employ a woman who could remain all day in the laboratory and continue in
> the position for many years, which are undoubtedly advantages. Perhaps one
> might say that a woman has no scientific knowledge; but while it is true that
> the scientific basis of the work is more or less complicated, the techniques are
> easy and require only meticulousness, patience and constancy, qualities that
> without any doubt women possess to a greater degree than do men. It has not
> escaped my attention that the promiscuous mixing of employees of both sexes
> presents its inconveniences; but that can be avoided with a careful selection
> and with the warning that at the first sign of incorrect behavior they will
> be inexorably dismissed. Besides, when the current first assistant leaves we
> have already agreed with the Señor Rector of the Universidad that he will be
> replaced by a señorita; thus soon the two laboratory assistants and the servant
> will all be of the female sex.

Gallegos went on to explain that a young woman had been assisting at the laboratory on a voluntary basis for several days; it was a common practice when seeking state employment to provide unpaid services for a period to prove one's aptitude. He observed: "She has shown interest in the work, seriousness, and sufficient intelligence; she has presented very good references as to her conduct; she is a poor and orphaned señorita; and I believe it would be convenient to offer her the position. However, it would be necessary to authorize her to receive her meals in the Hospital, since otherwise with a monthly salary of only 25 sucres no one could satisfy the current necessities of life. Perhaps I should also remind the Honorable Junta that laboratory analysis involves working with saliva, fecal materials, urine, etc., which most people find repugnant, and that it is a true act of abnegation for someone to dedicate themselves to this kind of work." Many of the issues touched on by Gallegos echo throughout the pages of this book, including women's aptitude for applied scientific work, the importance of single-sex workplaces, and again the idea that the state should provide employment particularly to unprotected and unattached women.

These points can be further appreciated by examining two snapshots of female employment in state institutions. The first picture comes from a census of the affiliates of the state pension system, Caja de Pensiones, which covered professional employees and office workers (the Caja del Seguro established in 1937 extended state benefits to additional groups of public and private employees).[44] It is clear that the most important area of government employment for Ecuadorian women was in the expanding education system. By 1935, according to this census, the Ministry of Public Education was the leading employer of women within the national government: 2,040 women worked for this ministry, constituting almost half of its employees; and 1,357 of them, or precisely two-thirds, were single. Some women did continue to work in this profession after marrying: there were 588 married women (29 percent of the female employees) working for this ministry but also 87 widows and 8 divorced women. The Ministry of Public Works, Agriculture, and Development (where postal employees and telegraph and telephone operators worked) was the second largest employer of women within the federal government, with 283 female employees, again about two-thirds of whom were single.

The number of women working for the Ministry of Government and Social Welfare—where women in the allied medical professions would have worked either in medical institutions or in the public health service—paled in comparison: in early 1935 only 111 of the ministry's 4,723 employees, or 2.4 percent, were female. Of those 111 female employees, 99 or 89.2 percent were single. That is not to say that the remaining 12 were married: while 6 of them were married, 5 were widowed, and 1 was divorced. In other words, 95 percent of female employees in the Ministry of Government and Social Welfare did not have husbands. Although the absolute numbers working in this area were not high, this ministry was the third largest employer of women within the federal government; and these numbers would increase with the establishment just two months later of a new program of maternal-infant health care, which employed midwives and nurses. In addition to the predominance of women without husbands among government employees, among both federal and municipal employees nation-wide, about 11 percent of *single* female employees were supporting dependent children. Not only did government employment provide support for women without male providers; it also allowed them to support other dependents.

A second snapshot of female employment provides additional insight; it comes from a listing of the employees of Quito's Hospital Civil San Juan de Dios in October 1949.[45] Among the seventy-seven employees of the hospital, forty-three were women (56 percent). There were no professional nurses em-ployed by the hospital: the Hermanas de la Caridad (Sisters of Charity) who ad-ministered the hospital were not considered employees and were not included in this list. Of the forty-three women on the hospital's payroll, only four earned more than 150 sucres per month (which was the recently established minimum government salary), leaving the other thirty-nine with this wage regardless of whether they were laundrywomen, cooks, assistant cooks, nursing aides (*asis-tentes de sala*), pharmacy assistants, switchboard operators, or the sole female medical intern. Five of the female employees were married, one was a widow, and the other thirty-seven were single. Of those who were supporting their own minor children, four married women and the widow had legitimate chil-dren, the other married woman had two legitimate children and an illegiti-mate daughter, and four single women had illegitimate children. Interestingly, the latter included the female medical intern: at the time she would have been about thirty-four years old, having persisted in her medical studies despite in-terruptions—perhaps related precisely to her pregnancy outside of marriage—which did not stop her from becoming one of Ecuador's first twenty female physicians.[46]

Some female employees were also supporting two elderly parents (in two cases), or just their mothers (three women, one of whom also supported two nieces). Some maintained other family members, such as the woman who sup-ported three minor siblings, another who supported four cousins, one who supported her six-year-old sister, and another who supported a twenty-five-year-old unmarried sister. These situations suggest that women employed in state institutions were able to take on support of otherwise unprotected depen-dents (some of whom may have been orphaned). Dependents might include minor male or female children, unmarried female relatives of any age, and el-derly parents. The legislation did not seem to contemplate the possibility that a woman might define a husband as a dependent. Still, it is striking that this legislation was not simply used to enforce the boundaries of legitimately consti-tuted nuclear families. Rather, it formally recognized a wider family network, including practices such as economic support for cousins and nieces as well as for illegitimate children. The names of these dependents were included in this document precisely because as recognized dependents of employees, the latter had the right to claim certain state benefits for them.

This discussion of political and social rights suggests that in Ecuador there was a strange mix of early achievements for women in some areas and quite late achievements in others. The vote came to women early in Ecuador, yet in the absence of a female suffrage movement. Divorce, too, came early, although again without significant female participation in the debate. In contrast, professional education came late. Matilde Hidalgo was not only the first female physician but the first university graduate in any field who completed the same curriculum as men did.[47] Twenty years earlier in Argentina a female physician had written a 1901 doctoral dissertation about feminism, following an undergraduate thesis in the early 1890s on women's health.[48] Female university graduation came much earlier in the southern cone, and these are early dates unparalleled in Ecuador for discussions of both feminism and women's health. Brazil's first female physicians and lawyers completed their training as early as the 1880s, although the historian Susan Besse has pointed out that few actually practiced their professions given the social obstacles to doing so. It was only in 1899, for instance, that a female lawyer was first permitted to defend a client in a Brazilian court.[49]

Some of the profound processes of social change that affected some other Latin American countries in the early twentieth century—with important implications for women's roles—were less evident in Ecuador. These included the industrialization of the southern cone countries that drew large numbers of women into factory work (directly prompting questions about their economic rights), large-scale European immigration to Argentina and Uruguay, and political changes such as the Mexican Revolution. In those countries feminist movements emerged to press for specific kinds of women's rights. Explicit discussion of feminism was strikingly absent in Ecuador. There was little in the way of organized feminist movements and no female political parties as there were in countries like Argentina, Chile, and Uruguay. Indeed, while there was some tentative participation in public discourse by female writers and teachers, there was little such participation by female medical and paramedical professionals, with the exception of Matilde Hidalgo. This should not lead us to think, however, that such women did not participate in Ecuadorian political processes. Rather, a review of primary archival sources shows the importance of their participation in the modernization of key services offered by the Ecuadorian state.

This strange combination of achievements that came early to Ecuadorian women with achievements that came late poses a puzzle: was it simply that leading state actors granted Ecuadorian women rights without any kind of action on their part? Ecuadorian historiography has emphasized, for instance, that female suffrage may have been promoted by conservatives working under the assumption that women tended to be more conservative than men and therefore that this would shore up conservative power.[50] The historian Raquel Rodas has contested this interpretation, pointing out that Zoila Ugarte wrote publicly in support of women's suffrage when it was under discussion by the 1910 Congress, and in 1924 Congress received three petitions signed by women urging a consideration of female suffrage.[51] Still, these efforts did not add up to a collective movement. Eloy Alfaro, too, seems to have provided opportunities to women in the absence of a sustained movement that demanded them. Situations of this kind may have been what Ecuadorian literary figure Piedad Larrea Borja had in mind when she wrote in 1943 that:

> The golden dream of the English feminists was realized by Ecuadorian women through a spontaneous recognition of all of her political rights. And all this occurred easily, naturally, as in the unfolding of a biological cycle. This liberated the woman both from the degrading attitude of the slave, and from the anti-aesthetic combative attitude. Ecuadorian feminism never suffered the horrible extreme: the masculine haircut, sunglasses and gym shoes. . . . Women of yesterday's generation . . . arrived naturally, elegantly, in the field of intelligence in all of its manifestations. And it was thanks to the serene grace of this attitude that prejudices were erased that had been deeply rooted in our medium. Softly, without the fatigue of dubious, repetitious speeches . . . , they demonstrated that the glory of contemplation, of knowledge and of work need not destroy the charms of personalities formed in the attributes of true femininity.[52]

Some of the struggles engaged in by the women considered here suggest against the ease of access to public space portrayed by Piedad Larrea. The quotation does, however, capture nicely the conundrum they faced of how to pursue new opportunities without contravening gendered codes of behavior. The full history of women's struggles for social rights is yet to be written in Ecuador. This book nonetheless aims to offer insight into questions such as: What was the lived experience of the women who took advantage of new opportunities? And how did their actions transform those projects?

Certainly Ecuador—especially in the highlands—has been seen as a deeply traditional and conservative society, and in Quito in the early twentieth century it was still the case for women from elite families that attending mass was the most acceptable reason to leave the confines of the home. Women who began to publish their thoughts in venues such as the woman's magazine *La mujer* (founded in 1905) focused on how women might contribute to the nation in ways consistent with their special qualities as members of the fair sex.[53] The covers of the magazine are striking in their depictions of women holding books, richly evoking their intellectual inclinations but also portraying the serenity and grace that Piedad Larrea highlighted.[54] Some of the women involved in that literary and journalistic work were also active in women's education. As teachers, they participated in a female public sphere where women worked together to plan curriculum, write textbooks, and participate in female workplaces. This book looks beyond the small group of women who were publishing their ideas, to examine, through archival documents of institutions that intervened in women's lives or in which women studied or worked, groups of women who did not write publicly but nonetheless participated in political processes and projects. In so doing, they stretched their limits. While the research results offered here are partial given that gender history is still relatively undeveloped in Ecuador, the use of institutional archives does reveal dimensions of women's actions and experiences that are not currently well known.

### Frameworks, Perspectives, and Sources

The areas examined include different kinds of intimate activity: child rearing, sexuality, birthing, and nursing, which involved care and treatment of other people's bodies. The Foucauldian concepts of biopolitics and governmentality illuminate these processes, drawing our attention to the highly political and power-laden ways that administrative practices and policies were forged in these areas of bodily activity. In a relatively early formulation, Foucault characterized biopolitics as focusing on "the species body, the body imbued with the mechanics of life and serving as the basis of the biological processes: propagation, births and mortality, the level of health, life expectancy and longevity, with all the conditions that can cause these to vary. Their supervision was effected through an entire series of interventions and regulatory controls: a biopolitics of the population."[55]

Foucault contrasted this biopolitics of regulation that operated at the level of population with anatomo-politics, the disciplining of individual bodies again with attention to what he called the processes of life. One might expect that child welfare and health, in which children were seen as human capital, would involve biopolitics, while policies around sexuality might constitute anatomo-politics. However, the specific ways that venereal disease control programs operated articulated notions of danger to the nation rather more than intimate regulation of sexual life with an individual focus. In any case, for Foucault an important shift in forms of governing came with the move from sovereign power where the sovereign exercised the right over death, the right to kill, to biopolitics where power operated diffusely via the administration of bodies and the calculated management of life. Increasingly these ideas came together in his concept of governmentality, where power is deployed via the "conduct of conduct."[56]

A key insight of Foucault and his followers is that state formation involves not only repressive mechanisms of policing and disciplining but also the more productive processes of management of the population. One significant dimension of how this is accomplished is when people internalize norms in such a way that they become self-regulating subjects.[57] As the historian Paulo Drinot has recently argued for neighboring Peru, the management of the population is more successful at sites where the interests and aspirations of the population come to be aligned with those of state agencies (although this may also generate discontent where programs fail to deliver).[58] This is especially clear when new opportunities were offered to women who already had a yearning for intellectual and professional challenges. But even Quito's antivenereal programs entangled women in quite specific ways, offering them new means to identify themselves as responsible members of society even though they were in the vulnerable position of having to prostitute themselves to survive economically. It was the partial alignment between state projects and individual aspirations that enabled novel forms of behavior in the context of a range of new choices, although those alignments were both unstable and had unintended consequences.

The concept of reproductive governance also offers useful ways to ground these issues, as it points to constellations or assemblages of specific institutions and actors who intervened in these areas. The anthropologists Lynn Morgan and Elizabeth Roberts have defined reproductive governance as "the mechanisms through which different historical configurations of actors—such as state institutions, churches, donor agencies and NGOs—use legislative controls, economic inducements, moral injunctions, direct coercion and ethical enticements to produce, monitor and control reproductive behaviors and practices."[59] An exploration of some of the everyday engagements with and consequences of these projects helps to inject a sense of the contingent, partial, and negotiated nature of such interventions into Foucault's diffuse notion of power. Moreover, those negotiations were not only between the clients of state programs and those who designed and operated them. Many other negotiations occurred, including both within and between state institutions. For instance, the terrain on which child welfare programs were delivered was an intensely populated and heavily contested one.

While "the state" insinuated itself into people's lives, it certainly didn't succeed in fully determining how they lived or saw the world. In the early-twentieth-century Ecuadorian highlands, even in the urban center of Quito, there was not the intense "statization" of everyday life that scholars have identified for North American and European countries.[60] Ecuadorian state agencies' success at monitoring and intervening in people's lives was quite partial. Not only were state agencies underfunded and competing with other forms of social control, but also people often experienced the world in ways that were in tension with dominant representations and could not be contained by them. At the same time, new state programs and agencies did succeed in aligning themselves with the aspirations of some Ecuadorian women, who as a group had not previously been taken into account significantly in political discourse and in and by public administration. Those programs helped to generate new aspirations in those they engaged, but the programs and agencies were also changed via those engagements.

Studies in both the anthropology and historical sociology of the state have emphasized the everyday and mundane character of the activities through which state formation occurs.[61] Moreover, they have challenged dominant representations of the separateness and neutrality of the state, which is often portrayed in spatial terms as standing above and apart and then acting on society.[62] Increasingly, ethnographic studies have explored the specific ways that those images have been socially and politically constructed, as an element in the cultural construction of stateness, turning an analytical eye on how the state comes to seem present and real to people.[63] Other studies have highlighted the often blurred boundaries between state and society.[64] In Ecuador, state and society were intimately intertwined in a range of ways in different program areas. This occurred in arenas like child protection, where a complex constellation of public and semiprivate institutions participated and in which state actors themselves might also take on allied roles as private individuals. In another example, midwives brought their social backgrounds into their work activities for the public health service in ways that changed the delivery of its programs, and physicians with whom they interacted also brought their own gendered and class assumptions to their interpretation of midwives' activities. In myriad ways "the state" showed itself to be an assemblage of multiple agencies with often conflicting agendas, and even within a single state institution it was not unusual for employees to be pulling programs in different directions. Informed by an eclectic mix of studies of state formation and power relations, the book's primary goal is to deepen our understanding of Ecuadorian society rather than to refine our understanding of theoretical concepts.

A recurring theme, in common with other studies of gender history, is honor. While this is not a theme that initially guided my research, the evidence of its importance could not be ignored. There is a large literature on honor, some of which links the importance of this notion in Latin America to Mediterranean cultural heritage. Recent studies have explored the ways that notions of honor are colored by various class experiences.[65] Works that have scrutinized the meaning of honor in specific historical contexts and emphasized change over time have also furthered our understanding considerably.[66] For instance, in a study of the late colonial and independence period in Quito, the historian Chad Black has shown how quickly the social relevance of notions of honor could change.[67]

Following the 1765 Rebellion of the Barrios, when popular groups rose up against Bourbon tax reforms, there was a concerted effort by colonial administrators to exert control over popular neighborhoods by regulating private life. New state agents and legal frameworks were developed that allowed people to denounce moral violations of their neighbors and permitted state entry into private residences to police such behaviors. No doubt this was simply another set of tools that could be used when people came into dispute, but it is striking how often it was used, and the extent to which it was gendered. Black's analysis of arrest statistics and court cases reveals an intensified surveillance of women's bodies and sexual behaviors, activated by accusations against their honor, which were central to the exertion of monarchical state control over popular neighborhoods. In the 1820s, as Ecuador was caught up in the uneven process of gaining its full independence, these frameworks were transformed again. While local officials were charged with monitoring public morals in a range of ways, sexual improprieties were specifically excluded from this list as domestic spaces were reconstructed as private and inviolable. Although women were not arrested nearly as often for moral improprieties in this decade, they also lost the mechanisms for redressing their partners' infidelities and mistreatment, as a new private sphere of gender and sexuality was constructed. Black's work reminds us that notions of honor and morality are far from timeless and are linked to political changes and state practices. Evoking a shared cultural heritage thus does not go very far in explaining the social significance of honor for people of different social groups in particular moments.

In the early twentieth century, Ecuadorian men served as guarantors and protectors of their women's honor, whether of daughters, wives, or sisters, and indeed they had legal responsibility for their women. The prevalence of this value within the elite could be institutionalized in laws and state practices, both concrete ways that dominant groups projected their values over other social groups. While the theme of honor appears repeatedly, it does so in a very specific way. To access particular kinds of government resources—from placements for one's children in institutions of care, to scholarships, to employment, to being removed from a prostitution registry, and more—women had to prove that they were honorable and therefore deserving of support. What did this mean for the kinds of women who populate this book's social landscape? Most important, how was honor preserved or proven when men were absent from women's family lives? Although the images of proper womanhood emphasized women's role as wives and mothers, there were in fact large numbers of women who were neither and many others who were the latter without being the former.

The apparent prevalence of such unattached women in the archival materials is borne out by the data collected in Ecuador's first national census, taken in 1950. The census showed, for instance, that while women married younger than men, they were less likely to remarry if they were widowed or divorced. Among elderly Ecuadorians, there were many more widowed women than men, both because men more often remarried and because of women's longer life expectancy. Among Ecuadorians age eighty-five and older in 1950, 55.8 percent of men were married but only 18.3 percent of women. Women without partners accumulated in older age groups. However, they also accumulated in urban areas. By the time age eighty-five was reached, almost a quarter of urban women were single—that is, they had never married. Similarly, about a quarter of urban women in the thirty to thirty-four age group were single in 1950, suggesting that the likelihood of ever marrying dropped sharply after age thirty. The census also indicated a disproportion of women of an economically productive age in urban areas, most markedly in Quito. This was due to short-range migration strategies, which led demographer John Saunders to conclude that rural-urban migration was primarily a female phenomenon in Ecuador.[68] There were also two male migration streams clearly evident by 1950: from the highlands to coast and from the highlands to the Amazon, both considered longer-distance migration strategies. The result was that by 1950 there was a surplus of women in urban areas in the highlands in general, and as Saunders noted: "Quito particularly appears to be a mecca for the female population in the productive ages."[69] This information helps to contextualize the large number of women who appear in this book who did not have male partners.

The census also showed that while there was a slightly greater tendency for both men and women to be single in the coastal provinces than in the highlands, much more marked was the large proportion of common-law or consensual unions on the coast compared to the highlands. In coastal provinces 26.2 percent of men and 27.1 percent of women were living in common-law relationships, while in the highlands the percentages for each group were 2.1 and 2.4 (although it is possible that consensual unions were underreported by those enumerated given the relative social stigma of such unions in the highlands).

On the coast the number of persons living in common-law unions was in fact greater than those formally married. This indicates a considerable difference in attitudes toward marriage in these two regions of the country, undoubtedly linked in part to the historical influence of the Catholic Church on highland society compared to the coast. Saunders further noted that subsequent data indicated that across the national territory, 33.1 percent of all Ecuadorians born in 1955 were illegitimate; however, the overall proportion of couples living in common-law marriages was only 11.9 percent, which he identified as a significant discrepancy. On the coast, where slightly more than a quarter of all men and women of marriageable age were living in common-law relationships, the proportion of births registered as illegitimate was twice that, at 56.5 percent. In the highlands, however, while only slightly more than 2 percent of men and women of marriageable age had common-law partners, it was more striking that over 14 percent of all births were illegitimate.[70] The figures suggest that many such children were not born into sustained relationships.

Given the significant numbers of unattached women, then—including many who might have children to support—just how did such women demonstrate that they were honorable? Social capital was crucial in doing so. The sociologist Pierre Bourdieu defined social capital as social obligations, networks, connections that could sometimes be converted into other forms of capital (economic and cultural).[71] In Ecuador, in the first half of the twentieth century, it was a routine part of seeking government services to provide certificates from respectable men vouching for the honor of the female petitioners. In such certificates, hard work and support of children (or other dependents, including elderly parents) were presented as measures of women's honor, notions that appear to have been shared to some extent by the women themselves and their sponsors. For women of the popular sectors (a general social category including all those whose economic situation was not secure, regardless of specific livelihood activities), this required cross-class as well as cross-gender social networks, which were often readily available as Quito had limited spatial social segregation in the early twentieth century. Not only was there considerable residential mixing in Quito's colonial center, but many poor women provided domestic service in elite or middle-class homes.[72]

Large houses in the center of Quito were often inhabited by wealthy families in one wing and included additional patios off of which poor families rented rooms; first-floor rooms facing onto the street might also serve as commercial venues. This began to change with the geographic expansion of Quito as the twentieth century progressed, including the construction of new residential neighborhoods for the wealthy and middle classes to the north of the old city center and the increasing settlement of the poor population to the south.

Certainly notions of honor and morality took on different shadings when they were articulated by and around poor women seeking help for their children, women seeking a change in their status in the prostitution registry, women who became midwives, and young women traveling to Quito to live apart from their families as they trained to become nurses. Still, all of these women in different ways had to prove their honorability, although many of them could not recur to the easiest answer: that a man both supported them economically and was in a position to guarantee their conduct. To provide any answer at all, they needed to draw on wider social networks of male sponsors.

Historians have found the records of courts and notaries to be useful for examining gendered rights and perspectives. Court records can be used to trace not only patterns of infractions and changing definitions of what constituted a crime, but also the ways that women and men used civil courts to defend their reputations. Notaries produce documents around land transfers, divisions of property, and inheritance that reveal gendered economic rights. The documentation that underlies this analysis is different. The detailed, everyday correspondence within and between state institutions reveals a world of contradictions in their operations, intentions that pulled in different directions, and both the processes underlying policy formation and the difficulties encountered in implementing programs. The principal archives drawn on are of the Servicio de Sanidad and the Junta de Beneficencia/Asistencia Pública (Social Welfare Board) and to a lesser extent the documentation of Quito's public Hospital San Juan de Dios. These sources were then enriched with documentation of the Faculty of Medicine at the Universidad Central and administrative documents of the National Nurses School, both important venues where female medical professionals trained.

This project grew in an organic way, as surprises evoked at one archive suggested interesting new routes through other archives to answer emerging questions. Historical anthropology, like anthropology itself, is especially open to seeing what the evidence suggests rather than following predetermined questions. Anthropology characteristically works up from social data rather than down from theoretical debates, following an inductive model. Anthropologists have long distinguished, too, between etic and emic research strategies, where the etic approach seeks to understand patterns in the evidence that may not be apparent to anthropological or historical subjects themselves, while the emic approach aims to capture people's own experiences and understandings. I move between both approaches, although it is admittedly more difficult to capture women's own perspectives from this kind of documentation.

The historical anthropologist Ann Stoler has identified a series of ways that one can do ethnography in and of the archives, suggesting especially that "the ethnographic space of the archive resides in the disjuncture between prescription and practice, between state mandates and the maneuvers people made in response to them, between normative rules and how people actually lived their lives."[73] There are myriad examples of those kinds of disjuncture. At the same time, the analysis also explores how those state mandates and normative rules emerged, sometimes out of intense discussion and negotiation and often in rather nonlinear ways, full of stops and starts, advances and reversals. In other cases there was no discussion, with state actors simply invoking and institutionalizing what seemed obvious to them and their peers.

One issue that was apparently obvious to leading state actors in highland Ecuador in the first half of the twentieth century was that none of the forms of government monitoring of, intervening in, or enabling intimate life explored in this book were relevant to indigenous women. While in this pre-census era indigenous people were believed to constitute about 40 or 50 percent of the national population, most of them living in the highlands, the absence of indigenous women from the various policy areas considered is striking. As the anthropologist Mercedes Prieto has argued, indigenous people were an important object of observation, analysis, and imagination among Ecuadorian intellectuals and politicians throughout the early part of the twentieth century, although the ways in which they were perceived changed over that period.[74] The historian Marc Becker has noted that within the history of the Ecuadorian left, too, indigenous activists and labor organizers—including illiterate peasant women such as Dolores Cacuango—held a central role, from at least the 1920s.[75] As the historian Erin O'Connor has pointed out, however, when Ecuadorian liberals wrote, spoke, and developed policy toward two disadvantaged groups—women and indigenous people—often indigenous women specifically were discursively erased from these processes, as liberal forms of paternalism overlapped with indigenous Andean gendered understandings to create dueling patriarchies that marginalized indigenous women.[76]

In the institutions and policies developed to address infant morbidity and mortality, seen as threats to future national prosperity, indigenous populations or individuals were rarely mentioned; as the anthropologist Esben Leifsen has argued, the population on which the nation's future was thought to rely was an urban and mestizo population, precisely what was considered the "national" population.[77] The Sanidad's maternal-infant health program established in 1935 also was not extended into rural areas to include indigenous populations, and given that a state midwife could only be in one place at a time, it was mostly limited to women of modest resources who sought their services in provincial cities. However, it is also evident that these services were of less interest to women in smaller population centers, where midwives found it more difficult to recruit clients for this state program. Neither the midwifery nor nursing programs offered by the Universidad Central had indigenous women among their students during the first half of the twentieth century. Entry to those programs required basic education and rural populations and the poor population—and women in particular in both of these groups—were considerably less likely to be literate.[78]

The disregard for indigenous women in social policy areas likely resulted from their association with rurality, a space primarily of interest to dominant groups in the form of productive resources or male labor. O'Connor notes, too, that the liberal period saw a masculinization of the ways that indigenous communities could communicate and interact with state institutions and agents. At the same time, indigenous communities had their own practices that shielded indigenous women from some forms of interaction with the state, including greater community protection for women experiencing conjugal violence and generally greater ability to withdraw from dysfunctional relationships so that it was less necessary to turn to state institutions for protection. As indigenous men began to embark on labor migrations out of their communities as the twentieth century progressed, indigenous women became even more tied to rural areas as they took on additional subsistence work that would allow their families to cobble together a livelihood that included subsistence agriculture and wage work, often straddling different regions of the country. They increasingly became the gendered guardians of indigenous identity as they maintained indigenous ties to the countryside and to community life in an era of considerable social change affecting these communities.[79]

While Stoler has highlighted for the colonial archive ways that silences were actively produced about some areas of social life, evidence was not found in the Ecuadorian archives of a deliberate erasing of indigenous women from the policy areas considered. They simply were not taken into account as significant social actors in the health-related areas explored here, suggesting an even more profound marginalization of this population in the early twentieth century. State projects oriented specifically toward indigenous women date to a later period, such as the projects of the Misión Andina in rural areas in the 1950s.[80] With the move toward agrarian reform from the 1960s, additional state programs began to target rural communities, where indigenous women had become increasingly important actors with the seasonal migrations of community men. If the various processes discussed here made urban mestiza women amenable to state action in a variety of ways, one could also say that in the first half of the twentieth century the lives of indigenous women were simply not as knowable, and as actionable, by the state.

· 2

# Gender, Class, and State in Child Protection Programs in Quito

Child health and welfare is a classic terrain of gendered social policy.[1] In chronological terms, this was the first arena in which Ecuadorian liberal governments at the turn of the twentieth century developed their capacity to inquire into the conditions of and administer the national population, and they did so first in the country's principal cities such as Quito. The terrain of child welfare was populated by many different groups, and over those decades shifts can be identified in forms of governance, which became increasingly more technical, targeted, and secular, even as Catholic women continued to participate in these programs under changing conditions. This was a gendered terrain in that mothers were considered to be key actors in their children's lives but also in how other groups of women took on important roles in child protection activities. Men also intervened in new ways in child welfare issues, casting the problems as an arena of technical expertise and secular state action, in which the state itself took on a gendered hue as its institutions were depicted as paternalistic actors, most notably where other male protectors were absent. As the state sought to modernize the activities of various women who intervened in these areas, so too was the state itself modernized. Although we can only occasionally discern the perspectives of poor women and girls in the documentation about child protection and welfare, it is nonetheless possible to tease out some patterns of experience and agency among them. The period explored here is roughly the four decades before the 1938 passage of Ecuador's first Child Code (Código de Menores), which centralized and harmonized various child protection programs and institutions.[2]

Two state institutions with rather different profiles oversaw issues of child health and welfare in Quito in the early decades of the twentieth century, sometimes directly intervening in specific areas of child protection, and at other times monitoring, coordinating, or partially funding subordinate institutions of public, private, or mixed character, both secular and religious. A year after the Liberal Revolution, the public Junta de Beneficencia was created in Quito by an executive decree, modeled on the active but private Junta de Beneficencia already existing in Guayaquil.[3] The members of the Junta were prominent men appointed by the government who undertook their activities on an unpaid (pro bono or ad honorem) basis. Together they oversaw various social welfare institutions: medical treatment facilities such as the Hospital Civil San Juan de Dios, the Maternidad (lying-in clinic), and the Lazareto de Pifo (lepers' colony); the Hospicio y Manicomio, linked facilities for the destitute poor and the mentally ill; and institutions dedicated to the care of orphans (San Carlos and San Vicente), as well as orphanage sections within Catholic facilities such as El Buen Pastor, La Providencia, and Los Sagrados Corazones. Members of the Junta were appointed as subinspectors of these various facilities, which were administered by Catholic nuns on behalf of the state, or in some cases the state sponsored children in special sections within Catholic institutions. The Junta included some physicians but also lawyers, landowners, merchants, and a range of other local notables.

The funding available for the Beneficencia's projects was extended in 1904 by the Ley de Cultos, which—in the midst of conflict over separation of church and state—turned the administration of rural landed estates owned by foreign religious orders over to the state and dictated that such orders must submit an annual budget to the government detailing the monies needed for their activities. After deducting the amounts approved for these annual budgets, whatever profit margin remained from productive activities on these properties would then be invested in urban social welfare institutions by the Junta de Beneficencia. The October 1908 Ley de Beneficencia went further than the 1904 Ley de Cultos, actually expropriating and nationalizing the properties of religious orders, including the many rural agricultural estates that had provisioned the urban convents. Those properties then became the state-owned *haciendas de asistencia pública*, which were rented out to private individuals, generating rental fees that partially funded the Beneficencia's programs of urban social welfare and health care.[4] Another result was that the urban real estate of religious orders became the property of the state. Thus, for instance, in 1910 the minister of the interior and beneficencia authorized the Junta de Beneficencia to freely celebrate a contract with an individual or corporation to establish an asylum for poor girls. In doing so, it was "authorized to occupy the nationally owned building currently inhabited by the Reverendas Madres de los Sagrados Corazones."[5] Just a few years earlier, that real estate would have been the private property of the order.

The activities of the Beneficencia were from the beginning established in ambivalent relation with religious institutions. The state's sphere of action was strengthened by the separation of church and state not simply by increasing the responsibilities of state welfare institutions vis-à-vis Catholic ones but quite literally doing so at the expense of religious orders. At the same time, the state delegated to one specific female religious community—the Hermanas de la Caridad, or Sisters of Charity—the administration of many of its health and welfare facilities. Thus in the midst of the conflictual process of separation of church and state, the liberal cabinet minister responsible for the Beneficencia portfolio could nonetheless express the sentiment in his 1899 annual report that "the Hermanas de la Caridad are every day more deserving of our gratitude and respect."[6] Indeed, the Hermanas de la Caridad had a special relationship with the state, as a religious community that had been contracted by the García Moreno government in 1870 specifically for the administration of its hospitals and allied institutions, rather than being longtime owners of extensive rural real estate, as were several other religious orders whose activities were more autonomous.

The second state institution with a leadership role in the area of child health and welfare was the Servicio de Sanidad, or Public Health Service. Initially established in Guayaquil in 1908 in response to the first infection of the port with bubonic plague, the Sanidad sent Dr. Carlos Miño to Quito in August 1913 as a delegate of the Guayaquil main office to consult on infectious disease control measures. Shortly after his arrival, he was converted to a subdirector of the service with the stable establishment of a Subdireccion de Sanidad in Quito effective January 1914, making the capital and the port the only two cities in the country with permanently stationed public health employees paid by the national government. Funds for public health activities were earmarked in the national budget, supplemented by the fines collected by the service for various public health infractions. In general, the Sanidad was kept busy during World War I fighting contagious diseases in Guayaquil that triggered international quarantine measures against the port, at a time when the institution's funding was also reduced because of economic constraints resulting from disruption of trade during the war. For the Sanidad's operations in Quito the result was that the central government reduced its promised monthly funding of ten thousand sucres for the Subdirection of Sanidad to merely two thousand sucres, and in some months only seven hundred sucres were actually paid out by the treasury.[7] Nonetheless, the Sanidad as an institution—and the more technical and medical approach to child welfare issues it pursued—increasingly invaded the space of other actors in the arena of child protection.

In the area of health care in general, the division of labor between the Beneficencia and the Sanidad was constituted as curative institutions falling under the authority of the Beneficencia, while the Sanidad was tasked with campaigns against infectious diseases and preventative health measures. Physicians worked for health-care institutions run by the Beneficencia as well as for the Sanidad, which increased its staff and the programs it offered in significant ways from the 1920s on. However, in the case of the Sanidad, the decision-making instances were firmly in the hands of physicians, employed by the government to dedicate themselves full-time to public health programs. The decision-making body for the Beneficencia was drawn from a broader group of professionals and notables, and the physicians in health-care institutions— again, administered for the Beneficencia by Catholic nuns—might provide their services partly on a pro bono basis and partly as a component of their teaching duties for the Faculty of Medicine, giving the Beneficencia in general a less technical and secular profile than the Sanidad. The prominence of lawyers among Beneficencia leaders was likely due to the many contractual negotiations it entered into with private individuals over the rental of its rural estates, which generated a significant proportion of its archival documentation. Following the 1925 Revolución Juliana, the renaming of the Junta de Beneficencia as the Junta Central de Asistencia Pública (with parallel institutions in the south centered in Cuenca and on the coast centered in Guayaquil) marked a shift from its roots in notions of charity to a new sense of public entitlements to state services encompassed by the notion of public assistance.

### Defining Child Protection and Children's Value in Quito

What constituted protection of children? Who was best qualified to define that protection and to carry it out? What were the various kinds of value ascribed to children in early-twentieth-century Ecuador? And in all cases, how were the answers to these questions gendered? The first statements about child welfare in the liberal period—and the first institutions—focused on the care of marginal and vulnerable children including but not limited to orphans.[8] This arena was gendered in at least three ways: there were more marginal girls than boys that came under institutional care; work in this area was delegated by the Junta de Beneficencia to female religious communities; and poor mothers facing crises of care were the secondary targets of programs of child protection.

Principal among Quito's orphanages were the Casas San Carlos and San Vicente, administered for the state by the Hermanas de la Caridad and consistently housing more girls than boys. Although some of the orphanages' inhabitants were classified as *huérfanos* (orphans), others fell under the label of *expósitos* (abandoned children). In 1901 there were 179 expósitos under care in San Carlos, whose distribution reflected the gender imbalance among abandoned children: there were 74 boys and 105 girls.[9] Nuns also operated, in San Carlos and in an adjacent facility in La Recoleta, two primary schools that served girls from the larger urban population. By 1903 there were three such girls' schools—San Carlos with 650 girls, San Gabriel with 250, and El Labrador, still under construction but nonetheless educating some 600 girls—while the interned children at San Carlos fell into the categories of 54 male expósitos, 71 female expósitas, 9 orphaned boys, and 29 orphaned girls.

Although there is no biological reason that parentless girls would be more common than parentless boys, there is likely a social reason: the perception that girl children were more of a drain on household budgets than a source of future economic support, itself a reflection of the gendered character of economic opportunities. As a result, orphaned boys may have been more likely to have been retained by their extended families when their parents died. Perhaps there was also a perception that girls were more in need of the forms of protection offered by state functionaries and nuns to whom they delegated some of these tasks, encouraging the channeling of girl children into institutions of care. In any case, many documents confirm that there was a disproportion of girls in the capital's asylums (*asilos*) or shelters (*casas*) for children early in the twentieth century. Still in 1922 there were a total of 194 orphans in the Junta's Orfelinato (orphanage) de San Vicente de Paul, in different sections by gender and age: by far the largest single category (numbering ninety-five) were girls ages five to twelve.[10] In 1928 the Junta's physician for the Casa San Vicente reported that in the orphanage the largest section was comprised of the group of girls ages seven to thirteen, who numbered 110.[11] The other two sections—of boys that age and of younger children of both sexes—together amounted to 107 residents.

The mandate of orphanages and other asilos for unprotected children was to offer shelter, food, and some basic education. The education provided was geared to be appropriate to the children's "class and condition," including gender. Boys learned carpentry, shoe-making, and other masculine trades that might allow them ultimately some economic independence following a period of dependence within artisanal workshops upon their release from the orphanage. Young girls, in contrast, learned skills that would prepare them principally for domestic service. This training was extended in 1903 when the Beneficencia's subinspector of San Carlos, Manuel Jijón Larrea, proposed formally establishing there a school for servants. He was worried both about the future of the interned children and about the deteriorating quality of domestic service in

Quito. Indeed, his concern for potential employers was expressed in his comments that at such a school girls could be taught "a class in morality where they could learn their duties to their masters as well as their rights; and classes in cleaning, laundry, ironing and cooking so that after completing a certain number of years of training they could receive a certificate and seek work, displaying their certificate as a guarantee to those who might solicit their services."[12] Within six months of his proposal, facilities had been adapted for a school of cooking to supplement the existing training facilities. By 1909 the ninety orphan girls sponsored by the Beneficencia at an allied institution, the Colegio de La Providencia, were receiving "a painstaking primary education; and they are also taught classes in sewing, embroidery, lace-making, and the confection of artificial flowers and other objects of fantasy; nor do we neglect to provide them with practical training in home economics, especially laundry, ironing, cooking, baking, etc. In sum they are given all the necessary tools to acquire a social and domestic education truly accommodated to their condition."[13] In 1922 the girls in San Vicente orphanage first received primary instruction "useful for the home," then advanced to occupational training where they acquired skills in sewing, ironing, laundry, cooking, housekeeping skills, and so on— "everything of practical use that a woman should know for her daily life."[14]

As orphaned and other vulnerable girls were being trained in these skills, their labor also helped to sustain the services they received. Although in principle the Beneficencia paid a fee or "scholarship" (beca) for each child it sponsored in orphanages, it was not always able to fulfill its financial commitments. As the Beneficencia's debts mounted in the mid-1910s, in one instance Sor Josefina, the superiora of San Vicente, communicated to the president of the Junta de Beneficencia her decision: "I absolutely cannot, and will not, admit any boy or girl into this Establishment given the Junta's failure to pay the indispensible amounts for the sustenance of the more or less 150 children who are already here. Please do not provoke painful and upsetting scenes with the families when I have to refuse entrance to so many boys and girls who appear with admission slips from the Beneficencia. I will gladly admit as many children as you wish once the payments are up to date."[15] When older girls in particular took up room in San Carlos, San Vicente, or the orphanage sections of Catholic facilities, as was often the case, Beneficencia subinspectors felt that these young women should be released to support themselves, making room for younger girls more in need of protection.[16] Given the age of many of the interned girls, following discussions with provincial governor Modesto Larrea Jijón during his visit to the Buen Pastor in late 1917, Superiora Sor María de San José looked into the costs of establishing "an industry that, within a year, could provide for the maintenance of the girls in the section of San José [that is, the older girls]. I have calculated that with 7,000 sucres including the necessary materials and adaptation of the locale, we could install an industry of weaving and manufacture of corsets."[17]

However, what could be seen as job training to ensure their futures could also be seen as exploitation: were these workhouses or protection and education facilities? In 1920 the director of education for Pichincha province (who had previously served as a member of the Junta de Beneficencia and in that capacity had been subinspector of various asilos for girls), argued:

> The Education Council (Consejo Escolar) is convinced of the necessity of guaranteeing the work of the orphaned girls of the Casas of San Carlos, El Buen Pastor, San Juan and San Vicente of this city, that is to say, so that such labor no longer continues in exclusive benefit of the [religious] communities assigned to their direction. We suggest the convenience of regulating it, taking into account the sad future that awaits the orphans when, after long and painful years of exhaustion, they are released from the Casas de Beneficencia without a penny of patrimony. It is evident that the communities exploit pitilessly the work of the orphans; and it is therefore urgent to oversee their welfare; for which purpose the Council believes that it would be opportune to establish *cajas de ahorro* [savings funds] following a determination of the percentage of profits that they should receive. I am also writing to the superioras of the above-mentioned casas; and it is to be expected that they will take up this suggestion, not only to protect their own good names, but also due to the sympathy they should have for these unfortunate daughters of work and misery.[18]

Not only was there a gendering of the skills taught to vulnerable children in orphanages, focusing on domestic skills for girls, but girls in particular were also seen as benefiting from the protections offered by private homes. Domestic placements in the homes of respectable families highlight the gendered contours of the economic value of marginal children. In the early years of the twentieth century, girls seem to have been released to private homes in a rather ad hoc way, leaving extended family members or even the Junta de Beneficencia to discover in surprise that specific girls were no longer at the orphanage.[19] The procedures by which children were channeled into domestic placements became more formal in the late 1910s and early 1920s. For instance, contracts began to be signed between the Junta de Beneficencia and respectable people (usually couples) who committed to receive wards of the Beneficencia. Thus in 1919:

Juan Francisco Navarro, president of Junta de Beneficencia of this capital and fully authorized by it, places under the shelter and protection of Señor Don Salomón Villavicencio and his wife Señora Doña Jacinta Andrade de Villavicencio, the minor M. D. aged thirteen more or less, from Tabacundo, expósita, without father or mother and raised at the expense of the Beneficencia pública, in order that the aforementioned spouses retain her in their power until she reaches the age of majority, providing her with food, clothing and education appropriate to her economic and social position. In the case of a serious failure in fulfilling their commitment, the Junta reserves the right to reclaim the above-mentioned minor from the Villavicencio couple at any time that there is sufficient proof of poor treatment or that they have ceased to provide her with proper education.[20]

The same couple solicited two more children in 1922—a girl age eleven and her three-year-old brother—although the terms of the contract had changed by then. Not only did they agree to provide education, clothing, and food until the children reached the age of majority, in exchange for light services that the children could carry out as appropriate to their age, but they made an additional commitment: "when the children reach the age of majority and express their will to leave the Villavicencios' house, they commit to offer each of the children one thousand sucres. If the Villavicencio couple dies before the children reach that age, they commit to include in their wills that amount in the name of each child. It is also noted that the minor girl has expressed her desire to leave the orphanage and to go with the Villavicencio couple. If the children abandon the Villavicencio couple the children will lose the right to claim the one thousand sucres."[21]

These kinds of arrangements could even include very young children. One orphan girl was placed in a home for domestic service at the age of two and a half.[22] In 1920, Obdulia Chiriboga de Araujo petitioned the director of Beneficencia of Quito that he "authorize Sor Teresa de la Caridad to turn over (*entregar*) under my responsibility and care the expósita L. L. who is currently in the power of the wet nurse Ambrocia Coyan, who received her on 18 April 1917. I will provide this minor, whom I receive in quality of domestic servant, the food, clothing and education corresponding to her class, until she reaches the age of majority."[23] The dates suggest that the child was three years old at the time of the petition. Three years later, Señora Chiriboga and her husband, Coronel Angel F. Araujo, contracted with the Beneficencia to take into their home another three-year-old orphan girl, providing her with education, clothing, and food in exchange for "light services appropriate to her age." Like the Villavicencios, the Araujos committed to provide a payment to the child when she reached majority, provided that she stayed with them that long. In this case, however, and in others in the archives, the payment was one hundred sucres rather than the extraordinary one thousand in the Villavicencio case.[24]

It should be noted that these were the only payments referred to in these documents. In other words, they could be seen as delayed payments for services rendered that replaced a regular wage, although they were only payable if the children stayed with their patrons until the age of majority. In the meantime they would simply receive shelter and sustenance in exchange for the services they provided. The anthropologist Esben Leifsen reviewed these archival sources for the period 1920 to 1948 and found only one contract from 1942 that mentioned payment of a regular wage. By then, however, the 1938 Child Code had altered the nature of family placements. As was indicated to someone who solicited an orphaned girl for his service in 1945, the new constitution of that year prohibited employing minors under the age of twelve in domestic service. Moreover, the Child Code authorized Tribunales de Menores to seek family placements for children who needed support and protection, but not in order to employ them as servants.[25] The sentimental or emotional value of children—rather than their economic value—was further institutionalized when Ecuador's first adoption law was passed in 1948.[26]

That the release of children to become dependents in households of higher economic standing was fully accepted in the early decades of the century was clear when in 1920 Quito's police chief requested a list of the orphans in San Vicente de Paul who lacked both parents and were of an appropriate age to be released, to make room for those with greater needs: "This Authority would be able to place those who are released in the houses of respectable and accommodated persons, given that in this office we are constantly receiving requests for the allocation (*consignación*) of minors."[27] Similarly in 1922 the director of the Junta de Beneficencia was authorized to arrange with the superiora of San Vicente de Paul to place orphans who had reached "a certain age" in honorable households, according to a notice that appeared in the press. Having read the notice, Señora Virginia V. v. de Pinto solicited "that the director [of the Junta] give the appropriate order to the superiora of that Establishment so that she provides me with a youth for my service, in exchange for which I commit to provide him with education, clothing, maintenance, and whatever else is necessary. I make this petition in view of the excessive number of children maintained by the Beneficencia in this Casa, thus making way for others who need the support of that Institution."[28]

By taking on responsibility for unprotected lower-class children, Quiteños of the middle and upper classes gained domestic help at a minimal cost and were able to fulfill a paternalistic role that helped define their own class identity as decent and respectable—even patriotic—residents. In doing so, they were participating in an established practice of cross-class child circulation, in which poor families sent young children (most often girls) whom they could not support economically to live in more prosperous households. Lola Crespo de Ortiz Bilbao, member of a notable Cuenca family, described this practice in her memoirs from the perspective of a recipient family: "Peasants would come from the countryside bringing their female children to leave them with known families [in Cuenca]. The idea was that they would learn urban customs, be fed and clothed, they would learn to read and write, up to their first communion, in exchange for providing services appropriate to their age in the house where they had been left 'in consignment' as it was called. . . . The patrons usually treated them well, educating them and clothing them, feeding them and taking care of their health, but the girls also soon had to sweep, to wash, to run errands, tasks that increased with age."[29] She further commented that some such girls remained their entire lives serving their patrons, others fled, others left these houses "with the consent of their patrons" to marry and establish their own families, and some as a result of a "misstep" ended up in the convent El Buen Pastor—a Catholic facility where young women could give birth to illegitimate children.

Parallel to the instances of domestic placements of orphans, there are other cases that appear much more like fostering for family formation in which sentiment was involved and which did not cross class lines to the same extent. The first petition that reads more like an adoption than a quasi-employment contract comes from 1917: "We have had the opportunity to get to know the expósito J. G. L. because Señora Doña Dolores de Estupiñan [presumably a wet nurse], to whom the Beneficencia entrusted the raising of this child, has lodgings in the same house as us. Since then, moved by humanitarian sentiments and the affection that we feel for him, we request that you grant us this boy, to act as parents to him [para hacer con él las veces de padres]. We thus request that you authorize the Junta to provide us with the boy in question, to raise him and educate him according to our position and circumstances."[30]

There was a wave of such petitions in 1927. With the founding of the Asistencia Pública's Casa Cuna for expósitos, the infants that had been in home placements with wet nurses were rounded up at the end of September to be raised collectively under more technical supervision. This led to several petitions from illiterate wet nurses (or commonly from their literate husbands on their behalf) to leave the children with them. For instance, carpenter Luis Rosalino Cruz wrote:

My wife received the orphan A. G. one day after his birth and has cared for him for nine months. Yesterday the Junta de Beneficencia ordered that all orphans be returned, and among these is ours. We love him as if he were our own son, so we have decided to petition the Junta de Beneficencia to return to us the child A. G., and we relinquish any salary or other benefits that the Junta might offer to raise the child, committing ourselves to adopt him as our son, to clothe him, care for him as we have been doing, educate him, teach him a trade, and from our small legacy grant him a portion when that becomes necessary. We beg that the Junta de Beneficencia accept our petition for the good of the orphaned child as well as for our own consolation.[31]

The following week, Carlos Ochoa wrote to say: "In my own name and as legal representative of my wife, Manuela Acijuela, I commit myself to raise, support, and educate the boy J. A. O., *niño expósito*, entrusted to my wife as wet nurse and who, from today, will remain our exclusive responsibility, without receiving any payment from the Junta de Asistencia Pública. If anyone can prove we have abandoned said child, we commit to paying a fine of one hundred sucres to the Junta."[32] And in a somewhat different case the following week, Genoveva Ortega petitioned that "as grandmother of the boy J. V. M. I receive under my responsibility and at my expense the abovementioned child. My lodgings are in the house of Señor Francisco Aguirre Nájera. The wet nurse María Velásquez will not charge even a cent to the Junta de Asistencia Pública."[33] Interestingly, these petitions all refer to male children, while the domestic placements for service most commonly involved female children. Perhaps having a son to whom they could teach their trades and pass on their small enterprises was of particular interest to these popular-sector couples, partly as a form of future support for the adoptive parents. Even these more affective adoption petitions were tinged with an economic consideration that expressed gendered expectations for how children might fit into a household over the long term.

These situations suggest that the predominantly economic valuation of children so clear when they were transferred to wealthier homes as dependents was not the only value that children had. The reference to consolation in the case of wet nurses suggests that these may have been women whose own infants had died at birth and for whom their wards represented an affective replacement rather than just a source of income. Another difference from the domestic placements across class lines is that in those other arrangements the patrons committed to educate and raise the children in conditions appropriate to the children's social position, while in these more affective adoption petitions, the receiving adults committed to raise the children to the best of their ability given *their own* economic and social situation (in other words, to treat them as members of the family). These documents suggest a very different vision of wet nurses that contradicted dominant views of how wet nurses "speculated" with children (by collecting a fee for feeding them with their "mercenary milk") and how lack of affection and care led to high mortality among orphaned infants entrusted to wet nurses.[34] Pediatrician Carlos Sánchez's warning was typical: "where the sentiment of maternity does not exist, affection cannot develop, and thus the orphans turned over to mercenary women die in the first months of their lives."[35] However, institutionalized infants raised under more technical care did not fare better than those fostered by wet nurses in their homes.

Just as poor women might claim their right to affective family formation via fostering or adoption petitions, they might also use state institutions when they encountered crises of care, which were particularly common for women without domestic partners. In doing so, they did not always relinquish their rights to their children and sometimes aspired to reunite their families when that became possible. Some institutions, including the sections funded by the Beneficencia within the Catholic facilities La Providencia, El Buen Pastor, and Los Sagrados Corazones, were oriented specifically to "providing girls whose parents lack the means of subsistence, with asylum, education and food in accordance with their class and condition."[36] In 1912, however, even in San Carlos—the orphanage—"both the boys and girls almost all have parents and even patrons, and I am unaware of why they were admitted as orphans," the Junta de Beneficencia's subinspector remarked.[37]

Thus state institutions represented one of the options that the poor could use, especially when they did not have sufficient social and kin networks to draw on. In 1915, Rosa Zumba v. de Latorre (the "v." standing for *viuda*, or widow) petitioned the Junta de Beneficencia for protection for at least one of her children, in her condition as an "unfortunate and poor [*desgraciada e infeliz*] mother." Her husband had recently died, "leaving me with six children in the most complete misery." She reminded the Junta of the severe economic crisis of the time, which weighed heavily in general on the disinherited class. If that was the case for the strong sex, "what might not happen to a poor widow, ill and without any resources but her own work which does not provide enough even to feed the six children of her heart?" This was the situation, she concluded, that had led her to solicit a placement for one of her children in any of the charity establishments administered by the Junta de Beneficencia.[38] Loss of a husband could also occur through abandonment. In 1923, Margarita Valencia de Valencia found herself in the situation of being left alone to support seven children, the oldest of whom was a sixteen-year-old who suffered from epilepsy and so was unable to help her support his siblings. The remainder were too young to work and should instead have been receiving some education. However, Señora Valencia explained that she was unable to provide this since, at a minimum, schooling required that the children be properly clothed and that they be fed at least once a day. Señora Valencia further declared "that I am married to Luis Valencia who, when after abandoning me he was officially served with my claim for support [*prestación de alimentos*], disappeared from this place without leaving a trace."[39] Her petition for asilo and protection for three of her children was supported with certificates from respectable men confirming that Margarita Valencia de Valencia was completely honorable and poor.

Loss of a wife could also cause the remaining spouse to seek protection for offspring from the Beneficencia. In 1922, José María Vera sought asilo for his two youngest children (one seven years old, the other two months of age) when his wife died, leaving him with five orphaned children to support on his own. "It is a true sacrifice imposed on me by the harshness of fate; but better this than to see them die of hunger and illness, misery and neglect, these pieces of my heart who are not to blame for having been born into misery and having lost their mother. In replacement of her, in replacement of all of the missing mothers [*madres desaparecidas*], is the Beneficencia and I approach her trusting that she will not refuse to save my two little children who are in such danger." José María Vera's hope was that in one of the casas administered by the Beneficencia, his children would "be able to form themselves into beings useful to themselves and to their family, receiving the quality education that is offered there, and cared for as if by their mother."[40] Striking in this petition is the gendering of Beneficencia itself as feminine and as a replacement for absent mothers.

Sometimes children came first into the custody of extended family members, and it was those relatives who then sought help to support them. For instance in 1911, Miguel Ortiz, given his financial situation, "was placed in the painful position of having to deposit in the Hospicio of this Capital, my legitimate niece M. L. L., aged eight, due to the simultaneous death of her parents; but only while the life-time pension that is due to her is adjudicated, as the legitimate daughter of Sub-lieutenant Pedro Juan López who was killed in action in the battle of Angoteros."[41] In a different kind of case a quarter century later, Emperatriz Escobar de Ruiz sought placements for her two grandchildren who had been left with her when her daughter and son-in-law had gone to the coast to seek work given the difficult economic situation. She had never heard from them again.

> The children were left under my poor protection, and my situation is such that I cannot even support myself in my condition of widow and with my work,

the work of a woman that is not even sufficient to support a single person, much less three. Although they are of school age I have not been able to even offer them basic knowledge of the alphabet, or even cover their little bodies adequately, except with some clothing donated by charitable people. I make a superhuman effort to attend to the most indispensable, to feed our exhausted bodies, and even our housing is given to me without payment in exchange for a few services that I am able to offer, in the time left over after my work.[42]

Thus Emperatriz Escobar de Ruiz sought placements for her two grandchildren in the orphanage, supporting her petition with certificates from three honorable men who were familiar with her difficult situation.

Some children ended up in institutions for more deliberate reasons, rather than as the last resort. In 1906 the police sent R. C. to the Hospicio for six months, at the request of her mother. The latter had based her petition on the fact that her daughter had not yet reached the age of majority (sixteen), her behavior was unmanageable, and "for the sake of morality and since I exercise *patria potestad* [parental authority over children] over the minor, I solicit that she be reduced to prison or to detention in another house of correction."[43] The police agreed that the (unspecified) reasons given were "very serious," signing the appropriate order and passing it on to the Junta de Beneficencia so that they could authorize admission to the establishment. The Hospicio was a joint house of correction, shelter, and madhouse (and indeed, sometimes inappropriate behavior could be considered a sign of mental instability).[44] As late as 1947, there was a disproportionate number of female over male inmates in this institution, especially among the indigent: on the Hospicio side of the institution (for the elderly, beggars, and those with incurable diseases), there were 94 men and 168 women, while in the Manicomio (for those with nervous and mental illnesses), there were 103 beds for men (with 152 occupants), and only 87 for women (but 157 occupants).[45] The deposit of this minor in the Hospicio echoes the practice of depositing women in protective institutions in the nineteenth century elsewhere in Latin America, where part of what needed to be protected was the honor and morality of others. [46]

Despite the case of R. C.'s mother, the rights of patria potestad were more often used against women than claimed by them. Indeed, for that mother to claim patria potestad, she must have either been a widow or a single mother; otherwise by law the girl's father would have had those rights over their daughter and by extension over her. Thus, for instance, in the first decade of the twentieth century María H. del Hierro petitioned the Junta de Beneficencia for the right to see her daughters, revealing another way that girls ended up in institutions: "It is unjust that after being completely abandoned by my husband

Don Luis del Hierro, he has given a rash and unnatural order that I not be permitted to see my daughters who are interned in the Colegio San Vicente de Paul and the Colegio del Buen Pastor. The Superior Mothers of those Colegios, obeying the unilateral order of my husband, deny me the consolation of seeing my daughters. On those rare occasions when I am able to go to the schools, I am always turned away."[47] As she was ill, she requested that her eldest daughter be granted a month's leave from the Buen Pastor to care for her and that her two younger daughters be allowed to visit her.

Finally, in an intriguing case from 1921, Rosario Vaca v. de Aguirre (an illiterate widowed woman of the popular classes) solicited asilo for an infant who had been abandoned in her lodgings. She explained that in April a casual acquaintance had appeared on her doorstep to ask for help in locating a live-in position as a domestic servant and had asked to stay with her in the meantime since she had no other shelter. A few days later to Señora Vaca's surprise, her acquaintance gave birth to an infant son in the middle of the night and as a charitable act Señora Vaca had cared for and fed her for a few days. However, ten days later her guest had stepped out "to warm herself in the sun" and hadn't been seen since. After months of caring for the infant, Señora Vaca sought his admission to an asilo in November, "in view of the calamitous era in which we find ourselves, and because it is not possible for me to conserve him given the cost of his food and clothing, and also because I have three daughters of my own; I cannot attend to the needs of this child named L. J. M. of unknown father."[48]

The child was indeed accepted in San Carlos, and two years later Señora Vaca attempted to reclaim him, arguing that her circumstances had changed sufficiently to allow her to support him financially and that she had developed affection for the boy while caring for him in his infancy. The president of the Junta de Beneficencia, however, denied her request based on the fact that she had not demonstrated that she was the mother of the child.[49] This case alludes to a number of relevant practices among the popular classes: mutual support among vulnerable women; informal networks of child circulation; temporary use of state institutions; and again the possibility that investing in the future of a boy child might ensure some long-term support (something that Señora Vaca lacked given that her own children were all daughters).

What these anecdotes suggest is that use of state institutions was a strategy employed by the popular classes of Quito to resolve difficulties of care, sometimes on a temporary basis. However, as both Señora Vaca and Señora del Hierro found in rather different circumstances, it was not always easy to reclaim children who were interned in these establishments. As a result, for instance, in 1936 several children were encouraged to escape the Orfelinato de San Vicente de Paul "at the instigation of their mothers . . . and they currently are with the latter."[50] Later that year, two more children fled and had taken refuge with their stepmother, while another was thought to have been taken in by a former wet nurse.[51] Women seem to have faced particular difficulties in both retaining and reclaiming their children, as they did not have the same rights of patria potestad over their children as men did, and their economic situation was often more tenuous.

While internment of their children in institutions was one option that poor women might use, employed women had an alternative option available after 1914: Quito's first daycare facility for the children of working women. In 1914 police intendente Antonio Gil was instrumental in establishing this daycare run by the semiprivate Sociedad Protectora de la Infancia, which became known as the Asilo Antonio Gil due to the intendente's leadership in founding and presiding over it until his death in 1917. As police chief, Gil was well aware of the challenges facing poor women and their children, since it was his subaltern employees who often encountered abandoned infants in the streets who then were referred by the police hierarchy to the Beneficencia's orphanages.[52] While in the official documentary exchanges involving abandoned infants there were references to those who abandoned them as unnatural mothers (*madres desnaturalizadas*), sometimes those mothers themselves explained in the slips of paper left with their infants that they took this step because they were not accepted for domestic service with their children, and because they received no support from the fathers. Established precisely to prevent child abandonments in this context, the asilo "offers shelter, food and instruction to the infant children of poor and honorable *sirvientas* [female servants], so that they can with some liberty dedicate themselves to the tasks proper to their trade: the children are taken to the asilo in the morning and collected in the evening, at the hour when these women rest from their labors as cooks, maids, laundrywomen, etc."[53] This institution catered preferentially to the children of Quito's female working poor, freeing up these deserving mothers so they could work—or seen from another perspective, so they could offer their employers their undivided attention during their long workdays—while providing various services to their children.[54] As in so many of the archival sources on which this chapter is based, fathers were absent from this formulation, as indeed they likely were from many of these families.

The Sociedad Protectora de la Infancia offers an illuminating example of the interweaving of public and private initiative and funding in the child welfare field in Quito. Although it was a private philanthropic project (led by a prominent liberal government official), Subdirector of Sanidad Miño in turn succeeded in obtaining some state funds to support it, indicating that it was considered to fulfill a public function. Moreover, the Sociedad Protectora also provided some scholarships for poor children to attend school once they reached an appropriate age; these were partially financed with funds from the Junta de Beneficencia as well as with direct funding by the national government. After the death of Antonio Gil, Dr. Miño himself assumed the presidency of the Asilo Antonio Gil, although like Gil, Miño took on this role as a private individual rather than as a public official. In 1922 this institution became even more closely linked to the state when the Congress ceded to the Sociedad Protectora de la Infancia a house that the government owned.

By 1926 some ninety boys and girls ages two through six were receiving daycare at this institution while their mothers worked. The establishment included a school operated under the authority of the provincial Department of Education, with two kindergarten classes and one first grade; the latter children spent the day receiving basic elements of primary education, gymnasium, and apparently even in music classes. All of the children received three meals before leaving at the end of the day, although they were modest (for instance, the bread that had been included in their breakfast had recently been eliminated because of the increase in its price, leaving only sugared milk for that meal). The institution was funded by a monthly contribution of five hundred sucres from the recently renamed Junta de Asistencia Pública and monthly donations from the society's members amounting to under forty sucres, together giving a rather meager annual operating budget of some sixty-four hundred sucres. By 1931 state support had been further deepened. By then, some 120 children were served by the institution, which was open every day of the year. Education was offered there in a kindergarten and the first two grades of primary school. Four female technical staff and two female servants received their salaries directly from the provincial budget for primary education. The wages of the remaining subaltern employees (two female assistants and a cook, plus a male servant and a gardener) were paid by the society, but from the five hundred sucres that they continued to receive on a monthly basis from the Junta. By then, the house that the government had ceded to the society—which had been in ruins in 1922, requiring substantial renovations to be serviceable—had further deteriorated so much that only the patios and gardens could be used by the children in the asilo. The ministerio de previsión social thus had rented an adjacent house for the use of the asilo. The society was also supported by the interest income from a private bequest of forty-five hundred sucres from the estate of Señora Carmen Muñoz v. de Vega (contributing about 540 sucres annually to the operating budget), plus occasional small donations from the members of the Sociedad Protectora de la Infancia.[55]

The forms of protection offered in the Beneficencia's orphanages were primarily shelter, food, and clothing as well as some rudimentary education. To a large extent, the Asilo Antonio Gil also followed this model. Ultimately, survival to an age at which they could be released to fend for themselves, with some education that would help them survive economically, was the best that marginal children could expect. However, an additional framework for defining children's value was increasingly prevalent from the 1910s on, which suggested that simple survival of children was not enough. If they were also healthy and strong, they could truly contribute to national progress—notions that sharpened the medical gaze on issues of infant mortality and childhood illnesses.

### Knowing the Population and Medicalizing Child Welfare

By the early 1910s the liberal state had come to identify population growth as a national priority for Ecuador. At the beginning of 1914, just a few months after taking up the newly established position in Quito of subdirector de sanidad, Dr. Carlos Miño expressed his concern about the situation of children in the capital city to the director of the Junta de Beneficencia. His review of vital statistics led to him to conclude that "the number of child deaths in the capital is very alarming, as too is the situation in the Republic's other population centers. The infant mortality statistics are out of all proportion with the birth rates, the result being the depopulation of the cities."[56] In fact, Quito was not undergoing a process of depopulation: urban censuses indicate that the capital's population was in a growth stage, increasing from 51,858 in 1906, to 80,702 in 1922, to 101,668 in 1936, and reaching 209,932 by 1950.[57] Nonetheless, there was an increasing perception that population growth was threatened and that correcting this trend by both improving the quantity and quality of the population should be a national priority. That same year, the minister of the interior identified the danger that "in regard to poor children . . . their increasing rate of abandonment and death . . . may lead to the depopulation of the country."[58] A decade after Miño's comment, a physician colleague echoed his concerns that "the growth of Ecuador's population is of such importance that all social efforts in this regard will simply be the practical comprehension of an undeniable necessity."[59] And as another physician noted a few years later, "human capital is the only kind that leads to the enrichment of peoples and their perfect state of development."[60]

The social theorist Michel Foucault has drawn our attention to the myriad ways that populations are administered through agencies, actors, discourses, and norms, regulating and producing forms of conduct.[61] In beginning to explore the possibilities of a national (or at least an urban) biopolitics, new state institutions and actors did not merely respond to preexisting problems but actively produced the realm of their action.[62] The very notion itself of "population"—an entity that would come to be characterized, for instance, by rates of morbidity and mortality—was also constituted in the process.[63] To think, analyze, and intervene at the population level, liberal public health reformers needed to generate opportunities to observe and analyze the health conditions and vital statistics of Quito's residents. They were able to do so because in their commitment to improve child health, they began to offer services that attracted large numbers of popular-sector mothers seeking help for their children. In the arena of child health and welfare, among the private and public institutions of various kinds that proliferated, two such institutions in particular came to comprise something akin to social laboratories in which medical reformers could observe children's health status, identify trends, and even experiment with alternatives (for instance, in regard to infant feeding practices). These institutions were the children's free medical dispensary opened in 1916 and a newly established Casa Cuna (section for infants) within the orphanage founded after much discussion in 1927.

The coming together of these ideas about the national population in the early twentieth century reflects a particular notion of this population as an object amenable to state action, a common theme in Latin American (and other) countries in this era. This was different from how the country's inhabitants had been perceived in the nineteenth century, when indeed the state did not even control basic information about the population, which was in the hands instead of the Catholic Church. It was different, too, from how population problems were defined after World War II, when concern with increasing the quantity and quality of the population gave way at the international level to a concern with runaway population growth, leading to a series of population-control policies promoted during the Cold War by the Population Council in which John D. Rockefeller played a prominent role. This would be associated with fundamental changes in notions of what responsible motherhood comprised, as researchers have shown for other Latin American countries.[64]

These early-twentieth-century notions of the national population as a source of wealth, as human capital, were consistent with the liberal governments' general emphasis on the importance of labor issues. In this agricultural nation the careful cultivation of children (through the teaching of the scientific precepts of puericulture) was sometimes seen as parallel to the raising of crops, with children portrayed as "the tiny human plant" by pediatrician Carlos Sánchez.[65] Sometimes the connection drawn between agriculture and child welfare was much more explicit: "infant mortality and morbidity continue to be, in Ecuador, the fundamental obstacle to progress, principally in agriculture due to the large number of potential laborers that are wrested away from the working classes by death."[66] In any case, while children represented the future potential of the nation, to ensure their health and well-being, it was necessary to influence the behavior of their mothers, even from well before they became mothers. In this context, "to teach future mothers [at school age] how to preserve the lives of children, and in this manner make our nation more populous and grand, is perhaps the most patriotic project that the State could . . . undertake in benefit of the protection of children and the enrichment of the country."[67] The flipside of this idea was that motherhood was also the most patriotic project that women could undertake, a notion that was widely accepted as just common sense.

Following the overthrow of the liberals in 1925 in the Revolución Juliana, the revolutionary coalition of nationalistic mid-ranking military officers and middle-class professionals proceeded to pass social legislation in a variety of areas. Indeed, the change in government only intensified the focus on such issues as children, labor, and health, with the emergence of a more active, interventionist state—and with it, expanding state programs and state employment—in the following years. Soon after the Revolución Juliana, for the first time a stand-alone ministry was created to deal with social issues of this kind: the Ministerio de Previsión Social, Trabajo y Agricultura (Ministry of Social Security, Work, and Agriculture). This consolidated a shift already in progress in forms of governing population: bringing technical expertise to bear on problems that were themselves increasingly understood through expert scrutiny; marking a move toward more secular models; and also reorganizing jurisdictions both among state institutions and between public and private activity.

As notions of population were being forged, statistical analysis began to be used to grapple intellectually with the nature of the national population and to define its problems in order to intervene in resolving them. This could not have been conceived of before the passage of the 1900 Law of Civil Registry, which made it obligatory to register births, deaths, and marriages with new state registry offices. This was also a key move in the separation of church and state, since previously such information was more likely to be found in the registries of the Catholic Church. Moreover, civil registry went together with the establishment of civil marriage considered as a contract between two parties before the state, rather than a religious sacrament before God. Following the passage of the 1900 law, the civil registry began to function in January of 1901. Despite delays in establishing some of the offices for this service, nonetheless during the first two and half years of the registry's operation some two hundred thousand registrations of births, deaths, and marriages were carried out.[68] Urban censuses also began to be undertaken in Ecuador's larger cities, although remarkably the first full national census was only undertaken in 1950 (and at that late date, still required mapping of remote locations by the military cartography service).[69] The Ecuadorian state's capacity to know its population was undoubtedly partial in the early decades of the twentieth century. Nonetheless, in the largest urban areas, one can observe an increasing density of various kinds of institutions that could act on the population, whose actions were informed by a deeper understanding of its characteristics and conditions. One of the earliest areas in which this occurred was precisely in regard to health issues of infants and children.

Although the establishment of civil registry was an important step toward state knowledge of the population, it was not in itself sufficient to render more specific kinds of information, such as causes of death. In mid-1914 in his annual report the national director of Sanidad expressed concern in general about the quality of mortality statistics and highlighted especially gaps in the state's knowledge of causes of stillbirths and newborn deaths:

> No one bothers to find out why so many children die at birth. . . . The Police are responsible for investigating the cause of violent and unknown deaths; among these should be included the cases of infants who perish at birth or shortly thereafter, when no physician has verified the cause or illness that led to that death. If the Police carried out the necessary investigation, more than once they would discover a crime, which today is simply authorized by two inexpert and unknown witnesses, in accordance with the existing Law of Civil Registry. More than laughable, this is shameful: the Congress must dictate a less deficient law in this and many other aspects which are of fundamental importance.[70]

Rates of illness that did not lead to death were also outside the mandate of the civil registry system. The director thus further noted the difficulty of determining the *movimiento hospitalario*, because no statistics were compiled in the hospitals either: there was simply a register of incoming and outgoing patients kept by a Hermana de la Caridad, often without updating the records with physicians' definitive diagnoses.

With the establishment of a subdirection of public health in Quito, Dr. Carlos Miño hastened to establish a statistics section within the office "for the comparative study of birth and death rates in the population, in order to attend to the causes that influence the disproportion between one and another of these phenomena."[71] His review of civil registry records revealed that there was no scientific basis to the causes of death noted in death certificates, making it impossible to formulate statistics about this important issue. He met with the national director of the civil registry, and they came to an agreement that no death would be registered without either a statement of cause of death by the attending physician or the presentation of a death certificate issued by the sub-direction of public health in cases where there was no physician in attendance. He then informed the physicians of the capital and the directors of the two hospitals (both public) then operating in Quito—the Hospital Civil San Juan de Dios and the Hospital Militar—of their obligation to report cause of death in accordance with the Bertillon system of nomenclature of illnesses, a copy of which he provided to them. Finally, he communicated these requirements to the president of the Sociedad Funeraria Nacional to ensure that no cadavers would be buried without the appropriate death certificates.

Some months earlier—indeed within weeks of his arrival in Quito as a delegate of the Guayaquil Direction of Sanidad—the issue of infant mortality in particular had been brought to Miño's attention by a request from Charles Baker, the U.S. vice consul general in Guayaquil, to provide him with information about the causes of infant mortality in Quito for the purposes of informing the U.S. Department of State. Without any numerical detail at that point, Miño was simply able to report that: "According to the statistics of the Office of Sanidad of Pichincha, digestive illnesses [enfermedades colibacilares] occupy the first place, due exclusively to the deficiency of childhood alimentation, the poor quality of milk, its lack of sterilization, etc. Bronchitis is in second place, due to the cold temperatures of this city. In the course of last year there occurred a strong epidemic of measles, followed by another of whooping cough, causing numerous victims. In addition to these principal causes, we could add the following that also produced some deaths: paratyphoid fevers, dysentery, congenital heart defects, anemias, cholera nostras and meningitis."[72]

Shortly thereafter, the acting governor of the province also drew Miño's attention to infant mortality, when he wrote: "From the death registries in this canton's civil registry office, I am aware of the large number of children who die daily of infectious diseases; and since almost all of them are members of the poor class, it is logical to deduce that the cause of death is above all the lack of medical attention due to the poverty of their parents. This matter is of enormous social transcendence, since population growth is one of the factors of economic progress; thus we must defend the lives of children by all possible means."[73] He proposed that a hospital ward should be reserved solely for sick children, organized by Miño. However, this area did not really fall under the Sanidad's mandate, leading Miño to propose to the Junta de Beneficencia that they install, minimally, a ward for sick children in any of the institutions of Beneficencia. When he referred to the possible effects of infant mortality on the depopulation of the cities, Miño further argued that children "almost always perish from lack of medical attention, and due to the negligence of authorities in establishing free dispensaries, where the disinherited can find shelter and assistance for children attacked by disease."[74]

A number of shared assumptions are displayed here: that childhood illnesses constituted a problem of national significance; as a consequence, that child health was an appropriate arena for state action; and that if population growth was to be assured, then the first task was to reduce infant mortality. These ideas were clearly circulating more generally at the time; however, the delay of some six months between the acting governor's suggestion and the Sanidad's suggestion to the Beneficencia that they establish a children's ward may have been due to the necessity of sorting out the areas of jurisdiction of these two entities in the initial period after the establishment of a public health office in Quito. Despite the fact that initially child health was not really part of his mandate, Miño did opine on the causes of infant mortality in his first annual report, attributing equal blame to lack of services offered by the Junta de Beneficencia and poor mothering. Thus he argued that "the majority of the infant deaths are caused by a lack of medical attention and above all, of the necessary medicine to cure them; not to mention the punishable lack of care [*descuido*] by mothers in the raising of their children and the poor quality of food or the actual lack of food."[75] Although there were indications of economic causes for poor child health, they were interpreted as mothers' negligence.

Given the growing perception of a health crisis affecting the children of Quito, as various officials examined the city's vital statistics records, the Beneficencia moved ahead in 1915 with a project to provide free medical care to Quito's children. In mid-1915 the locale for a free medical dispensary for children was being renovated adjacent to the Hospital Civil San Juan de Dios and the Junta was only awaiting the arrival of the equipment and medications on order from the United States to inaugurate it. "The examination and opportune treatment of the children, the distribution of sterilized milk to those in need, and above all the instruction that slowly but effectively will be given to the mothers about the hygienic precepts underlying the proper raising [*crianza*] of children, will make the dispensary a grand medium of child protection."[76] The *dispensario gratuito para niños pobres* (free medical dispensary for poor children) was opened in January 1916, offering both medical attention and medications free of charge to children under the age of six. In the first half of 1916 some 1,470 poor children were attended there by its physicians and medical students; in the same period a year later, a total of 3,726 children were seen. Among those children who died despite the care received in the first half of 1917, digestive illnesses stood out, along with measles.

Dr. Carlos García Drouet, the dispensario's first director, was persuaded by his initial observations of the dispensary's patients that the measure that would most reduce infant mortality would be the establishment of a service of sterilized milk, given the large number of illnesses of the digestive system.[77] In 1919 more than half of the deaths among the children attended were caused by illnesses of the digestive system. As Dr. García insisted again: "The greatest mortality is due to illnesses of the digestive system, because the mothers submit their children prematurely to a coarse and defective [*grosera y defectuosa*] alimentation; either because they do not have in their breasts a sufficient quantity of milk, or because many are occupied in work that does not allow them to offer to their children the quality and quantity of milk necessary to nourish them. To rectify this and reduce the mortality highlighted, it is indispensable to provide sterilized milk to the children who need it."[78] Although he alluded to a number of underlying economic and social problems facing mothers, the solution he proposed was a primarily technical one.

In 1923, when pediatrician Dr. Carlos Sánchez had taken over the directorship of the dispensario, the single most significant cause of death continued to be gastroenteritis, leading to about 20 percent of the deaths among the children seen at the clinic.[79] Despite the fact that almost twice as many patients arrived at the dispensario that year with Spanish influenza (1,211 cases) than with gastroenteritis (662 cases), the former caused fewer than three-quarters as many deaths as the latter. In his annual report Sánchez highlighted the fact that while in 1922 the total rate of infant mortality in Quito when measured against the birth rate had been 29.3 percent, nonetheless among those sick children attended in the dispensario in 1923 a mortality rate of only 7.4 percent measured against the total number of patients indicated a "result worthy of taking into consideration."[80] While this suggested to Sánchez the effectiveness of the dispensario, the rates of infant mortality were quite striking: he pointed out that in 1922 the rate of infant mortality (deaths among children ages one day to five years) in Quito when measured against the total mortality in the city constituted over half (971 of 1,886 deaths in the city, or 51.48 percent).[81] In Sánchez's comments one can imagine him turning the figures around and looking at them from different angles to try to extract the appropriate meaning from them.

Increasingly, medical reformers were able to place Ecuador in a larger comparative context as they tried to develop those meanings. Thus international figures from 1925 indicated that Ecuador had the dubious distinction of placing third in the world in high infant mortality when measured against total population, following Chile and Costa Rica (although it should be noted that not all of the world's countries were included in the figures provided). Or in a different calculation, for every hundred births seventeen to eighteen Ecuadorian infants died; Ecuador again ranked third after Chile and Costa Rica. When pediatrician Carlos Andrade Marín presented these two sets of figures in a 1929 medical study of child welfare issues (written as he was completing his medical studies and first prize winner in a contest organized by the association of medical students), he did not indicate his source.[82] These figures were also of concern to Chilean researchers. The physician Salvador Allende presented similar rankings in a study of Chilean health, indicating for instance that Chile, Costa Rica, and Ecuador (in that order) had the highest rates of infant mortality in Latin America in 1929.[83] Allende cited the annual statistical reports published by the League of Nations, and the similarity in figures suggests that this might have also been Andrade Marín's source. Both Andrade Marín and Allende were part of a generation of physicians who had been trained to think statistically about the population and who read widely about health conditions elsewhere to better contextualize and interpret their local situations. A comparative source that began to be cited by Ecuadorian physicians at the end of the 1920s was the annual English-language publication the *International Handbook of Child Health*.[84]

As the account of the work of Quito's dispensario suggests, this clinic provided not only free medical care to poor children, a service that was apparently welcomed by their mothers, but also gave the physicians and functionaries of the Beneficencia and Sanidad a much clearer notion of the main health risks faced by the capital's children. What was most evident to them was that preventable illnesses of the digestive tract demanded urgent attention (table 2.1).

**TABLE 2.1. Patients and Mortality at the Children's Free Medical Dispensary, Selected Early Years**

| Year | Children attended | Deaths | Main causes of death |
|------|------|------|------|
| 1917 (first half only) | 3,726 | 293 | Gastroenteritis: 79 |
| | | | Enteritis: 49 |
| | | | (Digestive illnesses: 128) |
| | | | Measles: 71 |
| 1919 | 6,631 | 361 | Gastroenteritis: 78 |
| | | | Enteritis: 86 |
| | | | Enterocolitis: 24 |
| | | | (Digestive illnesses: 188) |
| 1923 | 6,851 | 510 | Gastroenteritis: 101 |
| | | | Influenza: 72 |
| | | | Bronchitis: 54 |

*Source*: Reports to the Junta de Beneficencia, AAP/MNM.

These required a combination of new services (such as provisioning of sterilized milk) and new behaviors on the part of mothers. A new institution in the capital aimed to achieve both of these goals. In early 1920, following an initiative of Dr. Enrique Gallegos Anda (the director of the clinical laboratory at the hospital), a group of prominent señoras organized the Sociedad de La Gota de Leche. By June the society's statutes had been approved, their executive elected, and they were preparing to install a milk depot.[85]

Modeled on similar institutions elsewhere, the activities of the Gota de Leche included: "registration, medical examination and vigilance of the child, distribution of age-appropriate alimentation, study of the development of the child, promotion of maternal breast-feeding and when this is impossible for some reason, regulated artificial feeding, etc. The señoras who form this society also visit periodically the mothers served by these dispensaries, with the aims of monitoring the care provided to the children in their homes and distributing some clothing to the mothers and children, taking advantage of such visits to disseminate notions of hygiene and puericulture and to promote breast-feeding." The women involved were characterized as "the señoras of the highest society of Quito, who have taken on the duty of exercising charity in favor of the most vulnerable members of the Ecuadorian family: nursing infants."[86] If the nation was a family, then it was not just the biological parents who were responsible for their children and who had a stake in their well-being. The nation's children could and should come under the watchful eye and philanthropic action of other concerned citizens, too.

The president of the Junta de Beneficencia welcomed the founding of the Gota de Leche and went so far to suggest that the Sociedad de La Gota de Leche broaden its work to take over various other projects of Beneficencia. Its leaders responded that this would not be possible not only due to lack of resources but because the society's purpose was clearly defined and limited in its statutes.[87] The Sociedad de La Gota de Leche's focus on the provision of sterilized milk alongside the promotion of breast-feeding may well have been due to the prominent role in this institution of the wives of modernizing hacienda owners from the Guaytacama area in Cotopaxi province, who took advantage of their proximity to the railway line (completed from Guayaquil to Quito in 1908) to intensify dairy production for urban markets. Those landowners, via their leadership in a highland association of large agriculturalists, the Sociedad Nacional de Agricultura (SNA), had recently worked collaboratively with government officials to design a law favoring the modernization of agricultural production in the highlands. This law was passed in 1918 as the Ley de Fomento Agrícola and aimed to help provision coastal markets for basic foods given the difficulties of importing such goods during World War I. They also lobbied successfully for a tax on all large highland landowners, which was used to support and promote the SNA's activities.[88] Although the Sociedad de La Gota de Leche was protective of its rights as a private institution to set its own mandate, in 1920 the Ecuadorian Congress passed a special law dedicating 60 percent of the proceeds of a tax on inheritances to child welfare institutions specifically of this kind (the other 40 percent supported children in another way, through investment in the construction and repair of school facilities).[89] Perhaps the leaders of the Gota de Leche had learned some skills in political lobbying from their husbands. Access to these government-mandated funds allowed the Gota de Leche to quickly expand its activities, founding a second locale in short order.

The Gota de Leche represented one approach to child welfare, involving the philanthropic activity of elite women. It can be compared with another association of philanthropic women that had a very different approach and arena of activity: the Sociedad de las Señoras de la Caridad, working together with the Conferencia de San Vicente de Paul.[90] These associated organizations had been founded in Quito in the 1860s—that is, during García Moreno's government—as private charitable associations. Their purpose was "charity, support for poor families; [their] resources are the weekly and monthly donations by [their] members and the legacies and bequests from pious persons who wish to distribute their property to the poor via the Conferencia." In 1931 these associations were assisting some 370 families, providing them with food items on a weekly basis and occasionally in emergencies with small quantities of money. The Sociedad de San Vicente de Paul welcomed "all young Catholics who wish to take part in works of charity. . . . No act of charity should be considered outside the Sociedad's mandate, although the principal activity consists of visits to poor families." Each member was expected to visit poor families who were deserving of aid and then at regular meetings of local units of the society report on each family's needs so that the society could decide what kind of support to provide; following these reports, each member would make a donation to the funds used to provide such support.

The Sociedad de San Vicente de Paul also received bequests that, although they required payments of significant probate fees and inheritance taxes, could provide considerable income: in 1931 the society anticipated that it would be left with some fifty thousand sucres after taxes from the estate of Don Manuel María Casares Rivera. Señora Doña Carmen Muñoz v. de Vega had also left the majority of her estate to the Conferencia de San Vicente de Paul and the Asociación de las Señoras de la Caridad. This indicates the prevalence of an older model of private Catholic charity toward the deserving poor (and association members visited poor families regularly to ensure that they deserved aid) that coexisted with increasing state oversight of and intervention in the care of poor children, both directly and via semiprivate institutions receiving various kinds of state support. Still, even this older model had specific historical roots in a more activist and interventionist approach to Catholic religiosity that was later promoted as Catholic action.[91]

The early 1920s also saw the establishment of the Cruz Roja Ecuatoriana, with an active women's committee dealing with children's issues.[92] This was so much a women's domain that the pre-printed form the Cruz Roja used in late 1925 to solicit donations of materials for a *canastilla maternal* (layette) was addressed to "Sra. Doña _____," even when the name filled in was that of a man. The contents of the canastilla included linens and clothing for the infant as well as a nightshirt for the mother, and the communication included a copy of the Geneva Declaration of the Rights of the Child passed in 1923 and adopted by all Red Cross organizations worldwide.[93] This was an early expression of a rights-based approach to children's issues, something that did not become widely prevalent in Ecuador until 1990.[94] Still, the means by which this concept of rights was operationalized in Quito in 1925 was based on a model of private charity, albeit a modernized one.

Together these institutions created many contexts in which women of different classes interacted, usually with the stated goal of helping at-risk members of the national family: in other words, poor women's children. Many such programs were welcomed by poor mothers who sought ways to use them for their own purposes. They also generated opportunities for elite women to engage in public activities, given that child welfare was an acceptable sphere of gendered social action, where they could enjoy a certain degree of decision-making autonomy (something the leaders of the Gota de Leche, for instance, clearly enjoyed). And in some cases these programs generated opportunities for employment for women of the middle sectors as well as arenas of work for female religious orders. Some institutions could indeed fulfill all of these functions simultaneously.

While the establishment in early 1920 of the Gota de Leche was an important contribution to preventative health measures for children, later that year the situation of child health in Quito was such that the minister of the interior promoted a joint meeting of the Sanidad and the Beneficencia to discuss ways to address the situation. Together they examined the statistics of mortality and morbidity, including the resurgence of Spanish influenza and of whooping cough. The Sanidad's Dr. Miño argued energetically for the establishment of a service of hospitalization for sick children:

> It is time to put an end to the disproportionate infant mortality, which suffers from abandonment by administrative action [the state] as well as by social

action [private philanthropy], whose effectiveness is felt in other civilized centers.[95] Today I insist especially on the importance of the hospitalization of sick children, and not in a precarious way but as a permanent public service; if we combine the lack of public assistance with the ignorance of the population and its lack of economic resources, the depopulation of the country will be the immediate consequence, not to mention the discredit we will suffer as a civilized nation.[96]

The Beneficencia, in turn, was already working on a collaborative effort between the Hospital Civil and the Gota de Leche to adapt a hospital ward for sick children. However, it was hampered by an economic situation in which it had accumulated so much debt that it needed to first reestablish its credit before engaging in new activities.[97] (This may explain why the Beneficencia had been eager to have the Gota de Leche take over the delivery of some of its programs; the Sanidad showed itself to be considerably less amenable to offering up control of its own programs.) Again, the mixing of public and private was demonstrated when the subdirector of public health—who in his private life was the director of the Asilo Antonio Gil—facilitated the provision to the hospital of cots that the Asilo Antonio Gil had lent to the Gota de Leche when the latter had aspired to itself establish a clinic for sick children.[98]

Meanwhile, the rector of the Universidad Central hoped that the Junta de Beneficencia might be able to obtain from the Gota de Leche some children's nightshirts that they had confected in preparation for establishing that planned clinic. Dr. Alfonso Mosquera Narváez (who later that decade would be named general director of public health) offered to provide medical attention without remuneration in the Junta's children's ward under these urgent circumstances.[99] An in-patient children's ward was indeed decreed by the Junta de Beneficencia in 1920 and was established under precarious conditions as a dependency of the Hospital Civil under the direction of Dr. Antonio Bastidas.[100] From the early 1920s plans were also under way for the foundation of a children's hospital following bequests from the estate first of Señor Héctor Baca and then of his widow Dolores Ortiz, but this project encountered considerable delays before it was inaugurated as the Hospital de Niños Baca-Ortiz in 1948.

The mid-1920s saw efforts to reorganize this terrain of private, semiprivate, and public institutions in a climate of considerable administrative energy. Just a few weeks after the 1925 July Revolution, a decree of August 5 reorganized the structure and mandate of the Ecuadorian Public Health Service, affecting the Sanidad's relation with private institutions such as the Gota de Leche as well as with other public institutions. In mid-September, public health physician Dr. Alfonso Mosquera communicated with the Sociedad de La Gota de Leche that the Gota had become a dependency of the Sanidad, making the medical chief of the Sanidad's child welfare service, Dr. Luis Barberis, the technical director of the Gota de Leche. In the absence of the society's president, the Gota's vice president, Señora María Lasso de Eastman (from the prominent landowning family in Cotopaxi province into which liberal president Leonidas Plaza had married), took her time in responding. When she did so some weeks later, she expressed her surprise at his communication, explaining that the society was a private institution protected by the guarantees inscribed in the Ecuadorian Civil Code, that it had juridical independence, and moreover that the technical services of the society were under the expert direction of Drs. Isidro Ayora and Pablo Arturo Suárez.[101]

Following discussions between Dr. Barberis and Dr. Ayora, the Sanidad communicated their mutual agreement that a physician should be named immediately to oversee each of the two Gota de Leche locations, and the Sanidad nominated Dr. Barberis and his assistant Dr. Sergio Lasso for these two appointments. Señora Lasso de Eastman agreed to appoint Dr. Barberis given the recent resignation of Dr. Suárez, but only because this suggestion by the Sanidad coincided with her personal opinion. However, Dr. Lasso could not be designated since Dr. Ayora was director of Gota No. 2, and given his well-known personal and professional qualifications, it would not occur to her to replace him.[102] By December the Sanidad was reduced to explaining that its goal was simply technical cooperation, as a form of encouragement and support for the services the Gota de Leche offered, but if that was not possible then they simply wished to request the Gota's assistance in establishing a school of *nodrizas* (wet nurses) under the Sanidad's auspices, encouraging the mothers who benefited from the Gota's services to enroll in the classes that would be offered there in hygiene and puericulture (in this case, the "wet nurses" in question were the actual mothers of the nursing infants).[103] Señora Lasso graciously applauded this initiative.[104]

A battle of wills emerged clearly from these exchanges between the leaders of the Sanidad and the Gota de Leche. In contrast, a few years later the male leaders of the Sociedad Protectora de la Infancia expressed their view that they would welcome more frequent exercise of the Asistencia Pública's legal right to supervise the organization's activities.[105] Perhaps the fact that such leaders were often prominent men filling other public roles—in other words, with other arenas in which they could exercise their authority—made them less protective of their autonomy than philanthropic women who had fewer opportunities to engage in autonomous forms of public activity.

While the December 1925 communications between the Sanidad and the Gota de Leche seemed to indicate a truce, the Sanidad's attributions in this area were further expanded by a decree of the Juliana's provisional Junta de Gobierno at the end of that month. In Quito the director of public health via (*por medio de*) La Gota de Leche (and in Guayaquil via the Sociedad de Puericultura) was charged with establishing suppliers of sterilized milk for the feeding of infants who did not have access to breast milk from their mothers or a wet nurse. Such milk would be sold at cost to those who could afford to pay and free of charge to those who were able to demonstrate need to the director of the Sanidad. Where it was not possible to establish supply depots of sterilized milk under the Sanidad's direction, the Sanidad would monitor in general the sale of milk to ensure that to the extent possible (depending on local conditions), such sale respected the precepts of hygiene. No one would be permitted to sell milk without the permission of a public health official; such permits, however, would be free of charge.[106] By this means, part of the activities of the Gota de Leche did come under Sanidad supervision. Perhaps the appointment of Dr. Pablo Arturo Suárez as general director of public health in 1926 (with the headquarters of the national institution moved to Quito) helped to smooth the relations between the Sanidad and the Gota de Leche.

By the end of 1926, the Gota de Leche's technical services were being overseen by Dr. Gabriel Araujo (son of early scientific midwife Juana Miranda) on an ad honorem basis.[107] Alternating between the two locales of the Gota, he spent an hour each day on his medical visits to these sites. Meanwhile, the ongoing administration of the locales was carried out by three Hermanas Dominicanas (Dominican nuns), who oversaw the sterilization and distribution of milk and the weighing and bathing of infants. Milk was distributed to infants each afternoon, with Gota de Leche No. 1 serving eighty-four infants in its rented location on the first floor of a house on García Moreno street, and No. 2 serving another seventy infants a few blocks away in a "comfortable and hygienic house" on Avenida Colombia that was owned by the Sociedad de La Gota de Leche, together distributing some 110 liters of milk each day.[108] The society was financed at that point by state funds amounting to twelve hundred sucres per month and donations by its members, which amounted to some 100 to 110 sucres each month, while its monthly expenditures fluctuated between a thousand and thirteen hundred sucres.

For several months the national treasury had not provided its monthly payments, however, so the society had been unable to make the contributions it had budgeted for of 600 sucres for the Sociedad Protectora de la Infancia and 960 sucres for the Casa Cuna (the daycare center) of the Cruz Roja Ecuatoriana. The Gota de Leche's role in channeling funding to other semiprivate institutions of child welfare was due to its privileged position as prime beneficiary of the 1920 tax on inheritances. By 1931 the Gota's rented premises had been replaced with more adequate ones on the Carrera Loja, and together the two locales served some 170 infants.[109] In the mid-1920s the society was also considering the establishment of a Comedor de la Madre, which by feeding poor mothers would also help their children. Indeed, a principal way that poor women could access resources for themselves was via programs that were established to support their children, who were implicitly considered beings of greater public value.

The establishment of the Gota de Leche was one response to high infant mortality associated with digestive problems, which had become increasingly evident among the patients served by the dispensario. Another site where medical experts explored issues of infant feeding through medical observation and intervention was among the abandoned infants who were cared for by the Asistencia Pública, where physicians and policy makers debated the relative advantages of engaging wet nurses and of using artificial feeding methods (sterilized cow's milk) as well as of raising infants institutionally versus in family placements. An attempt by the Junta de Beneficencia to collect information on the health of its nursing infant population in 1916 had run up against the fact that among the wet nurses who were contracted to feed them, "some live far away and even in neighboring towns," although they brought the infants to Quito to be checked periodically by the nuns of the Casa de San Carlos. The Hermanas assured the Beneficencia that "the children in general are well cared for, and several are even robust; because we always take care to inspect the wet nurses to ensure that they fulfill their duties."[110] In 1922 infants continued to be confided to the care of wet nurses in their homes, but by then it was the physician subinspectors of the Junta who carried out monitoring during periodic domestic visits.[111]

Given the difficulties of oversight, in 1924 the Junta de Beneficencia conceived of the idea of finding a way to "exercise greater vigilance over the niños expósitos" of Quito, since offering "special care in an adequate establishment would be much more favorable for the preservation and health of these unfortunate infants than entrusting them to the care of wet nurses in their own homes."[112] The Beneficencia engaged in an initial consultation with the madre superiora of San Carlos to consider options. They also developed a draft budget for a projected Casa Cuna, including twenty sucres a month for each of twelve Hermanas who would administer the institution, plus monthly wages for eight female employees at twelve sucres each.[113] The latter were clearly wet nurses given the attention paid to how much it would cost to feed them appropriately (sixty centavos each, per day), such that the latter amount was significantly more in the annual budget than the amount of their wages. Milk and the fuel to sterilize it were also prominent items in the budget as well as supplementary foods for children over eighteen months of age.

When an internal regulation for the Casa Cuna was drafted later that year, however, it had a significantly more secular and technical profile.[114] It would be administered by a directora named by the Junta, overseeing one or two assistants and a sufficient number of wet nurses; and the medical service would be overseen by a physician member of the Junta, assisted by a junior physician (*ayudante*) who would ensure the fulfillment of the physician's instructions, monitor the healthy development of the children, give classes in puericulture to the wet nurses, spend at least three hours a day in the institution, and sleep on-site. The obligations of the wet nurses included eating the diet prescribed for them by the physician, wearing uniforms during their hours of service, maintaining personal cleanliness, and breast-feeding the infants assigned to them and generally attending the children with care and affection, "given that they have neither father nor mother." Each year coinciding with the civic holiday, the children would be entered into a contest and the wet nurses of the two most robust infants would receive prizes of fifty and twenty-five sucres. As well as being fed and clothed, the children were to be bathed every day in the temperature indicated by the physician, weighed and measured regularly, and vaccinated against smallpox.

In September 1925, Dr. Luis G. Dávila was named the director ad honorem of the Casa Cuna. An Ecuadorian physician who had been sponsored by Eloy Alfaro's government to study in Lyon, France, Dávila was active in various philanthropic institutions and boards of directors in Quito. For instance, in 1924 he was a member of the Junta de Beneficencia and a member of the planning board for the projected children's hospital; he was also a member of the Junta del Ferrocarril a Esmeraldas and a board member of the Sociedad de Crédito Internacional "etc., etc."—all of which prevented Dávila from accepting a position that year as a board member of the Sociedad Protectora de la Infancia to which the director of the Junta de Beneficencia wished to name him.[115] At the time he was appointed medical director of the Casa Cuna by the Junta de Beneficencia, he had also just been appointed the director of the Northern District of the Sanidad, following the initial reorganization of the public health service in early August 1925.[116]

Thus a week after accepting his position at the Casa Cuna for the Beneficencia (which he communicated on Sanidad letterhead), Dávila wrote again to the director of the Junta de Beneficencia to inform him that under the *decreto supremo* of August 5, the area of child welfare (*protección a la infancia*) fell under the authority of the Sanidad. He thus asked the director of the Junta to consult with the head of the Sanidad's child welfare service, Dr. Luis Barberis, to discuss appropriate regulation of the Junta's services with the aim of harmonizing the functioning of all of the state programs in this area.[117] In December, however, the Casa Cuna de Expósitos had still not been established by the Junta, leading Dávila in his role with the Sanidad to insist on its immediate establishment.[118] By then, he visualized its personnel as consisting of the medical director and a medical intern, four *muchachas cuidadoras* (nursery maids), and two laundrywomen—all six of whom would live in the institution—as well as a doorman (*portero*). Apparently the infants would no longer be breastfed; several items of the equipment to be ordered were for the sterilization and preservation of milk.

In the end, the Casa Cuna was not established by the renamed Junta Central de Asistencia Pública until September 1927. And when it was, it was indeed administered by the Hermanas de la Caridad as a kind of annex to the orphanage. This decision may have been made on the basis of the recommendation of Dr. Luis de la Torre (who was named its medical director) that "the directora should be a nun, for reasons known by all and therefore unnecessary to enumerate here."[119] (While that may have been obvious to him, it had not been obvious to all involved in the early planning stages of this institution.) The medical director, in turn, would oversee technical issues, such as indicating the amount of milk provided to each child, the number of bottles, whether it was pure milk or diluted with sugar water (and in what proportion), the feeding schedule, and other details.

Some of the clients were expected to be infants with mothers, who should leave work during the day to nurse them if such infants were very young (the superiora of San Carlos also sought a wet nurse for service in the Casa Cuna, however). In his recommendations on how the Casa Cuna should be operated and what kinds of services it should offer, de la Torre referred frequently to research conducted in France on related issues (like many of his colleagues, he likely had undertaken advanced training in France). Moreover, the doctor provided more general reflections on medical problems of infant health and welfare, reminding the Junta that in Ecuador "infant mortality is largely due to gastroenteritis and other digestive disturbances caused by being deprived of the maternal breast, premature weaning, and the lack of hygienic feeding methods: the fatal triad of infant mortality." In other words, the three principal causes of infant mortality were all linked to inadequate maternal behaviors. Paradoxically, however, according to French experts cited by de la Torre, children separated from their mothers died four times more often, and of every hundred infant deaths, eighty-five were among children fed artificially, twelve had been nursed for only a short time, and only three were breastfed. Thus "it is our duty to inculcate in mothers that the only way to ensure the life of their children is maternal lactation."[120]

Nonetheless, for those abandoned infant expósitos who had been placed with wet nurses in their homes, the Asistencia Pública decided to gather up such infants from their domestic fostering placements in September 1927. Three months later de la Torre summed up the experience of the first months of functioning of the Casa Cuna by emphasizing the difficulties of raising children collectively, again with a thorough review of French and other European views on the matter. Most pediatric experts, he argued, systematically rejected child rearing in common (that is, institutional care) under the age of one year. In Quito he argued that the Casa Cuna should continue to operate for children over a year of age, but that infants should again be entrusted to wet nurses in their homes, under regular supervision by physicians or visiting nurses. Indeed, after three months of operation of the Casa Cuna, only those children over a year had survived the experience: all of the younger infants had died.[121] The following year, he had to report that the mortality rate of orphaned and abandoned babies that entered the Casa de Expósitos in 1928 was 100 percent, leading him to insist that infants under a year of age be turned over to wet nurses to be cared for in their own homes, as had been done previously. If the situation continued as it was, he remarked that very soon Ecuador would have no more orphan infants to worry about, since they would all die.[122] As their colleagues elsewhere in Latin America, Ecuadorian physicians were discovering that something was missing from the most carefully planned technical environment. In Mexico infants in foundling homes were recognized as suffering from a syndrome known as hospitalism, resulting in them "dying of sadness."[123] Perhaps the political climate of postrevolutionary Mexico lent itself more easily to formal recognition of the virtues of the working-class family environment.

By 1935 the Asistencia Pública was running two Casas Cunas that served orphans but also one that provided daycare for the children of workers, where needy children could receive the benefits of their family context at night combined with the benefits of state services during the day. These institutions were referred to as "Casa del Niño" No. 1, No. 2, and No. 3—more technical-sounding names that only slightly masked the fact that No. 1, for instance, was a renaming of San Vicente. There was also a Casa Cuna daycare being run by the Cruz Roja that by 1937 had capacity for some 150 children; the Cruz was planning a second Casa Cuna to be installed in the southern part of the city in the more industrial area. The Cruz Roja established a prenatal clinic that year as well.[124] Dr. Cesar Jácome, who communicated these developments as the secretary of the Cruz Roja, was also the director of the Asistencia's Maternidad clinic at the time.

In addition to bringing children into various kinds of institutional care, state physicians began to provide free medical care to children in their homes.

In months of significant infectious diseases affecting children, the Asistencia Pública began to operate a program of free medical assistance via house calls. In 1929 the general director of public health, Dr. Alfonso Mosquera, asked that the Asistencia Pública not allow children with infectious diseases such as bronchitis and whooping cough to seek medical attention at the dispensario but rather for the mothers of such children to request home visits from the Asistencia's physicians.[125] A similar system had already been established the previous year during the same season (June and July), when Dr. Braulio Pozo i Diaz of the Hospital Civil conducted 574 home visits to attend 463 sick children, of whom that year 75 percent were ill with measles and 25 percent with whooping cough. Of those, only twelve children died, most of whom were suffering from both diseases and as a result experienced serious complications such as broncopneumonia. The doctor took advantage of his visits to "attempt to inculcate in the families the most elemental principles of hygiene and prophylaxis."[126] Given the importance of this kind of measure to avoid the spread of contagious diseases, the Sanidad itself formally expanded its office of child welfare in 1930, to monitor statistics of child mortality and morbidity as well as to visit and inspect the various institutions of child welfare operated by the Junta de Asistencia Pública, part of the broader process of providing more technical and medical monitoring of those facilities.[127]

By 1931 house calls were a regular part of the duties of the dispensario medical staff, such that physician Eduardo Batallas felt that the work was beyond what he was physically capable of handling. He was seeing some fifty to sixty sick children at the dispensary every day as well as making house calls and working night shifts, leading him to request that the latter at least be removed from his unmanageable workload.[128] Batallas worked with two other physicians and a medical intern, together attending 11,354 children at the dispensary in 1931, with a mortality rate among their patients of 5.5 percent.[129] Injections and treatments ordered by the on-duty physician were given by nurse Señorita Inés Carrera, who two years earlier had formed part of the first cohort of formal graduates of the nursing school operating out of the Maternidad.[130] Given the crowded nature of the space used, at the beginning of 1932 the outpatient services of the dispensario were expanded into some additional space, although the hospitalization of sick children was still impeded by lack of appropriate space in the old hospital. However, by then physicians were looking optimistically toward the upcoming 1933 inauguration of the new Hospital Eugenio Espejo to solve the chronic need for inpatient services for children.[131]

With a new outbreak of measles in Quito in 1933, two physicians were assigned by each of the Asistencia Pública and the Sanidad to collaborate in providing home medical attention to sick children.[132] By 1937 the Sanidad was running its own Dispensario Infantil, which in a single month saw 1,031 children, among whom only 10 died, mostly of bronchitis.[133] The increasing direct involvement in child health by the Sanidad in the second half of the 1930s may have been informed by an Executive Decree of April 25, 1935, that established two programs of child protection conceived of as preventative rather than curative, placing them squarely under the authority of the Sanidad rather than the Asistencia Pública. One was a program of prenatal, natal, and infant care that entailed the employment of scientific midwives and visiting nurses in an outreach program of maternal and infant health in poor neighborhoods of Quito and in provincial capitals and county seats (this project is discussed in detail in chapter 4). When nurses working for the Sanidad began to visit the homes of Quito's poor to provide advice and monitoring of the health of newborn infants, they also began to channel child clients into other child welfare establishments. For instance, the service identified a number of women who were unable to breast-feed their infants, who were recommended to the Gota de Leche for their services. Once social workers began to undertake home visits in the late 1930s and 1940s—under the provisions of the new Child Code—channeling of children into care was further enhanced.[134]

The second project initiated under the Sanidad's auspices in 1935 involved the establishment of *colonias infantiles sanitarias* south of Quito in the countryside outside Machachi, on a section of the state-owned *hacienda de asistencia pública* Tolóntag. The colonia sanitaria was aimed at children age ten and younger from Guayaquil who were determined to be at risk of tuberculosis. They were selected by public health officials in the port to be sent in groups of one hundred for three-month stays in the healthier climate of the highlands. These colonias began to operate with the first group of children embarking on the train from Guayaquil less than a month after the passage of the decree; two years later, the eighth such group was en route to Machachi from Guayaquil. In 1936 medical oversight was carried out by the head of the Sanidad's department of child welfare, Dr. Rafael Quevedo Coronel, a pediatrician with particular expertise in tuberculosis (who a few years later would be appointed to the Consejo Nacional de Menores). By September 1937 a similar colonia infantil for boys only was being established in the state-owned hacienda Santo Domingo de Conocoto.

## Shifting Contours of Child Protection

On the eve of the passage of the 1938 Minors Code, physician Pablo Arturo Suárez (professor of hygiene at the Universidad Central, a former general director of the Sanidad, and founder of the medical-social branch of the Instituto Nacional de Previsión) and lawyer Gregorio Ormaza (director of the

Junta Central de Asistencia Pública) summed up the situation of child welfare in Quito in a report written to inform the new code. By 1938 they reported that twenty-five hundred pregnancies annually out of an approximate total of thirty-one hundred in Quito received prenatal care or medical attention during the birth, either in the Maternidad, through outpatient consultations, or from private physicians. Approximately five thousand children were also served by various institutions oriented toward the protection of children, including the Casas Cunas and the free dispensario, out of a total preschool urban population estimated at twelve thousand at that time. School children in turn received some health monitoring, especially vaccinations and dental examinations, through the Department of Education's offices of Higiene Escolar. While this 1938 report suggests a story of increasing coverage of Quito's population by state medical and other child welfare services over the four-decade period considered in this chapter, the main thrust of the report was to indicate to the minister how inadequate the coverage was. The authors hoped that with proper funding and harmonization of child protection services, within five years "a good portion of Ecuador's proletarian children would be under the protection and custody [amparo y custodia] of the state. A large-scale social program of this kind would imply an increase in the population and improvement in the quality of our nationality's future man."[135]

The processes examined here also tell other interconnected stories. One of them is a story of shifting jurisdictions among different state institutions—primarily the Junta de Beneficencia/Asistencia Pública and the Servicio de Sanidad—and between those institutions and philanthropic societies and female religious orders. The latter two kinds of groups were closely associated with state institutions. Private societies such as the Gota de Leche and the Sociedad Protectora de la Infancia functioned largely with state funding of one kind or another. In the relatively small circles of dominant society in Quito—including as the twentieth century progressed not just the traditional aristocratic landowning families but also prominent professionals of the middle sectors—state officials might also play leading roles in private voluntary associations. Administration of various health-care and child welfare institutions was delegated by the state to female religious orders, foremost among them the Hermanas de la Caridad, whose very presence in the country was due to a state contract to administer public hospitals. The Sociedad de La Gota de Leche also contracted Dominican nuns to undertake the daily administration of their locales.

While institutions like the Asistencia's three Casas del Niño continued to be administered by nuns, a serious conflict erupted in 1940 between the Hermanas de la Caridad and Dra. Alicia Sternberg, a German Jewish immigrant who had been appointed technical director of one of the casas in 1937. The

Hermanas felt that they could not continue working there under the supervision of a secular directora, an experience that convinced them "yet again" that "an establishment whose direction is entrusted to a woman is not appropriate for Hermanas de la Caridad."[136] There are parallels between this incident and problems that emerged in the 1940s after the establishment in Quito of the National Nurses School, where we see conflicts in jurisdiction between technically trained women and nuns, sometimes expressed there (as here) as conflicts between Ecuadorian women and foreign ones. On the terrain of child welfare, state functionaries continued to work to define an appropriate division of labor between themselves and female religious communities, as the latter struggled to maintain their foothold as providers of child protection services under changing conditions.

Alongside a partial process of secularization of these institutions as the first half of the twentieth century progressed, there was an allied movement from more ad hoc collections of unprotected minors to categorizing children and applying expertise to address their problems by creating institutions increasingly targeted to specific problems or populations. For instance, in the early twentieth century, vulnerable children were interned not only in orphanages but also in general asylums such as the Hospicio (administered for the Beneficencia by nuns). In 1900 the minister of beneficencia characterized its residents as: "in addition to madmen, orphans, lepers, idiots, the elderly, etc., the Hospicio has also been destined as an asylum for incurable drunks and those suffering other forms of social pestilence," opining that the inclusion of the latter was inappropriate.[137] In 1914 the number of girls in the orphanage within the Hospicio who were receiving "not only corporal sustenance but also the necessary spiritual instruction" was approximately one hundred.[138] It was considered unfortunate that the front patio of the institution was accessed daily by the poor lunatics from the madhouse, since it was considered inhumane to keep the latter locked up in their cold and damp locale.[139]

In 1915 the Junta decided that the girls interned in the Hospicio should be released to relatives where possible or transferred to another institution for the two months of school vacation, to "preserve the children, at least during the vacations, from the painful spectacle of so many unfortunate wretches interned there, such as lunatics, idiots, degenerates, etc." In this case, though, the minister of the interior had grave concerns about whether their impoverished families would be in any position to receive them, whether there was space or resources to house them elsewhere, and not least, "what opinion the public might form on seeing so many children released to the streets from establishments of Beneficencia"—something he feared would reflect poorly on the government.[140] Similarly in 1915 the Junta's subinspector of the Colegio del Buen

Pastor noted that in addition to the 160 girls sponsored by the Beneficencia in the Colegio, there were numerous other categories of women interned in the Buen Pastor, which "does not offer the amenities desired, perhaps because it is largely occupied in services unrelated to the objectives of the Institution and the desires of the Junta. In addition to the Colegio that occupies a small portion of the building, other sections are used for asilos for orphans, religious novices, reformatories for women of suspicious conduct, an area for fee-paying lunatics [*pensionistas dementes*], and this establishment has even been used to lodge some women accused of conspiring against the current Government."[141]

Over this period institutions became increasingly more targeted to children with specific needs, and this was particularly the case after the 1938 Child Code set up tribunals in each province to channel children into appropriate institutions of care depending on the diagnosis of their situation. By the early 1940s such institutions included in Quito a Centro de Re-educación Femenina, or girls' reformatory, which was considered an appropriate place to intern underage prostitutes, since institutions of Asistencia Pública were in contrast populated by "innocent" girls. There were other establishments of child protection, such as the Hogares de Protección Social operated under the auspices of the Consejo Nacional de Menores. The Consejo Nacional de Menores itself embodied a range of technical expertise in various dimensions of child welfare: its members included one pediatrician, one psychologist, one psychiatrist, and two educators, appointed precisely because of their specialist training in different kinds of children's issues.[142]

There is evidence of the changing nature of general public attention to vulnerable children over the first half of the twentieth century, at first (like state policy) often expressed specifically in relation to orphans. In December 1915, coinciding with the end of the races in the Nuevo Hipódromo (horse track), a "Meeting de Gala" was organized by its owner, César Mantilla, for December 25. The proceeds were fully dedicated to a special charity fair the next day for the poor children of the city.[143] In 1918 the officials of Quito's military academy formed a Comité "Pro Infancia" that among other things held a special fête for the children interned in the San Vicente orphanage as part of their celebration of the August 10 civic celebrations of independence, explicitly linking nationalism and the fate of the country's orphaned children.[144] The undertone of charity in these events was increasingly displaced by service organizations that had a more eugenic tone to their activities and that aimed to influence poor children in general rather than orphans specifically. For instance, in 1935 the Rotary Club of Quito proposed that wherever there were vacant lots in the city, playgrounds should be developed, and they solicited collaboration in this project from both the Asistencia Pública and the Sanidad.

In the program of Rotary activities figures in first place the protection of children, and the observation of our social reality has shown us that children inhabiting rooms in the lower floors of houses in this and other densely populated cities lack the necessary space and liberty to access more or less pure air, light, the warmth of the sun, and movement, which are so indispensable for the healthy and normal development of these small beings. On the other hand, impelled by a biological necessity, they seek places to breathe more deeply, to warm themselves, to play, and as they cannot find them within the dark, narrow, antihygienic houses that, in our large cities, serve as habitation for the majority of Ecuador's urban proletariat, they insist on going into the street, where they find not only inconsiderate adults and the rude attitude of the police agent, but sometimes also death, caused by the transit of vehicles, and in any case they are at risk of being injured by the intense mechanical transit [streetcars].[145]

This is also a story about the ways that state institutions entered into popular coping strategies. Many of these cases involved women experiencing economic hardship, who sought assistance for their own children when they faced crises of care or when the children fell ill. There were an increasing number of petitions from popular-sector men, too, seeking resources to support a broader group of children, often expressed in broader class or nationalistic terms. For instance, a rural schoolteacher in Chillogallo in the countryside south of Quito solicited the Asistencia Pública in 1932 to provide milk from the nearby Asistencia haciendas to his students, since "the students of this school are the children of impoverished peasants who barely subsist, and are unable to provide their children with even a drop of breakfast."[146] Two years later, a similar request was made to provide the schoolchildren of the Canton Pedro Moncayo with a school breakfast from the products of the nearby nationalized estates given that "in this county there are haciendas of great value corresponding to the Asistencia Pública and these properties should also be of use to the population."[147]

Artisans and workers in Quito, too, felt they had a stake in the provision of free hospital services for sick children of the popular classes. As the year 1933 approached, they expressed considerable concern that the bequests from the estates of Héctor Baca and his widow, Dolores Ortiz, might be partially lost if a hospital for sick children was not founded within ten years of the 1923 death of the widow Ortiz (the concern was not misplaced, since in the end it took a full quarter century after 1923 before the Hospital Baca-Ortiz was opened). In 1933, however, the Hospital Eugenio Espejo was being inaugurated, and leaders of the artisans' and workers' association the Sociedad Artística e Industrial de Pichincha felt that their members were among those with the greatest stake in the planned hospital for poor children. Thus they urged that the children's ward in the Hospital Eugenio Espejo be named for the Baca-Ortiz couple as an interim measure to fulfill at least nominally the terms of the inheritance.[148] They weren't the only workers with an interest in the new pediatric ward: the Hermandad Ferroviaria (railway workers' brotherhood) took a collection among their members to provide a four-hundred-sucre donation to help equip the ward.[149] Meanwhile, continuing the tradition of women's voluntary work in support of children, the female-led Comité Pro-habilitamiento del Pabellón de Niños del Hospital Eugenio Espejo (presided by Agripina de Suárez, the wife of physician Pablo Arturo Suárez) obtained a donation from Quito's municipal council for the ward, including the fourteen-hundred sucres remaining in its budget for celebrating civic holidays and ten children's bathtubs worth one hundred sucres each.[150]

In 1935 on the inauguration of the Asistencia's Casa Cuna daycare, the leaders of two male workers' associations, the Sindicato de la Madera and the Sociedad de Carpinteros Union y Progreso, communicated their congratulations and appreciation for the establishment of this institution to protect proletarian children.[151] The male leaders of the mixed-sex Asociación de Trabajadores del Fósforo Libertad y Justicia in turn solicited various positions for the children of widowed female members in the daycare in 1937: in one instance, because "attendance to her factory work obligates our *compañera* to abandon her little daughters [*pequeñuelas*] without care from anyone, so in this sad situation we solicit your valuable help to mitigate her suffering"; in another case, "our *compañera* . . . must abandon her little daughter every day to seek her necessary livelihood and within her difficult work the fear that something terrible could happen to her little one makes the burden of her daily tasks even heavier."[152] While the concerns of women of the popular classes were oriented toward the safety and survival of their own children, men of these same classes had more leeway to project broader collective interests in discussions of child welfare.

At the same time, political constructions about the nature of collective responsibility for social welfare were also changing. Initially such responsibility was expressed when Beneficencia was linked to private philanthropy and charity—as it was in Guayaquil—with the state simply filling in where private initiative was not sufficient. Thus in 1910 interior minister Octavio Díaz characterized this relationship as follows:

> If something demonstrates that man was born to live in society, it is the spontaneous fact of cooperation and help that he offers to another man who lacks the means to attend to his own subsistence. Charity is the consequence of fraternity, and this engenders sociability. Reciprocal aid, the mutual support

that men offer each other, is the corollary of the equality of human beings. If beneficiencia—which is no more than the altruistic manifestation of the free activity of man, in the sense of doing good for the simple reason of being a man—is a duty of the individual, it is also an obligation of the state. . . . And this duty of the state presupposes that individual activity, private philanthropy, is not sufficient to attend to the misery of some social classes. When man cannot aid the indigent, then the state must do so: this is the rule.[153]

By 1938 such collective responsibility was expressed very differently, when a supreme decree of January 27 provided for the establishment "throughout the republic, of Casas Cunas, Colonias de Recuperación Física, Hogares Infantiles . . . etc." To fund the expansion of these child welfare services, one day's wages annually would be deducted from the salary of all state and municipal employees, bank employees, members of the military in active service, and those receiving pensions.[154] In other words, this applied to all salaried employees eligible for benefits from the national pension system, who in this way returned something to the nation's children.

There was a clear gendering of child welfare programs, as an arena in which women held a central role in the everyday lives of their children. Mothers were ubiquitous in the materials on which this chapter is based, even where they were absent from their children's lives: it was always mothers, for instance, who were assumed to abandon their infants, while fathers seemed to have little connection to or responsibility for their children's well-being. The bond on which projects to better the health status of poor children was centered was not the family itself but the mother and child. State physicians often emphasized the role the state should have in protecting national health, but this was combined with regular commentaries on how ultimately the prevalence of preventable illnesses such as those of the digestive tract, which so often proved fatal, was due to ignorance and lack of care by mothers of the popular classes. These women too needed to be modernized then, as the state modernized itself and its services, through advice and monitoring received whenever they turned to a state institution for assistance or when state or quasi-state functionaries visited their homes to provide medical or allied services.

One arena where mothers' responsibility and state responsibility for child health were identified in shifting proportions was in regard to breast-feeding, an issue that gained in importance as the threat of digestive illnesses became clear and where a broad consensus was built. In a 1914 pamphlet of advice to mothers (published with government funding and distributed across the national territory), Guayaquil sociologist Alfredo Espinosa Tamayo defined motherhood itself as breast-feeding. As he advised mothers: "Breast-feed your child: only in this way will you be a true mother, when you not only give your child life but also the strength of resistance from your breast so that he can face the dangers that threaten him."[155] Physician Emiliano Crespo from the southern city of Cuenca argued that the failure to breast-feed was almost a criminal act: "The mother who does not feed her child with the milk of her breasts commits an offense even more criminal since it is against the laws of Nature, who wisely placed those fountains of life in the organism of the mother."[156] Similarly, a Catholic clergyman who wrote a pamphlet published with ecclesiastic authorization argued that a mother's first duty was to breastfeed her children; her second duty in his opinion was to provide a Catholic education.[157]

Quito pediatrician Carlos Andrade Marín showed more empathy with the difficult economic situation of many poor women, leading him to suggest that mothers should be financially rewarded by the government for breast-feeding their children: "Every mother should be the paid wet-nurse of her child."[158] Andrade Marín's view of state responsibility for Ecuadorians' health ultimately gained an outlet when he became the first director of the medical services of the state social security institution Caja del Seguro in 1938; he also held prominent public roles as mayor of Quito in the late 1930s and again two decades later, and minister of social welfare for two different governments in the 1940s. Any sympathy that was expressed toward poor women who had difficulty combining their livelihood strategies with their maternal duties was not, however, extended to mothers with greater economic resources who might seek opportunities to engage in activities outside of the domestic arena. Dr. Luis Dávila, for instance, condemned wealthier women for avoiding breast-feeding to preserve both their liberty and their beauty, preferring to "confide the fruit of their wombs to the care of mercenary hands," irrespective of the consequences.[159]

The crucial connection between mothers and their children was especially clear in situations of illegitimacy, which frequently implied the absence altogether of the father. The mother-child connection was both highlighted and reconfigured when Dr. Antonio Bastidas offered a public lecture to medical students about illegitimacy and child health in 1932, in his capacity as *profesor de medicina legal* at the Universidad Central.[160] As a pediatrician and director of the Hospital San Juan de Dios's children's ward in the early 1920s, Bastidas was well aware of the health dangers facing children, many of them preventable. He calculated, however, that whatever the general risk to children from such causes, the risk to illegitimate children was probably twice as high. Illegitimacy had a role in congenital weaknesses and infant mortality: "The children of poor abandoned mothers who work until the last day of pregnancy, girls who have been seduced and live in lamentable hygienic conditions often trying to hide their state, such pregnancies end in miscarriages, in still births, or often in the birth of a weak being that succumbs to the most minor infection or digestive irregularity." Bastidas calculated that about a third of all births in Ecuador were illegitimate, with higher rates in the coastal provinces and lower rates in the highlands, nonetheless amounting to about 24 percent in Pichincha province in 1929 and 1930. He cited approvingly the notion that there are no illegitimate children but only illegitimate parents—in other words, children should not have to pay the price for errors they did not commit—and joined his colleagues who wrote about prostitution and venereal diseases in noting the hypocrisy around sexuality that contributed to illegitimacy. Although he spent considerable time reviewing different legal models dealing with illegitimacy, his discussion of the biological underpinnings of parenthood is more significant. In his comments he chose to foreground the results of Mendel's genetic research, which he used to argue forcefully that father and mother contributed equally to the biological make-up of the child: that is, a child's underlying genetic constitution would inevitably reflect the recessive and dominant genes offered by each of its parents in equal measure. Bastidas hoped that in the future this might offer ways for women and their children to prove paternity.

These were arguments that could potentially reorient the widespread assumption that mothers were more closely tied to their children than fathers were. The Ecuadorian social reality, however, was that mothers were seen to have a much more intense and direct connection to and responsibility for their children. Indeed, as the daughter of public health physician Dr. Eustorgio Salgado commented in an oral history account, only the children of the mother were seen as siblings: "We had a brother by our father who we never saw, because that is what it was like then. Your siblings were only those with the same mother. Now I see that things have changed, but in those times, my goodness! I did not even know I had a brother, I did not find that out until I was twenty years old."[161] That mothers held primary responsibility for their children's welfare—and that women were first and foremost mothers—were widespread beliefs that were continually stressed in the provision of state services for children as well as in general commentaries on child welfare.

# Governing Sexuality and Disease

**W**hile Ecuadorian women's actions as mothers were of interest and concern to state actors who intervened in child welfare issues, other intimate activities of women were seen to pose a different set of challenges and dangers for state and society. Just as having a child required a man and a woman, so too the spread of venereal disease involved the activities of both sexes. Nonetheless, for social rather than biological reasons, state programs to control venereal disease came to focus on monitoring the sexual health of women in particular. In 1911 an initial attempt to regulate prostitution and venereal disease was established in Quito, setting the stage for future programs by bringing together medical and policing efforts to constitute "a penal and curative system among the women subject to surveillance."[1] Indeed, before the establishment of a stable Subdirection of Sanidad in Quito in 1914, the 1908 Ley de Sanidad (Law of Public Health) allowed for the rather precarious founding of what was also called a Subdirection of Sanidad within the Oficina de Higiene Municipal, funded and overseen by Quito's municipal government.[2]

In 1910 oficina director Dr. Francisco Martínez Serrano began to explore the possibilities of using the law's provisions to address the venereal diseases being spread by Quito's prostitutes. Although no additional funding was available to expand the oficina's services in this direction, the director thought that perhaps the salary of an additional staff member could be paid with the fines collected for infractions of a new *reglamento de profilaxis venérea* (venereal prophylaxis regulation). The identification of women whose health status might need to be controlled was a joint effort of the Higiene Municipal and the police: the police might initiate this by asking the Higiene Municipal to inspect the hygienic conditions of brothels, or hygiene officials might ask the police to look into accusations of prostitution received by their office. This early attempt to control venereal disease via the control of prostitutes functioned only for a few months in 1911. Despite its short duration, the project nonetheless set a pattern that continued to be relevant as state institutions began to pursue more comprehensive policies to control some of the health consequences of sexual acts: most importantly, coordination between medical authorities and police functionaries, and a focus on controlling the health of female prostitutes first and foremost. The gendering of problematic sexuality as primarily female may have been due to the fact that only among prostitutes could the state justify monitoring of sexual behavior—or at least its health consequences. State functionaries had much less latitude to reflect on the sexual activities of other groups of women, or for that matter most men. Nonetheless, they did make some attempts to reach groups of men associated in particular with state institutions.

## State Services and Antivenereal Campaigns

In August 1913 there was hope that a more sustained campaign against venereal diseases might be undertaken, with the arrival in Quito of public health specialist Dr. Carlos Miño as delegate from the main Guayaquil office of the Servicio de Sanidad. He was converted a few months later to a permanent subdirector of the national public health service under the auspices of the central government rather than the municipality. The acting governor of Pichincha province (who elsewhere expressed his concern about the effects of infant mortality on the nation's future) took on the task of explaining to Miño the dire situation existing in the nation's capital:

> Without exaggeration, the newspaper "El País" writes that the brothels located in busy central streets of the City are almost too numerous to count. It seems to me that if these Establishments must exist, at least they should be monitored preferentially by the Policía de Higiene y Salubridad, to avoid the spread and contagion of the worst of all diseases: syphilis. I have heard many physicians, and I have heard them with horror, say that this affliction has taken root in Ecuador to such an extent that if the Authorities don't combat it the future of the Republic will be bleak, since its population will be made up of sickly and degenerate people. If respect for the rights of Man goes so far as to respect his freedom for vice, then at least this should not come saturated with an exterminating poison for his offspring. I hope, Señor Delegate, that you dedicate yourself to science's most important enterprise: venereal prophylaxis. If we must be poor, let us at least be healthy, not poor and sickly.[3]

The acting governor was alluding to the notion that syphilis constituted a racial poison, transmitted biologically to future generations and weakening them. This was a common understanding of syphilis's lasting effect on the population through much of the first half of the twentieth century, and dovetailed with concerns over child health and with notions of the national population as a form of human capital. As with those concerns, here too future children would be affected by their parents' behavior, but men had a more central role in discussions about venereal diseases than in child protection policies, as those seen as most compelled to express their biological impulses via sexual activities. Still, concern with the health of the nation's future children was implicitly attached to women here, when female prostitutes became the primary targets of state programs to control venereal disease. Articulating the view of venereal diseases as a racial poison, several decades later a public health official argued in 1943 that venereal diseases were "infiltrating all social classes with serious risk for infant mortality, because hereditary syphilis is found in a great proportion of our population, and it weakens infant organisms, making them easy prey to other illnesses regardless of how insignificant they seem, especially tuberculosis and gastrointestinal diseases. Similarly, neurosyphilis is making itself felt in an appreciable percentage, a complication that should attract the attention of the public powers, if we do not wish to see our welfare institutions filled with the mentally ill, invalids, beggars, etc. But the greatest danger that threatens us is the degeneration of the race."[4] That year, however, was also marked by the discovery that penicillin was an effective treatment for syphilis, leading to shifts as the decade progressed in how the social dangers associated with syphilis were understood.

Although Miño agreed with the 1913 concerns of the acting governor, he pointed out that to dedicate himself effectively to this and to "a thousand other projects of equal importance, it is first necessary to have the financial resources to do so, without which all of our good intentions, all of our noble initiatives, will remain mere illusions."[5] And mere illusion this did indeed remain for the rest of the 1910s, as the meager funding dedicated to the Sanidad—in an era of economic crisis precipitated by the paralysis of international trade during the First World War—was used above all to fight contagious diseases that threatened Ecuador's prosperity in much more immediate ways. Sustained campaigns against bubonic plague and yellow fever were undertaken, primarily in the port city and its environs (but for plague also along the railway line toward the interior). Not only did these diseases constitute a threat to life; they were also a threat to livelihood, as the nation's principal port suffered international quarantine measures because of the prevalence of those diseases.

Although Miño designed a regulation on "Enfermedades Venéreas, Reglamentación Sanitaria de la Prostitución" in November 1916 that did not come to much, this issue had gained more momentum in Quito by 1920. That year functionaries of the Subdirection of Sanidad and the provincial office of security and statistics began to discuss ways to coordinate their work to deal with what they perceived as an alarming increase in venereal disease and in prostitution. The chief of the provincial office had become aware of the increase in these diseases not only from his own observations but also from a review of health statistics, which had begun to be compiled and examined more systematically within just the past few years. The chief felt that it was probably too much to hope to regulate prostitution, but his office had at least begun to register habitual prostitutes in preparation for monitoring their health. In a telling slip that gendered the problem as female, he discussed the alarming increase in prostitution such that "at present there are even minors of ten or twelve years of age of both sexes who are already *enfermas* [sick, in its female form] and who need to be isolated to avoid further spread of these terrible diseases. This should not only be seen in terms of social morality, but rather it should be considered from the perspective of public health, which is the prime law and the most primordial necessity."[6]

Miño was pleased to have such an energetic ally and assured the chief that in fact he had every intention of adopting a system of prostitution regulation to combat disease: an amended Reglamento de Profilaxis de la Prostitución harmonized with a new Reglamento de Vigilancia de la Prostitución were already in the process of being approved by the ministers responsible, respectively, for public health and for policing.[7] The passage of these regulations was facilitated by the active interest taken in this issue by the new national president, José Luis Tamayo. Perhaps it was Tamayo's support that helped secure the funds necessary to establish and maintain the Sanidad's new Servicio de Profilaxis Venérea (SPV, the Venereal Prophylaxis Service) in Quito, in the form of taxes on the introduction into Quito canton of imported alcoholic beverages and both foreign and national cigarettes and cigars, assessed when such merchandise arrived in the train station in the capital. Thus taxes on one vice were used to combat the effects of another vice. While a 1912 legislative decree had authorized the use of such taxes for a similar purpose, no enabling regulation had been passed to establish procedures by which they would be collected. Finally, this occurred in May 1921, allowing for the launching of the SPV in late August once the treatment facility had been renovated and equipped.

While Quito followed the lead of other Latin American jurisdictions in making prostitution legal and regulated, in different countries quite different social anxieties and social relations were expressed through prostitution control policies.[8] The historian Donna Guy has discussed the importance in Argentina of debates emanating from Europe over white slavery and ambivalence within Argentina about European immigration. In addition, in Buenos Aires prostitution regulations were engaged in such a way to remove women from certain occupations that were subsequently reserved for men (such as in restaurants and shops).[9] In Brazil prostitution control policies were part of a campaign to reorganize urban space in Rio de Janeiro, as some areas were cleared of the poor and reserved for the use of middle classes and the elite. These policies were also associated with concern over the images of Brazil being disseminated in Europe.[10] The continuing existence of prostitution in the capital of postrevolutionary Mexico, in contrast, became a much-debated arena for discussing the challenges the revolutionary government faced in improving the living and working conditions of the lower classes, as well as articulating the state's concern with regulating private life.[11] Finally, policies toward prostitutes in Guatemala City were one arena within which coercive policies were brought to bear on the population, indicative of the constitution more generally of a coercive state apparatus in Guatemala.[12]

According to its designers, Quito's regulation drew eclectically on other countries' legislation to create a regulation that was appropriate to Ecuador.[13] Indeed, public health functionaries were in periodic contact with international organizations and colleagues working in this area. For instance, in 1925 they responded to a survey from the France-based Unión Internacional Contra el Peligro Venéreo with information on Quito's venereal prophylaxis program, taking advantage of the opportunity to dialogue on how best to combat clandestine prostitution and to promote eugenic marriage policies.[14] In Quito one of the most distinctive traits of prostitution control policies was that after the creation of the SPV, public health authorities registered individual women, rather than brothels. Elsewhere, licensed brothels became institutions of social control, and there were provisions by which women could be sent to such brothels as punishment for various kinds of transgressions; this was an important cause for criticism of regulated prostitution elsewhere in Latin America as well as in Europe. Because prostitution control did not focus on brothels, there was no formal *zona de tolerancia* or red-light district in Quito as there was in many other Latin American cities. Moreover, the historian Judith Walkowitz has argued for Great Britain that as long as the nature and transmission of venereal diseases were not fully understood by physicians, they emphasized changing social and moral norms to control these diseases.[15] In Ecuador the fact that venereal disease control policies were established relatively late, after Neosalvarsan (a considerably more effective remedy for syphilis) came into use, may be one of the reasons that in Ecuador the emphasis in prostitution control was on medical intervention rather than relying first and foremost on a discourse of moral danger.[16]

The work of Quito's SPV focused on monitoring the health of Quito's registered prostitutes by examining them each week and, if necessary, treating them for venereal diseases. Registered prostitutes were not charged for medical services or medications, nor did they pay registration fees. The funds to pay for the medical treatment of prostitutes came from various public health fines as well as the taxes dedicated to this program. In addition to free medical treatment, the SPV staff "had the obligation to give each woman an individual consultation detailing the danger of venereal diseases for the women and their descendants, how to avoid contracting these diseases and infecting others, how to recognize when someone was in an infectious state, and finally, what procedures they should follow, prior to sexual intercourse, to avoid passing on the infection, indicating to them the responsibilities they had . . . according to the terms of the Regulation."[17] Indeed, the SPV provided registered prostitutes with vaginal *irrigadores* so that they could maintain sexual hygiene between clients. The results of their weekly exams were recorded in individual *libretas*, which prostitutes were to show to clients, police, or public health employees on request.

In addition to regular medical examinations of registered prostitutes to assess their health status clinically, the work of the SPV was based on laboratory verifications of venereal disease infections. SPV physicians knew that infections could exist and be transmitted even when there were no clinical manifestations, so the use of bacteriological analysis was central to the office's activities. Initially Ecuadorian bacteriologist Benjamín Wandemberg was appointed *médico bacteriólogo* of the new service, and to set up his laboratory, he was able to obtain a loan from the municipal government of equipment that had been previously used in their Laboratorio Químico Municipal (they had recently eliminated the position of municipal bacteriologist for budgetary reasons).[18] Miño's position as an elected member of the Municipal Council likely facilitated the provision of these items to the Sanidad. Given the demands of running the laboratory, a second physician, Dr. Eustorgio Salgado Vivanco, took over the operations of the SPV (initially on an ad honorem basis), freeing Wandemberg to concentrate on bacteriological work to confirm not only venereal diseases but also other contagious diseases affecting Quito's population. Salgado was assisted by two medical students, one of them Pedro Zambrano who on completing his medical studies and a thesis on the social and medical dimensions of prostitution in Quito would go on to direct the SPV for many years. When public health officials emphasized the fact that their program was scientifically based, they meant first and foremost that it was based on laboratory analysis, so that both clinical and bacteriological manifestations of disease were monitored and controlled to the extent possible. Among the 246 women registered by the Sanidad between the inauguration of the SPV in August 1921 and the end of June the following year, the service's bacteriological analyses and medical examinations showed that 208 were infected with venereal diseases: 75 with syphilis, 75 with gonorrhea, and 58 with both diseases.[19] While the main goal of the SPV was to control the spread of syphilis, it also offered treatment for the less serious but widespread gonorrhea.

Once the SPV began to function, the Sanidad hoped to expand their prophylactic services quickly to serve a larger population, both by establishing dispensaries for free treatment of syphilitic infections for the general population and by agreeing with the Sanidad Militar to found antivenereal services in the army.[20] The first step in expanding antivenereal services was indeed to begin with the members of state institutions, the armed forces and the police. In the spring of 1922 joint meetings were held by the Sanidad with both the military surgeons and the police's medical staff, to develop a unified campaign against venereal diseases. The consultations led to the design of a military venereal prophylaxis regulation submitted to the military high command for approval, "with the objective of obtaining at least a reduction in the excessive proportion of venereal diseases among members of the troops, which also prevent soldiers from undertaking rigorous marches and in general contributing to military campaigns."[21] In late 1925 this project gained additional momentum, following the Revolución Juliana—a movement that precisely brought together military officials and professionals, including physicians, in a program of national reform. The Sanidad sought to offer lectures to the troops about venereal prophylaxis as well as designing a program to establish dispensaries of venereal prophylaxis in each military unit.[22]

Not only were venereal diseases widespread among soldiers, but in principle the military structure lent itself more easily to the imposition of sanitary measures than would be the case among the general population. However, it was only in April 1927 that, at the urging of the Sanidad, an executive decree by newly appointed president Dr. Isidro Ayora formally created a venereal prophylaxis program within the armed forces, and a regulation establishing medical posts within each barracks was agreed to and formally approved by the general director of public health, the director of sanidad militar, and the minister of social welfare and public health.[23] The reasoning underlying this program included the fact that the main medical problem among the troops was venereal disease; that such diseases were rarely cured given the conditions of troop movements and lack of appropriate treatment and repose; a suspicion that some soldiers even contracted such diseases deliberately to avoid their military duties; and that it was more economical to prevent than to treat such infections (with the availability of easy preventative measures that had a 60 percent success rate).

The regulation established a health post within each military unit and the selection of two orderlies per unit who would be trained in the principles and practice of venereal prophylaxis to assist the army surgeon. Each soldier upon entering and leaving active duty would undergo a prophylactic treatment, and fines were established for any soldier who contracted a venereal disease and did not seek treatment. While this seemed a comprehensive new start for dealing with venereal disease among soldiers, half a year later the general inspector of public health (a position created to coordinate the Sanidad's campaigns against contagious diseases at a national level, to which Dr. Carlos Miño was appointed) discovered just how inadequate the procedures were in those health posts. In a visit to one of Quito's barracks, Miño found that instead of a true prophylactic treatment, soldiers were simply offered "a little soapy wash in an inadequate form since the locale created for this service has neither running water nor individual wash basins. Besides, according to the records of the post, very few soldiers have received even this treatment, since it is limited to those who voluntarily seek it."[24] Apparently even within this hierarchical state institution, there were obstacles to combating venereal diseases comprehensively.

The Sanidad also sought the opportunity to present information to young men in other state institutions in late 1925—namely, secondary students at the Instituto Mejía and the Colegio Normal Juan Montalvo (the men's teacher-training facility), "in order to warn them from the first years of adolescence against the dangers of venereal contamination, through an adequate instruction making systematic use of pamphlets, posters, cinema, and especially lectures presented wisely and discreetly by physicians of recognized scientific authority."[25] By 1932 the Sanidad's antivenereal activities had been extended considerably at the men's Colegio Normal. Zambrano carried out medical examinations of all of its students and identified some thirteen infected youths in a contagious state, drawn from each and every grade at the school, in need of confidential treatment from the SPV.[26] These medical examinations of the Colegio's student body by SPV staff became an annual event. Perhaps the age and the aspirations of these students made them more receptive to state monitoring of their sexual health. After all, they constituted an emerging middle sector with hopes of achieving upward social mobility via education and ultimately state employment.

At the same time, the situation of male inmates in another state institution (who had no such aspirations) showed vividly the flimsiness of state control even in a context where we might think officials would be well positioned to exercise their authority. In the mid-1920s there was a group of prostitutes who plied their trade among the prisoners in the penitentiary. Such prisoners were engaged regularly in hard labor outside the walls of the prison, such as in the transport of construction materials for public works projects, at which point they apparently had an opportunity to use the services of prostitutes under what were no doubt precarious conditions. These moments also constituted the only opportunity for the Sanidad to formally notify such prostitutes, of no fixed address, of their obligation to undergo medical examinations. However, public health agents found that the guards and policemen overseeing the prisoners were more likely to side with the prostitutes and hostile prisoners than to cooperate with the Sanidad's employees.[27] Likely the prison guards were closer to the social class of the prisoners than to that of public health officials, despite the fact that both guards and officials were ultimately state employees. In any case a 1930 medical examination by the SPV of the prisoners in Quito's penitentiary, the Penal García Moreno, indicated that of sixty-two infected prisoners, forty-eight had been infected before their incarceration, but fourteen more had contracted their diseases while in prison. Zambrano pointed out that the "contagion occurring in the Penal is caused by the fact that the prisoners go out into the street and are infected there, while others have been infected within the prison itself."[28] Indeed, documentary evidence shows that not only could prisoners meet up with prostitutes when they were engaged in labor outside the prison walls, but also prostitutes freely entered the jail to offer their services to its inmates.[29] The fact that public health officials expressed no surprise about this suggests that this was part of the normal functioning of the prison rather than, for instance, the result of bribery. The walls of the prison seem to have been rather permeable, figuratively speaking, allowing both prostitutes in and prisoners out.

In 1925 the Sanidad began to reach beyond the participants in state institutions, opening its antivenereal services to members of the general public. In June 1925, Quito's SPV expanded its facilities and services. An evening service for men was established, in the same facility where women were treated during the day. The daytime service was extended to include not only treatment of prostitutes but also other women who attended voluntarily to treat infections transmitted to them by their partners. SPV staff members were concerned to convince the public that those infected with venereal diseases would find at the clinic not "criticism and insults . . . [but] patriotism, humanity, and well-being, [and treatment] undertaken out of love for the generations to come."[30] In March 1927 the Sanidad established two additional medical posts for venereal treatment for the public as well as to promote preventative measures. To facilitate the latter, the Sanidad contacted the leaders of a wide range of associations that brought men together—the presidents of the *gremios* (guilds and unions) of car and truck drivers, the Sociedad Bar de Pichincha, bakers, tailors, shoemakers, porters, bootblacks, barbers, the Asociación de Empleados (for white-collar employees), the Sociedad Artística e Industrial de Pichincha (for artisans and workers), the police chief, the directors of the police academy and the military academy, and the commanders of the troop units stationed in and around Quito—to inform them of the services offered in these new health posts as well as to ask them to arrange a time when a public health official could provide a succinct lecture to their members about venereal prophylaxis.[31] Moreover, by August that year short talks on venereal prophylaxis were being offered by medical students every week night from 8:30 to 9:00 in one or the other of the two venereal dispensaries.[32]

Although the Sanidad thus did seek to reach men in state institutions early on, and increasingly members of the general public as well, it was primarily through systematic treatment and monitoring of prostitutes—seen as key nodes in the spread of venereal infections to the larger population—that the Sanidad hoped to achieve its goals in combating such diseases. By the end of 1925, there were 444 prostitutes registered with the SPV. Each prostitute was required to carry a registry card in which the date of her last medical exam as well as her current state of contagion were recorded. Moreover, in June 1925 a new office of *identificación dactiloscópica* (fingerprinting) was established within the police institution, and they began to register and fingerprint prostitutes using these new techniques to issue personal identity cards to them. The Sanidad agreed to cooperate but asked that a functionary of the fingerprinting office go to the SPV to process the prostitutes so that these women wouldn't lose trust in the SPV as might occur if its officials forced them to go the police station.[33]

Prostitutes were also required to have a photograph on their registry cards, and public health officials argued to the police that registered women should be exonerated from paying the cost of the photo, since they were mostly women of very scarce resources.[34] In 1928 the police went further, with a project to issue individual and unfalsifiable identity cards to members of a number of groups (such as workers, office workers, and so on); among such groups, they thought it would be particularly useful to have registered prostitutes carry personal identity cards including their names, addresses, ages, and a photograph to ensure that such cards were nontransferable.[35] While the Sanidad was concerned with monitoring the health of prostitutes and ensuring that police measures posed neither obstacles to their own work nor additional difficulties for those prostitutes who were fulfilling their obligations under the regulations, some-times police functionaries seem to have been using this group to try out new forms of personal identification that might eventually help them monitor the population more generally.

The information registered about prostitutes was thus individual but also allowed for cumulative and comparative analysis as researchers searched the data for explanatory patterns. For instance, his experience at the SPV showed Dr. Pedro Zambrano, who became one of the principal medico-social research-ers of prostitution in the city, that the typical profile of the registered prostitute in Quito was a young, illiterate, single, mestiza woman, with little education. In his doctoral thesis he analyzed the 325 prostitutes registered in Quito as of 1924 (table 3.1).[36] Zambrano understood the causes of prostitution among different ethnic groups to be somewhat different. Among mestizas, he attributed pros-titution generally to their lack of economic opportunities; in contrast, among white women, while he recognized the lack of appropriate work, he highlighted their desire to maintain a luxurious lifestyle, pointing out that there wasn't an absolute lack of employment opportunities, but instead few that offered suf-ficient earnings to satisfy this group. Zambrano pointed out that there were very few indigenous women in the registry of the SPV; this despite the fact that indigenous people were commonly considered to make up about half of Ecua-dor's population during this period and lived predominantly in the highlands. Zambrano's explanation was that "the indigenous race can more easily secure various kinds of work, is less likely to engage in certain kinds of relations, and lives in a world with fewer artificially created needs."[37]

TABLE 3.1. **Profile of Registered Prostitutes in Quito, 1924** (total number = 325)

| Ethnicity | Mestiza 191 (58.8%) | White 122 (37.5%) | Indian 8 (2.5%) | Black 4 (1.2%) | |
| --- | --- | --- | --- | --- | --- |
| Birthplace | Quito 177 (54.5%) | Neighboring towns and provinces 137 (42.1%) | Foreign 11 (3.4%) | | |
| Age | Under 18 60 (18.4%) | 18–24 178 (54.8%) | 24–30 49 (15%) | 30–40 28 (8.6%) | 40–50 10 (3%) |
| Marital status | Single 301 (92.6%) | Married 14 (4.3%) | Widowed 10 (3.1%) | | |
| Literacy | Literate 158 (48.6%) | Illiterate 167 (51.4%) | | | |
| Employment | None 202 (62.2%) | Employed, low income 123 (37.8%) | | | |

Source: Zambrano, *Estudio de la prostitución en Quito*, 21–28.

Zambrano attributed the relatively few prostitutes in Quito of Afro-Ecuadorian descent simply to the reduced size of this ethnic group in the city. The small number of foreign prostitutes generally came from Colombia, with one white woman from Italy and one white woman from Guatemala registered. In regard to occupation, Zambrano found that about two-thirds were unemployed, while the other third worked precariously as seamstresses, cooks, laundresses, waitresses (*cantineras*), or domestic servants. He proposed that the remainder "have obtained luxury through prostitution, and it is almost always this ambition that drags the majority of the poor into this most degrading life."[38] It should be noted that in fact, according to the figures given, no registered prostitutes were in this third category (the other two categories add up to 325). Apparently there was nonetheless a perception that a small number of prostitutes had indeed prospered. Table 3.2 summarizes the main causes of prostitution in 1924, as offered by the prostitutes themselves (although the range of possibilities was no doubt suggested by Zambrano). Economic difficulties and various kinds of failures of social support networks both figure prominently. By 1937, according to a study by Dr. Enrique Garcés (who would go on to become the regional director of the Sanidad for the northern highlands the following decade), the main changes in this profile were that there were significantly more mestiza than white women registered (72.3 percent were mestiza, and only 15.2 percent were white), there were slightly more women from the provinces than those born in Quito, and public health officials were concerned that there was a great increase in the number of clandestine prostitutes.[39]

Many of the registered prostitutes attended the SPV clinic regularly, both gaining access to free medical care and suffering less harassment in their livelihood activities. Those who did not were cited by *notificadores* (notifiers) work-

**Table 3.2. Causes of Prostitution in 1924** (total number = 325)

| Cause | Number | Percentage |
|---|---|---|
| Poor and unable to obtain work | 77 | 23.7 |
| Poor and seeking luxury | 49 | 15.1 |
| Conquered by madams | 48 | 14.8 |
| Encouraged by their friends | 47 | 14.5 |
| Lack of parental care | 31 | 9.5 |
| Deceived by boyfriends | 30 | 9.2 |
| Orphans | 17 | 5.2 |
| Obligated by their parents | 10 | 3.1 |
| Seduced by their employers | 8 | 2.5 |
| Abused by their husbands | 8 | 2.5 |

Source: Zambrano, *Estudio de la prostitución en Quito*, 21–28.

ing for the Sanidad, whose main task was to keep track of the many prostitutes with no fixed address and also to identify clandestine or unregistered prostitutes. Such women could be cited or detained by public health employees and taken to the SPV for examination. If they were habitually *remisas* (remiss in being examined and seeking treatment), they could be fined. Because most of them were unable to pay fines given their lack of resources, they were incarcerated instead in a facility attached to the Hospital Civil, where they could work off their fines in the hospital's laundry service. Attached to this Camarote or Santa Marta was an annex for the hospitalization of women who needed sustained treatment for syphilis in its most contagious stages, a small (and poorly equipped) twelve-bed *sifilicomio*. According to the records of the SPV, there might be up to ten women hospitalized and ten incarcerated temporarily in any given month.

The SPV generally appeared to take seriously the confidentiality of their prostitution registry. In the first decade of operations they repeatedly refused to respond to police queries about whether particular women were registered, unless they received a judge's order to give out this information. Indeed, to be successful in their work, public health officials felt that they had to do everything possible to "always inspire the greatest possible trust among the women who should frequent this office."[40] Thus in 1923, even when the police contacted the Sanidad for a copy of their registry with the goal of properly controlling brothels, which often became sites of "scandal" as well as transmission of venereal diseases, the subdirector applauded their intention but regretfully declined to release this confidential list to assist them in their campaign.[41] Moreover, when a husband tried to defend himself from his wife's case against him for economic support (*juicio de alimentos*), he sought confirmation that she was a registered prostitute to prove that he owed her nothing; despite a judge's order that the Sanidad confirm her status, they refused to do so, based on the confidentiality of their files.[42] In other words, while her husband tried to make this woman's legal rights contingent on her moral conduct, at least some state officials were unwilling to collude.

Although this was the practice throughout most of the 1920s, by the middle of 1929 the Sanidad had changed its procedures when it came to official requests from police authorities, answering such queries by providing information on specific registered women. They provided a complete list of their registry three times to high functionaries of the police between May 1933 and October 1934 (perhaps a result too of the frequent change of senior police functionaries during years of great political instability).[43] In 1935, however, the Sanidad continued to apply the procedure requiring a judge's order to confirm information about specific women, whether such requests came via formal channels or were made by private individuals.[44] By 1945 the Sanidad sought a legal opinion on whether they were obligated to release the contents of the prostitution registry, even with a judge's order. They had found that frequently such orders were transmitted in the context of women's support cases against their husbands or the fathers of their children (and indeed the archival record indicates precisely that). Public health officials did not want to be party to a process by which, if indeed the woman involved was registered, her partner could use this as a pretext to deny her any economic support.

As Dr. Enrique Garcés (at the time the senior public health official in Quito) pointed out, "this creates an atmosphere of distrust in the Sanidad among the women who attend the Profilaxis Venérea, since they know that their registration records can be turned over and with this their personhood is annulled in any lawsuits they launch. The most disgraceful example is the following: a woman has a child fathered by Señor X who, upon being sued for support for that child, defends himself by arguing that she is a public prostitute which is proven by her registration in the Profilaxis Venérea."[45] Not only was the Sanidad concerned to maintain the trust of the women served by the SPV, but they had no interest in colluding in processes that would keep women in prostitution when they had the possibility and right to seek other forms of economic support.

When prostitutes left the capital for any reason, they had to inform the SPV, whose officials would note them as "absent" in its register. Given that Quito was the first city in Ecuador to regulate and monitor prostitutes, some left, especially for Guayaquil, to avoid surveillance.[46] This was considered to be especially dangerous when their infections were in a contagious phase. This problem was addressed in part when by 1925 similar regulations had been passed in both Guayaquil and the provincial city of Riobamba. However, venereal prophylaxis was difficult to pursue in a place like Riobamba, where neither the Asistencia Pública nor the Sanidad was in a position to establish venereal treatment as part of their services; the Sanidad sought, instead, to obtain free train passage for infected prostitutes to travel to Quito for treatment in the SPV.[47] Unlike in Quito, for several years the Guayaquil office of public health charged prostitutes for their obligatory medical examinations, until they eliminated these fees in 1928, having learned that this practice only led prostitutes to evade registration.[48]

Even within the Sanidad there was disagreement on how best to combat prostitution and venereal diseases. In 1925, Dr. Wenceslao Pareja, director of public health in Guayaquil, argued against regulation of prostitution, expressing his preference for "the modern system of abolitionism, which is the one that has been adopted in the most advanced countries, eliminating regulation which has not offered the anticipated results, and which simply constitutes legal authorization for prostitution. . . . In this area the same occurs today as with alcoholism, which everywhere is combated by prohibiting absolutely the use of alcoholic beverages and not regulating their administration by the State, as if their use were inevitable."[49] His colleague in Quito, Dr. Luis Dávila, responded that to his knowledge no country had succeeded in abolishing prostitution, but only in abolishing *regulated* prostitution—with the possible exception of Uruguay, where the transmission of venereal diseases was a criminal offense. Moreover, "the criteria of tolerance towards prostitution, as an escape valve to avoid worse sexual depravations which experience has taught us always appear when prostitution is repressed, is a necessary evil, still, for Humanity. For these reasons, in the campaign against regulation, we are in complete agreement and in terms of how to best combat prostitution I believe that we should take a prudent approach penalizing only the spread of disease due to negligence in seeking medical treatment."[50] In other words, despite assuring his colleague in Guayaquil that he agreed with him, in fact Dávila recommended a contrary approach: he was interested in defining prohibited behavior in the narrowest terms, only where medical danger resulted.

With the establishment of the main office of the Sanidad in Quito in 1926 following the reorganization of the public health service (and many other government services) after the 1925 Revolución Juliana, officials in Quito were in a better position to promote their own approach to venereal prophylaxis. This was an era of intensified attention to health issues in general, when physician Isidro Ayora took on first the position of minister of social welfare and then the national presidency, including a variety of attempts to unify and harmonize public health practices across the national territory throughout 1926. In this context the new Dirección de Sanidad in Quito designed two regulations— one of venereal prophylaxis and one of surveillance over prostitution—that not only were projected to apply nationally (although lack of facilities in the end impeded this) but were carefully designed to clarify the roles of the Sanidad and the police.

In the new regulations the police were the main agents responsible for the *vigilancia de la prostitución* (surveillance of prostitution), while the Sanidad was charged with carrying out the provisions of the *reglamento de profilaxis venérea*.[51] Once police issued an operating permit to a prostitute, she was required to register with the SPV within twenty-four hours. The police were responsible for monitoring various conditions of public morality, such as ensuring that the lodgings of registered women did not house any girls under the age of eighteen, women who were not themselves registered, males under the age of twenty, habitual drunks, or men lacking productive occupation (that is, who might be pimps, *rufianes*). Similarly, a prostitute was required to lodge any children she might have over the age of four somewhere other than her habitual place of business, and she could not employ as a domestic servant any woman who was herself unregistered, unless she was over fifty years of age (and regardless of whether she were registered, such a servant's health would also be subject to monitoring by the Sanidad). No one other than employees of the police or Sanidad on official business could insist on entering a registered woman's lodgings against her wishes; if anyone else outstayed their welcome, prostitutes could request the assistance of the police in removing them. Police were also responsible for enforcing the provisions against rowdy and noisy behavior in brothels and indiscreet public displays by prostitutes (such as presenting themselves in windows and doorways to entice clients).

Meanwhile, under the new 1926 regulations the Sanidad's sphere of responsibility was more clearly articulated in terms of health and hygiene. If a registered woman did not attend the clinic regularly for medical examinations, the Sanidad could solicit assistance from the police in ensuring her compliance. Even with a clean bill of health, a registered prostitute could not exercise her trade if her lodgings did not meet a sufficient standard of hygiene and if she did not use the *neceser* (hygienic supplies) provided by the Sanidad to ensure her ongoing sexual hygiene. Women could petition to be eliminated from the registry for good conduct, provided that their behavior for six months following such a petition merited it; in cases where they were infected with syphilis, their health would continue to be monitored by the Sanidad. Registered women who wished to marry could do so if they first obtained a clean bill of health from the SPV, and then following the marriage could petition to be eliminated from the registry. Registered women were responsible for informing both the Sanidad and police of any change of address. Both regulations stipulated that a woman who caused a serious venereal infection due to her own negligence in following the Sanidad's prophylactic measures could be required to pay financial compensation to the infected person.

As the economic crisis precipitated by the global depression and the decline of the coastal export economy deepened, financial constraints led to difficulties in expanding the venereal prophylaxis services offered by the Sanidad. In 1932 with merely a hundred sucres per month in funding for the SPV, only the most basic supplies could be purchased, including a very insufficient quantity of Neosalvarsan to treat syphilitics. This led the director of the SPV to ask patients to purchase their own medications when they were in a position to do so, so that he could reserve the Neosalvarsan provided by the Sanidad for only the most destitute among the infected. With this measure he had been able to supplement the fifty series of Neosalvarsan doses provided by the Sanidad and another thirty-four from the budget of the Hospital Civil (for its small vene-real treatment ward) with an additional thirty-two series. He was particularly concerned about the number of syphilitic patients who arrived from the prov-inces, seeking care in Quito to "repair their health lost in a moment of sexual impulse, giving in to their natural instincts." A proper system of hospitaliza-tion was needed, because if such patients were able to find accommodations with relatives or acquaintances in the city, that only led to the risk of further contagion; and if they were not, "they would return to their homes in the same state as they arrived in the city, to continue serving as inexhaustible sources of contagion in all the corners of Ecuador."

Without a system of proper isolation for sustained treatment, prophylaxis efforts amounted to nothing, and many people who did obtain treatment for syphilis or gonorrhea suspended it when their clinical symptoms disappeared, regardless of the latent bacteriological infection. Zambrano warned that such infections could then reemerge as a nasty surprise, for instance after such peo-ple had married. "All of the ill resist public health efforts: some due to a lack of resources to meet their basic needs, others due to ignorance. To counter the spread of venereal diseases, it is necessary to isolate forcibly and obligatorily the infected population, without regard to their social position; it is enough to know that they are not following the treatment prescribed by public health functionaries—but always only when that is based on scientific principles."[52] Despite all of these constraints, from the end of April 1931 to the beginning of May 1932 the SPV had operated a busy day service (for both prostitutes and other women from the general population) amounting to 2,317 examinations; 11,813 treatments of various venereal diseases; 475 doses of Neosalvarsan in-jected; 3,541 injections of mercury biniodide; and some 1,655 citations of regis-tered women who were remiss in seeking regular examinations and treatments, as well as 109 women captured for treatment when the citations were not suf-ficient. In the night service some 8,260 treatments had been provided to men.[53]

In 1937, Zambrano was still urging the establishment of a proper facility for venereal inpatient treatment and lamented that only two series per month of Neosalvarsan—twenty-four series for the year—were funded by the Sanidad. Moreover, in recent months there had been a multiplication of sites of prosti-tution in the city—cabarets, inns, brothels, and so on—and given the growth of the city, many of them were distant from the city center, making it even more important to monitor them especially at night, when clandestine prosti-tutes evaded the Sanidad's efforts at control (leading Zambrano to request at least free passes for his notificadores on the tram lines). Meanwhile, increasing numbers of infected persons were arriving in Quito from the provinces, full of hope that they might find something to mitigate their afflictions in the state's free dispensaries.[54] Indeed, provincial delegates of the Sanidad regularly contacted the Quito offices of the institution to see whether the latter could provide treatment for either members of the general population infected with venereal diseases or prostitutes who were key nodes in the transmission of such infections, given the lack of resources to provide effective treatment in other cities and towns.

The problems continued to deepen. By 1942 the economic constraints had led Zambrano temporarily to suspend the free medical treatment of prostitutes, to offer treatment to some members of the general population who particularly needed it:

> Given the small supply of medications that we receive on a monthly basis, we have only been able to satisfy a very few patients who have voluntarily solicited our services, whom it has been necessary to prefer for treatment because, besides being very poor, they are artisans and female domestic servants who need to be in good health to be able to work since the majority of these women have positions as cooks. Many of these women have been infected by *carabineros* [a new unit of soldiers established in the early 1940s] under the action of alcohol and other fermented substances which they have imbibed to a state of drunkenness.[55]

An obligatory service like the control of prostitutes' health required many more resources than were available. As Zambrano concluded: "With a simple medical exam preventative hygiene is not achieved. For a true control of venereal diseases . . . it is necessary to cure and to isolate the ill, in order to protect the healthy; to destroy the sources of contagion is the true mission of the *sanitario* [public health expert], where this is lacking any effort is futile." After more than two decades working continuously in the SPV, he was losing confidence in the possibility of achieving an effective service.

Zambrano hoped, however, that the American Commission might take into account this area in its planning. Indeed, that year a comprehensive health and sanitation agreement was signed between the governments of the United States and Ecuador. For the Sanidad, an important result was the construction of the first Centro de Salud adjacent to the Hospital Civil San Juan de Dios, a modern facility where the preventative health services of the Sanidad as well as its facilities to treat infectious diseases were brought together in 1945. Indeed, a new start was made that year, with another reorganization of the Sanidad and the elevation of the antivenereal campaign to a national program (*campaña nacional antivenérea*). It helped, too, that the *seguro social* (social security system) was by then also offering medical services to its affiliates. In 1946 the Sanidad asked the director of the medical services of the Caja del Seguro, Dr. Carlos

Andrade Marín, to consider whether the Seguro could extend treatment to the family members of its affiliates who were infected with venereal diseases. If the police medical staff did the same thing, then the Sanidad could focus on serving members of the population who had no connection with the Seguro, the police, or the military.[56]

The project to transform the SPV into a clinic for sexually transmitted diseases under the auspices of the Sanidad in 1946 indicated a considerably broader mandate beyond the earlier focus on prostitutes.[57] Public health officials continued into the 1950s trying to combat venereal diseases with both specifically targeted measures and comprehensive medical and social programs. However, by then the era of antibiotics was well established, revolutionizing syphilis treatment. Indeed, when a legislative project to declare venereal contagion a crime was discussed in a congressional committee in 1950, after much delay they recommended against the proposed law based on the fact that the latest advances of medical science had reduced its relevance.[58] While the advent of penicillin certainly did not mark the end of sexually transmitted diseases, its effectiveness in treating syphilis changed notions about the degree and nature of danger posed by such diseases for the individual, the family, and society as a whole.

In their portrayal of state services to prevent and treat venereal diseases, a number of the documents of the Servicio de Profilaxis Venérea raise the question of what constituted the line between prostitution, being sexually active, and simply being out on the street. And perhaps of greater immediate concern to state agents, who was in a position among state functionaries to interpret this line? What, for that matter, constituted protection of prostitutes by male state employees: offering them medical care, or defending them against the Sanidad's programs? These issues were brought to the fore when a major conflict erupted early in the registration process between the police and the Sanidad over the latter's attempt to cite a woman to appear in the SPV for registration. The police refused to cooperate, prompting the Sanidad to complain to the minister of government about the actions of the police. An internal investigation undertaken by the provincial police *intendente* (chief) revealed that a public health inspector had encountered a woman seated on a bench, alone, in Alameda Park at 9:30 at night. He suspected her of prostitution and thus tried to take her to the SPV.

Since she resisted, he whistled for help, and the police constable on patrol appeared on the scene. The policeman recognized the woman, knew that she was married and pregnant, so he believed her when she said that she was just waiting in the park for her elderly aunt to return from making some purchases. This was his reason for refusing to arrest her. The police chief suggested that

such problems could be solved if the Sanidad limited itself to using the police's own list of registered prostitutes. While the subdirector of public health
believed the sincerity of the chief, he assured him that the police report was
inaccurate in most of its details and that Sanidad officials were accustomed to
encountering hostility in carrying out their work. Moreover, some of the most
notorious prostitutes in Quito had appeared in the Sanidad offices petitioning
to have their names removed from the registry with signed statements certifying their honorable conduct.[59]

This was not the only time, by far, that "the state" demonstrated that it was
made up of many different agents who were not always in agreement. In 1927
a Sanidad notificador was impeded in his work by a soldier in Alameda Park
in the company of two registered women (who were negligent in their duty to
undergo regular medical examinations). The director of the SPV requested that
the director of public health ask the battalion leaders to impose some kind of
a punishment on soldiers who presented obstacles to the work of the Sanidad,
since "on many occasions they oppose themselves scandalously to the concur-
rence of such women for their exams or their treatment, thus interfering with
the operations of the service. This kind of opposition by private individuals
and especially by soldiers leads registered women to evade their obligation to
be treated."[60] Often, police too refused to assist public health authorities to detain prostitutes to register them, and the Sanidad attributed this problem to
the fact that there were so many policemen who were "friends and allies" of
the prostitutes.[61]

On multiple occasions in 1945, too, the Sanidad was impeded by members
of the Civil Guard from carrying out their duties:

> The Inspectors of this Service are making an effort to capture clandestine
> prostitutes who hang around the streets, especially at night, engaged in sexual
> commerce. However, they are confronted with the serious obstacle that such
> women are sheltered by their friendships with the Guardias Civiles, who re-
> fuse to offer aid to my Inspectors, refusing also to show their badge numbers
> to avoid having to take responsibility for their actions. Moreover, constantly
> these police agents present themselves in this Office posing as the legitimate
> husbands of these women in order to frustrate the efforts of the Inspectors
> and nullify the work of the Dispensary. I should also report that the Guar-
> dias Civiles take advantage of any opportunity to exploit this class of women,
> whether in their person or economically [that is, sexually, or by profiting from
> their sexual commerce].[62]

Not only should such police agents be punished, this official argued, but medical examinations should be conducted among suspicious women associated

with the Guardias Civiles, since the occurrence of venereal diseases among the police was very alarming. Given the repeated incidents of Guardias Civiles refusing to assist the Sanidad and indeed protecting prostitutes from public health inspectors, in August that year the provincial director of Sanidad activated the legal provisions that authorized him to demand the dismissal of police agents who did not fulfill their obligations to support agents of the Sanidad.

Indeed, some of the men most likely to be infected with venereal diseases were precisely employees of the state—policemen and soldiers—who were also very likely to be clients of prostitutes (and might even marry them and solicit that their names be removed from the registry). Among the men treated for venereal diseases by the SPV, there were men of all classes, occupations, and marital status. However, those who were identified as most affected by these diseases were policemen and bus and truck drivers, followed by significant numbers of artisans and workers: shoemakers, carpenters, shop workers, mechanics, day laborers, and factory workers are mentioned, in this order.[63] The dispensaries were not the main treatment option for soldiers, so they are not mentioned on this list. By 1939 there were 972 women who had been registered as prostitutes, while 854 other women were treated for venereal diseases that year, as well as more than four thousand men. Venereal prophylaxis information was provided to working-class men not only when they attended the dispensary but also collectively in public lectures to the associations that they formed.

Thus, for instance, in 1930 the director of the Hospital San Juan de Dios, Dr. Alberto Correa (one of about a dozen physicians in Quito who were specialists in the treatment of venereal diseases) offered a series of lectures to the members of the Centro Católico de Obreros. Given his audience, it is not surprising that Correa emphasized the responsibility of men to control their sexual urges, arguing against the widespread belief that men needed to exercise their sexual impulses with prostitutes and that a moral education could help them to channel those energies into noble pursuits.[64] While physicians might urge Ecuadorian working-class men to sublimate their sexual energies rather than expressing them with prostitutes, they weren't particularly successful even with encouraging state employees to do so, as suggested by the evidence of policemen and soldiers. Even some of the people over whom we might think physicians would be able to exercise considerable moral authority and persuasion didn't always act in ways that their mentors hoped.

In 1924, when the Hospital Civil experimented with establishing its own outpatient clinic for venereal diseases, its operations were suspended the next year due to unspecified problems with medical students at the hospital.[65] Two decades later, the provincial director of the Sanidad had to prohibit medical students from hanging around the offices of the Servicio de Profilaxis Venérea trying to make contact with the women who received treatment there. By then the service was employing two graduated nurses along with one carefully selected medical intern, which helped to ensure that its services were offered with the right tone of delicacy and respect for the office's clients.[66] In sum, there was considerable variability in "the state's" approach to prostitutes, if we take the state to mean not only its formal programs but also its highly diverse agents.

## Women, Male Protectors, and the State

This account of the Servicio de Profilaxis Venerea outlines the kinds of services offered by the state to combat venereal diseases in Quito. The files of the service also allow us to explore a broader set of issues about gender ideologies and women's lives, through this service that focused the state's gaze on sexuality, disease, and women's behavior as embodied in prostitutes. One issue that emerges clearly is that although prostitutes may have been the only people whose sexual health was directly subject to ongoing state scrutiny, public health officials communicated preferentially with specifically situated men regarding the status of prostitutes: especially employers or patrons, fathers, and husbands or *convivientes* (cohabitors). Respectable male employers had not only a gender but also a class advantage that made them acceptable guarantors of women's behavior, sometimes placing them in a position to negotiate with the Sanidad on behalf of subordinate women.

In a 1925 case the regional director of the Sanidad communicated with a Spanish diplomat about his domestic servant. Although she had been denounced as a clandestine prostitute, he had chosen not to register her out of deference to her employer, knowing that as long as she was a member of his household, he would ensure her good conduct. However, if the diplomat insisted on contesting the matter, then it would have to go through legal channels, including a medical examination to establish the state of his servant's health.[67] In another case the subdirector wrote to a woman's employer to explain that his domestic servant had been formally registered in the SPV, that she was infected with both syphilis and gonorrhea, that she was not fulfilling her obligation to undergo examinations and the treatment ordered, and that her patron should also be warned that it was risky to have in his household a servant in a contagious state.[68] And in 1927 a woman who had been interned for some three months in the Santa Marta for "infractions against morality" petitioned to be freed under the supervision of her employers, who had agreed to accept her back into domestic service and to guarantee her good conduct; she hoped that with these guarantees she could be eliminated from the registry since she had decided to reform her behavior.[69]

A certain amount of social capital in the form of a network of respectable men who could vouch for women was of crucial importance in these kinds of exchanges. In 1922 a woman collected certifications from respectable men to support her argument that she should not be registered by the Sanidad. One of her supporters explained that he had known her for four months during which time she had been working as a cook in his home; in that time he had not noticed anything resembling scandalous behavior on her part, and in her work she had shown herself to be reliable. The one irregularity he had noticed as her patron was that she maintained a relationship—*tiene relaciones*, suggesting a sexual relationship—with a soldier, but other than that "her moral conduct is not such as would invite censure, much less an accusation that she is a woman of a brothel [*mujer de burdel*]." Two additional certifiers agreed that they had observed nothing in the woman's behavior that could be described as scandalous or publicly immoral.[70] In a certificate signed by several men in support of another woman, they assured the Sanidad that she was a very hardworking woman who prepared food for sale in the Plaza Sucre, living honorably and taking good care of her daughters.[71] In this case the woman did not have a formal employer who could vouch for her, making her situation more tenuous; it is clear from the documents that she also lacked a male partner who could add his support to her petition. For both of these women, the men confirmed that they "did not behave in a way to attract attention [*sin dar nota de su persona*]," an important measure of honorability.

That inappropriate public behavior could put women in jeopardy of being accused of prostitution was clear in the provision that members of the public could confidentially denounce prostitutes to the Sanidad (provided that those communications were signed rather than anonymous and that evidence was presented to support such accusations), who would then notify them to register with the SPV. In 1921 as the registration process began, a father protested that his daughter had been inappropriately cited to appear in the Oficina de Profilaxis, "as if she were a woman dedicated to prostitution and thus subject to inspection by the Sanidad; no, Señor Subdirector, my legitimate daughter is a minor of fifteen years of age; she does not have such a low and indecorous occupation; and I, as her father, take care of her and of her education and honorability." He suspected that it was "an enemy or someone interested in seducing her" who had made such an unfounded accusation, and he was quite prepared to offer proof of his daughter's good and honorable conduct.[72] Two months later a very similar petition was submitted by another father whose sixteen-year-old daughter had also been cited to appear and register herself with the Sanidad. However, this was illegal since she was under age, and besides, she was his legitimate daughter and he could vouch for her honest and honorable behavior. Moreover, he believed that this must have been motivated by a "false accuser who undoubtedly did not succeed in persuading my daughter to respond to his heated affections; thus his revenge. How low! How miserable!"[73] Although the situations themselves might be parallel, the similarities between the two petitions might also be due to the fact that both were prepared and signed by the same scribe.

The scribe was quite correct in stating that the regulation did not permit the registration of women under the age of eighteen. While by law women could not be legally registered as prostitutes until they reached eighteen, from the beginning, the SPV did register minors, to provide them with free medical treatment. By 1924 sixty underage women had been registered. This technical issue aside, what is clear in these petitions is that three additional arguments were considered to be persuasive: that these young women were legitimate, that they were under their father's authority and protection, and that the accusations must have been precipitated by their rejections of the inappropriate advances of a man (that is, precisely by their virtuous behavior). The emphasis on the first two factors are particularly revealing: not only was there a belief that illegitimate daughters carried the stain of their mother's conduct (suggesting they too might be more likely to engage in sexual activity outside of marriage), but the absence of a father who could watch over a young woman's virtue and conduct could also imply a more unstable economic situation that might itself make prostitution more likely.

Although petitions of this kind are difficult to interpret, given the conflicting evidence offered, as suggested they do indicate what kinds of arguments were considered persuasive. In another case in 1928 a group of neighbors together wrote to the director of the Sanidad to object to the harassment suffered by a local couple at the hands of public health notificadores. They argued that the couple was married and that:

> Although it is true that [the woman] used to work for various people as a domestic servant when a group of women rented some rooms on this street, about a year ago she abandoned that kind of service and, reduced to living in an interior apartment of the house, surrounded by the owners of the house and by her immediate neighbors, we attest that under the shadow and care of her husband she has exhibited truly exemplary moral conduct, since in her lodgings there are neither suspicious gatherings nor friendships, to the contrary this household merits all respect and consideration.[74]

Zambrano, however, reported that for many years the woman in question had rented out rooms to several registered women where they plied their trade; the Sanidad had been motivated to contact her recently when it came to their attention that an unregistered woman with suspicious health was lodged with her, against the regulations. In any case, Zambrano suggested that it would be worthwhile to ask the couple to present both their marriage certificate and the supporters who had signed the petition, since most of the names there were entirely unknown in the neighborhood.[75] Although it is unclear what the underlying facts are, the importance in the petition of the evidence that she was living under the "shadow and care" of her husband is consistent with the emphasis elsewhere on men's simultaneously protective and supervisory role with women.

Certainly not all arguments that articulated these notions were considered persuasive. In one case a guarantor argued that a registered woman had resolved "to live a more serious life" and that he also wished to "have her close to me." Indeed, at the present she was in Guayaquil, where she was passing "honorably together with my family and soon she will come to Quito to accompany me, and I guarantee her fully; but, if unfortunately there is any future guilty conduct, then I will be the first to accuse her." This was an unusual petition in which her supporter did not clarify his relation to the woman involved. Zambrano reported that this woman had first been identified in the Cabaret La Violeta (a recognized brothel) and had since then been almost completely remiss in fulfilling her obligations to be examined and treated for her active gonorrhea. Given that she had left for Guayaquil without informing the Servicio, he could not offer any opinion on her current state of health. Moreover, he argued that "these petitions should only ever be accepted for a limited time of three or six months because many of these women simply wish to distance themselves from the control of this Office in order to exercise clandestine prostitution, under the signature and guarantee of some person who often has no moral or economic responsibility for her nor ability to control her behavior."[76] In another case a sponsor petitioned that a young woman be exonerated from the Sanidad's monitoring because "this señorita is currently under my care and protection, exhibiting honorable and dignified conduct, far from dishonor and shamelessness."[77] He assured the Sanidad that if she were to return to her past life, he would denounce her immediately to the SPV, since his honor would require him to do so. Although here too the sponsor's role is unclear, perhaps it was the fact that the woman was not contagious that tipped the balance in favor of her being eliminated from the registry.

From the beginning, prostitutes could petition to have their names removed from the registry when they married. The fact that by 1933, 113 of the 704 prostitutes who had registered with Quito's SPV had been eliminated from the list indicates that it was not unusual for them to move out of a life of prostitution.[78] When married women were eliminated from the registry, they passed from the responsibility of the state to the responsibility of their husbands, an authority with which the state normally did not interfere. Thus, for instance, in a 1923 petition to the minister of public health, a woman used her married status as the main argument against the Sanidad's right to mortify her with constant citations to attend the SPV clinic, since after all, "no law authorizes anyone other than the husband to accuse a woman of adultery."[79] In 1924 a man petitioned to have his wife released from detention, explaining: "Two years ago, under the influence of bad friends, this woman was registered in the Prophylaxis, the same woman who, twenty months ago, I made my wife as she proved herself to be faithful only to me, and with her I have a child." These were powerful reasons, he continued, justifying his petition that she be released, particularly out of empathy for his poor infant.[80]

The following year, a policeman petitioned that his wife also be removed from the registry. He commented that about a year earlier she had been registered due to the bad intentions of wrongdoers seeking revenge on her, but he had since married her. "My wife is dignified in all of her acts, and I, as a respectable man who knows how to look after my home, say to you that what she is accused of is false, very false, since I would not tolerate any kind of *picardía* [misbehavior] in my wife not only as a police employee, but because I entrust to her my entire monthly wage which I earn with hard work and long nights."[81] This petition highlights women's common role as managers of household resources; it also foregrounds the argument that as a married man, this petitioner was perfectly capable of monitoring the behavior of his wife and did not need the state to do so (despite otherwise being connected to the state as an employee). In a 1938 case, despite Zambrano's concern that a registered woman had in the past offered space to other prostitutes in her lodgings, the fact that she had recently married was sufficient reason to approve her request to be eliminated from the registry.[82]

Interestingly, men also began to petition for the removal of their partners from the registry even when they were not legally married. In one example from 1926 a man certified that he had been "living matrimonially" with a woman for several months, and she was "living a serious and honorable life."[83] Since the reasons that had motivated her registration had disappeared, he asked that she be eliminated from the registry. Similarly, the next year a woman and her partner together petitioned to have her name eliminated because she had "committed to live maritally" with him, and he would therefore "guarantee her future good conduct." The director of the SPV confirmed her noncontagious state at her last exam some months previous, recommending an additional examination to verify her ongoing sexual health.[84] And in another case the Sanidad agreed to remove a woman from the registry because of her partner's assurance that "she has marital relations only with the [petitioner] and she is under my responsibility"; furthermore, her recent medical examination indicated that she was not contagious.[85]

In a touching case from 1938, a woman was eliminated without formally marrying, since she was in a stable relationship and the SPV confirmed that she was not contagious. As she explained: "Since I found myself abandoned in life, without the protection of my parents, in a fatal moment I was registered in the Servicio de Profilaxis Venérea, without ever even having exercised the carnal trade, but rather as the *niña* [girl/minor] that I was I had to survive one way or another." Indeed, under the 1926 regulation, even if she herself were not a prostitute, this young woman would have been registered with the SPV for health monitoring if she were working as a domestic servant for an individual prostitute or a brothel. She continued,

> Happily after so much suffering, destiny favored me in finding a man who would care for me and redeem my situation, contributing with his honorability to the formation of a home. Now it has been more than eight years that I live subject to him [*sujeta a él*] and I have acquired my children, healthy and well. . . . Now that my children are growing—one of them is in the Instituto Mejía—they may find out that their mother has a fatal stain on her reputation, and this is why I solicit based on Art. 21 of the Reglamento de Profilaxis Venérea, in light of my good conduct, that my name be eliminated from the registry.[86]

In 1942 a woman and her *conviviente* together petitioned to have her name removed. As she argued, since 1936 she had lived a moderate and correct life as was well known, living martially with her partner "to whom I have subjected myself [*a quién me he sujetado*] from then to the present date and it is my intention to continue in the same situation." She wasn't at the time contagious, so the Sanidad approved her petition for as long as she continued to exhibit good conduct.[87] Several of these petitions point to situations in which stable long-term conjugal relationships were established, without being formalized by marriage. Although some former prostitutes did marry, for others marriage might simply not have been particularly relevant. Where the couple did not possess property, formalizing relationships to ensure transfer of property through inheritance was less important. Perhaps there were also limitations on women's autonomy or other disadvantages to marrying that were taken into account when deciding whether to formalize a conjugal relationship.[88]

What is clear in all of these cases is that the willingness of a man to take responsibility for a woman—and her willingness to subject herself to his authority—was the key not only to being removed from the registry but also in principle to being able to move out of a life of prostitution. While one role of a male guarantor and protector was to vouch for and ensure the proper behavior of a former prostitute, the economic support such a man could offer—whether as employer, father, spouse, or conviviente—was also recognized as an important safeguard for women who might otherwise have to recur to prostitution. Many women found themselves simply unable to survive economically, a situation that public health officials recognized and for which they exhibited some sympathy (for instance, when they preferred the poorest for free treatment or asked the police not to charge fees for prostitutes' photographs). In his 1924 study of prostitution in Quito, Zambrano emphasized the economic dilemmas facing prostitutes and highlighted the many registered women who also worked in other occupations on a precarious basis. He was particularly concerned about the growing numbers of women who occasionally prostituted themselves (thus operating as "clandestine" prostitutes), and in doing so, escaped the control of public health officials. Such women sold flowers or lottery tickets, were domestic servants, or engaged in other urban livelihood activities that did not provide them with sufficient funds to support themselves, which Zambrano considered to be an increasingly common situation.

While the numbers of registered prostitutes grew over time, in the 1930s the rapid growth of clandestine prostitution to supplement inadequate incomes grew much more rapidly. By 1933, 704 prostitutes had registered in Quito.[89] In that year it was estimated that there were about 600 clandestine prostitutes also working in the city.[90] By 1937 there were 909 names on the registry, while physician Enrique Garcés estimated that there might in fact be some 3,500 prostitutes in the city, with a total urban population of 105,000.[91] According to a 1939 estimate by Zambrano, the total number of women who prostituted themselves in Quito included at least 8,000 clandestine prostitutes, in addition to the 972 who were registered. According to his estimate, the clandestine prostitutes at that point included large numbers of day laborers and factory workers. Meanwhile, the vast majority of registered prostitutes gave as the cause of their prostitution, poverty and the difficulty in obtaining honorable work.[92] While the growing number of registered prostitutes might have indicated the persistent efforts of public health officials, the number of clandestine prostitutes may have reflected the deepening economic crisis.

Although many women faced difficulties subsisting in the early twentieth century, the general economic situation in Ecuador deteriorated with a crisis in the country's export economy that began due to trade disruptions during

World War I, then continued into the 1920s with the spread of crop diseases that undermined Ecuador's principal export product (cacao), and then the advent of the global depression. Indeed, the cost of basic foodstuffs in Ecuador increased 428 percent between 1921 and 1943.[93] In 1936, 60 percent of the households in Quito lived in one-room dwellings, according to a study undertaken by Dr. Pablo Arturo Suárez and his students.[94] A full 34 percent of the families had monthly earnings below sixty sucres, of which at least half was spent on food; 25 percent of Quito's families spent one sucre daily on food, while another 49 percent spent between one and three sucres. The minimum wage for factory workers had been set in 1934 at 1.2 sucres per day, although Suárez argued in that year that factory workers required a minimum of 3 sucres a day to support their families.[95] Few working-class families could survive on a single income, and women without partners (who often supported dependents) found it even more difficult to subsist.

Given the economic stresses on poor women, in many cases prostitution was one strategy that was combined with others to enable a woman to patch together a living wage. In 1939 prostitutes generally earned around fifty centavos (half a sucre) per client, but rates went up to five, ten, or more sucres "depending on the woman and the client."[96] Where we can capture the voices of prostitutes themselves explaining the reasons for their occupational choice, they stated explicitly that prostitution allowed them to provide for their families, usually highlighting their lack of a male protector. In 1951 the director of the venereal prophylaxis service in Guayaquil presented a project to congress for a law of sexual education.[97] With his supporting documentation, he included a sampling of individual prostitutes' responses to a questionnaire administered by his office. Thus one registered prostitute in Guayaquil explained that she became a prostitute "in order to maintain her household, because her father died, leaving her mother and a younger brother, both of whom she supports." This woman expressed her intention to continue as a prostitute until she was able to accumulate enough money to establish a small business. Another woman explained that "she used to be a domestic servant, but she did not earn enough to even pay her rent, so she registered herself as a prostitute, in order to support and educate her daughter." Another found herself abandoned by her partner, left to maintain two children on her own (two more had died). When asked if prostitution fulfilled her expectations, this woman answered "yes," because it allowed her to support her children. And another indicated that she had withdrawn from prostitution once when she had a partner, but when he abandoned her, she had no choice but to return; she indicated that she was unsure whether she would try again to change her livelihood strategy as she didn't know how else she could support herself and her child. These documents suggest that for many women, prostitution was simply a way to support their families in an economic situation that offered them few alternatives, probably a common situation of prostitutes in other regions and time periods, too. In Quito this was most likely to occur when women could not count on male protectors.

This was often the case elsewhere, too. Mexican archival documents for this period demonstrated "women's own insistence that they worked in prostitution because they were members of large social networks and bore responsibility for supporting numerous family members." For the Ecuadorian case, these social networks were short on adult men. However, the historian Katherine Bliss was struck during her Mexican research by how much women's own self-representation contrasted with physicians' portrayal of "prostitutes as deviant individuals."[98] The Ecuadorian evidence does not indicate the same kind of pathologizing of the behavior of women who prostituted themselves, at least among those physicians who monitored their health for the Sanidad. Such physicians were quite consistent in invoking pathology in its precise biological terms and found prostitutes' behavior dangerous only when they were negligent in complying with their legal responsibilities to seek treatment and prevent contagion. For women who were not *remisas*, the evidence suggests that Ecuadorian public health physicians showed more empathy toward prostitutes than their Mexican colleagues did. Perhaps this was also an important part of their own self-representation as medical experts who went about their work in a nonjudgmental and scientific way, rather than emphasizing the kinds of moral judgments that they felt contributed ultimately to the spread of disease.[99] It was also this attitude that dignified prostitution and allowed the women in the registry of the SPV potentially to be seen (and perhaps to see themselves) as responsible members of the national community.

## Sexuality and Venereal Disease at Midcentury

Two documents from midcentury demonstrate some of the collective experience acquired through the Sanidad's programs, proposing broad approaches to the control of venereal diseases and setting them in their social context: a 1945 comprehensive plan of action developed in Quito and a 1951 report to Congress prepared by the director of venereal prophylaxis in Guayaquil to support his proposal for a law of sex education. The 1945 plan emphasized the difficulties of public health work in general in Ecuador—in particular, the devastating problem of venereal diseases.[100] The author pointed out that some 95 percent of the population was ignorant when it came to hygiene, which was not surprising given that were at least a million illiterates in the population (frequently estimated at about 2.5 million total) and that "99 percent" of Ecuadorians had a very low standard of living. It was not unusual to have ten or more people living together in a single room, in a monstrous degree of promiscuity (meaning not only sharing beds but sharing dishes, and so on—in sum, exchanging germs). He argued that the Catholic Church had exercised its evil influence in everything related to sexuality, treating it as a sin and thus cloaking both sexuality and venereal diseases in secrecy.

Some private physicians had also contributed directly to the spread of venereal diseases by maintaining the confidentiality of infected patients, allowing them to carry venereal infection into the heart of the family. Moreover, government finances depended on alcoholizing the country's inhabitants (given the weight of the resulting taxes and government monopolies in the national budget), and there were few laws protecting women, preventing illegitimacy, and discouraging sexual promiscuity. Any plan to combat venereal diseases should include both preventative and curative dimensions, but in addition to targeted measures in those regards, a much broader approach should be taken. Education was necessary, starting at home where mothers should be well informed and willing to answer questions arising from children's natural curiosity, helping thus to uproot in Ecuador the notion that sex equals sin. Then teachers should continue along the same vein, treating sexuality as a natural function but also correcting the false belief that sexual abstinence was incompatible with men's physiology. And in schools, factories, unions, barracks, and elsewhere—anywhere people were gathered in collectivities—leaders should educate them about the prevention, the cure, and the consequences of venereal diseases. The state itself should promote coeducation from primary school on, to develop the character of the child through interaction with members of the opposite sex. In sum, educational efforts should take advantage of all possible arenas as well as all media, including radio, cinema, lectures, pamphlets, posters, and so on. It was also necessary to train medical and paramedical experts in this kind of work, expand state facilities of prophylaxis and treatment, and found quarantine facilities for those in contagious states.

The author further argued that perhaps it was the moment to consider eliminating prostitution, considering the failure of prostitution regulation in controlling the spread of venereal diseases. However, to do this would require confronting the fact that prostitution was "the economic support for thousands of people in Ecuador." The state should therefore provide reeducation services that included facilitating productive employment, echoing the words of liberal reformers from some four decades earlier who emphasized how women's virtue could best be protected through providing them with decent forms of work. Finally, women should be educated to better protect themselves—this in a context of suggesting how illegitimacy could be prevented—raising the provocative (but unanswered) question of whether the Servicio de Sanidad should recommend the use of contraception, a highly unusual suggestion for Ecuador in this era.

The 1951 project for a Law of Sex Education (Ley de Educación Sexual) emphasized many similar themes, seeing such education as the basis to combat both prostitution and venereal diseases. Its author, the director of the venereal prophylaxis service in Guayaquil, argued that:

> The union of the two sexes that is the physiological act called coitus, which is necessary for reproduction, is also a pleasurable act that is often embittered by: venereal contagion, excessive use (sexual degeneration and vices), and abuses. Very few people are not affected, legally or illegally, when the two sexes seek each other out in response to what nature demands, in spite of the shadows that can darken these acts. What matters is to know how to dissipate those shadows and it is Sexual Education that casts light over these matters, which should be offered to all human beings in programs of public education: men and women, children and adults.[101]

This was a more modern-sounding approach, to be sure, portraying women as well as men as compelled by sexual impulses and arguing for education of both sexes in these matters. The author went on to argue that "we must convince our compatriots that they should not see the sexual act as a sin or a shameful act, dispelling that hypocrisy and locating it in its rightful place: as an organic function, just like respiration, circulation, or digestion." Only thus would the shame of venereal infections be dispelled—rather than seeing them as punishment for sin—so that their sufferers would always readily seek medical treatment. If children encountered answers to their questions among their parents and teachers, framed in a prudent and progressive way, this would set them on a healthy path. If not, they would inevitably seek answers elsewhere: "in pornographic books, erotic magazines, libidinous pamphlets, and through practical instruction from perverts." In the sample survey answers that he presented in the appendix to his proposal, in contrast, he portrayed vividly the issues that led women to a life of prostitution: illiteracy, lack of economic opportunities, and rejection by their parents or by respectable society if they ever faltered in their moral (that is, sexual) conduct. When parents evicted young women from the family home on discovering some moral infraction, this led them directly to prostitution since such women were left without other options. A more forgiving attitude on their fathers' part could instead set them back on the path to a secure future.

In general, expressions of sexuality had a much more severe effect on the lives of women than of men, given that the consequences could be clearly marked on their bodies, particularly if they became pregnant; for that matter, medical examinations could also determine if women were still virgins. The assumed connection between women and their children that appeared in discussions of child protection had its expression, too, in regard to venereal diseases: while the SPV kept a record of its female patients' offspring, no similar records were kept for the service's male clients. This might express the notion that women were more likely to be living with their children, which might lead to transmission of diseases by sharing living quarters, eating implements, food, and so on. It might also capture the assumption that it would be difficult to trace men's descendants, considering the frequent expression of their sexuality outside of marriage.

This chapter outlines state projects dealing with sexuality and disease that were directed especially toward women and some of the strategies that women themselves used to deal with the limited options available to them. Some of the evidence presented here suggests that women might have used prostitution as a way to support themselves and their families, under conditions in which they had few other skills or resources with which to make a living besides their bodies. Other evidence shows how this might be a temporary strategy, with women leaving the occupation and the Sanidad's registry when they were able to establish more stable circumstances. The key to being able to do so was to develop relationships with men who could support them and who did not hold their past against them. The argument such women offered that they had "subjected themselves" to the authority of a man as a guarantee of their honorability was partly a rhetorical device. However, it also points us to a much harsher reality in which poor women had few rights and few opportunities, which might lead to extraordinary levels of abuse. One woman whose story forms part of the evidence offered to Congress in 1951 by the director of venereal prophylaxis in Guayaquil recounted a harrowing tale of her initiation into prostitution: she was invited by her boyfriend to attend a dance, at which he sold her for fifty sucres to a madam who locked her in a room and forced her to be with men, holding her down with the help of others during the first such encounters (that is, rapes). While this seems a world away from the women who combined prostitution with other forms of work on a temporary basis, or who moved from prostitution to married life or stable consensual unions, it could also be seen as the logical extension of a situation in which many women lacked economic opportunities and were, in both law and practice, subjected to men in a range of ways.

Chapters 4 and 5 move to an analysis of other areas of intimate behavior, but with a focus on women who provided (rather than received) state services.

Issues of honor and morality were also at stake for women who studied and worked in state institutions, seeking new professional spaces for themselves in the fields of midwifery and nursing. As with poor mothers and prostitutes, for midwives and nurses, too, the presence—or absence—of men was also a relevant factor structuring their experience.

# Midwifery, Morality, and the State

·4

I n 1929 university-trained midwife Consuelo Rueda Sáenz proposed to the director of the Servicio de Sanidad (Public Health Service) that an outreach program for maternal and infant medical care be established in the poor neighborhoods of Quito. Just as the state employed physicians to serve the poor, she wrote, it should also pay for the services of professional midwives. To ensure that poor women took advantage of such a program, it should be required that all birth certificates be signed by a registered midwife or physician. Rueda explained that her proposal "is aimed at serving those women who cannot, because of their poverty, go to clinics or pay for the services of physicians or licensed midwives, and who therefore prefer to die alone, or entrust their terrible moments to untrained hands that for a small fee present themselves as knowledgeable but that are ignorant of the difficulties of the issue and the consequences of their actions." Indeed, Rueda argued that infant mortality was caused solely by *empiricismo* (unlicensed practitioners) and that "obstetrics [midwifery] is one of the most interesting branches of medicine, and is a beautiful and dangerous science. As the mother of lives that should multiply, it should be practiced only by scientific hands."[1]

Six years later, in 1935, an outreach program of maternal-infant care, much like the one that Rueda outlined, was established by the Ecuadorian state. Rueda's letter emphasized many of the points that would later be highlighted in this state project: the need to reduce infant mortality, the effort to displace empirics with professionally trained and licensed midwives, and the notion of childbirth as requiring scientific management. Her letter also underlines how women themselves sought to broaden the arena of professional work available to them and to promote the state's goals in the area of public health. What she did not anticipate, perhaps, were some of the challenges that women like her would face once this project was established, particularly in their relations with other employees of the Sanidad.

Rueda was not a traditional midwife who had upgraded her skills at the university. Rather, she was part of a new generation of scientific midwives who had studied at the Universidad Central in Quito in the early twentieth century. Soon after the 1899 opening of the new Maternidad (lying-in hospital) in Quito, Rueda registered at the university in 1900 to study midwifery. She had been born in Quito in 1882, and at eighteen was the youngest of the three women who began university study that year in the only field open to women. She was a paternal orphan and lived with her mother during her studies. One of her two classmates was also an orphan (having lost both mother and father), and these were the two students who completed the program most quickly. They both graduated in July 1903, following three years of study; it took their class-mate some seventeen additional months to graduate. Rueda clearly had some intellectual inclinations, since she then formed part of the first female cohort admitted to the second field of university study opened to women, registering with five others in a preparatory year of study for pharmacy in 1904.

She went on to study three more years of pharmacy, although for unknown reasons she did not graduate in this field; four of her classmates, however, did become the first group of female pharmacists in 1909. Further evidence of Rueda's scientific inclinations appeared in her notes on her work as a Sanidad midwife in the late-1930s, where she described interesting cases she had attended and the challenges of childbirth conditions in the Andean towns and cities where she was posted. While she apparently shared with policy makers a series of notions regarding both childbirth and state responsibility, and indeed professional midwives can themselves be seen as the products of a state project to modernize childbirth, nonetheless the record of conflict over the work of government-funded midwives shows that they were not simply mechanical representatives of state goals in the towns and cities where they worked.

Maternal and infant health was an important topic in Ecuador at the turn of the twentieth century. Women of all social classes began their reproductive lives early and had numerous pregnancies. Infant mortality was high. From infancy to adulthood, mortality rates declined for every subsequent age group. The only exception to this rule was, notably, that mortality rates increased again for women in their childbearing years. The fact that at the beginning of the twentieth century the wife of an Ecuadorian cabinet minister died of puer-peral fever underlines how widespread was the danger to women's health posed by childbearing: no social class escaped.

Improved care of pregnant women and infants was not only a humanitar-ian impulse on the part of the liberal governments at the turn of the century. As was evident in programs of child welfare, they had begun to see popula-tion growth as a source of national wealth and prosperity, which was consis-tent with their overall interest in improving labor productivity and mobility. Equally important was the liberal project to provide forms of honorable work to women. Ecuadorian women in the nineteenth century called on the exper-tise of other women to assist them during childbirth. Indeed, it was almost unheard of to call in a male physician to attend a delivery, given the moral standards of the time. Most women who assisted at deliveries had achieved their expertise through years of practical experience. Increasingly, however, there was interest in normalizing the training of women for this work, with the growing confidence in medical science as the nineteenth century progressed (the cause of puerperal fever was only discovered in 1879 in Paris). In this con-text the training of midwives in the Faculty of Medicine at Ecuador's Univer-sidad Central was regularized and expanded significantly, well before women were permitted to study in any other faculty.

While the words "midwifery" and "midwives" are used throughout this chapter, it should be noted that this was seen, at least in principle, as a scientific profession and field of study, and in Ecuadorian Spanish the field was referred to as *obstetricia* (that term is not used here because of potential confusion with the medical specialty of obstetrics). Notably, however, the women who received university training in this field were referred to using the more scientific-sounding term *obstetriz* (more recently, *obstetra*) rather than the term *partera* (from the Spanish *parto*, or birth), which in turn suggested practical—literally, empirical—rather than scientific training. All of those who studied *obstetricia* (or midwifery) in the period under consideration were women.

## Midwifery Students at the Universidad Central

There is a spotty history of formal midwifery training for women in Ecuador that dates back at least to 1835.[2] This irregular process was briefly consolidated in the early 1870s, during the conservative (but modernizing) government of Gabriel García Moreno, as part of his larger project to develop scientific ex-pertise through such acts as the establishment of the Polytechnic School and his recruitment of two French physicians to reform the Faculty of Medicine at the Universidad Central. His government hired a French midwife to train fe-male students who would be licensed by the Universidad Central at the end of their three years of study and training at a small and short-lived Maternidad founded in Quito. After the assassination of García Moreno in 1875, this project stagnated with government disinterest and the departure of the French midwife. Throughout the 1880s there is only a record of one midwife graduating from the university. In 1890 concrete steps began to be taken to establish a new Maternidad, and simultaneously women began to study midwifery more regularly at the university. The Maternidad project received a further impulse in the 1890s, when some inheritances were willed to this project (including funds from the estate of Juliana Vallejo, who had graduated as a midwife in 1870). With the coming to power of the liberals, this project was further promoted. Finally, in November 1899, the new Maternidad was opened. It served both as a home for midwifery classes and as a place for poor women to give birth.

In the six decades from 1890 through 1950, the information in the registration records of midwifery students at the Universidad Central falls into five historical periods: 1890 to 1899, as this training was reorganized and preparations for the establishment of Quito's new Maternidad were undertaken; 1900, following the opening of the Maternidad, to 1911, after which no women registered to study midwifery for the better part of four years; 1915 to 1928, during which this study was revived; a hiatus from 1929 to 1938, during which only two women registered to begin their studies in the mid-1930s (and there is no record that either of them graduated), although some women already in the program continued their studies; and 1939, when the new School of Obstetrics (midwifery) became an independent unit within the Faculty of Medicine, to 1950 (the end of the period of study).[3] This periodization seems to be related to larger issues in the politics of midwifery. The status of the Maternidad was relatively unstable in the early years of the twentieth century. In 1900 the Maternidad was moved from its initial site to a somewhat larger (although still inadequate) facility on Pereira Street. In 1908 it was relocated from the Pereira site and entrusted briefly to the religious sisterhood Hermanas de la Caridad, in part due to the cost to the Universidad Central of running what was at least as much a health-care institution as an educational facility. For instance, in 1911 there were eight midwifery students being trained there, but 322 births attended.

In 1909 Dr. Isidro Ayora returned from receiving advanced medical training in Germany (sponsored by the liberal government), where he had become Ecuador's first physician to specialize in obstetrics. From his appointment as director of the Maternidad at the beginning of 1910, he fought to regain and improve the clinic's previous space on Pereira. In 1912 the Maternidad was brought under the control of the Junta de Beneficencia and was reopened at the Pereira site in late 1915 as women again began to register for midwifery study. It is unclear why there was such a prolonged hiatus in the training of midwives from the late 1920s—the records of the meetings of the faculty council of the Faculty of Medicine could not be located in the archive of the Universidad Central—but it may be relevant that there was marked political instability throughout the 1930s. There was also increased competition from physicians in the field of maternity care during this period.

Despite the irregular progress of the midwifery program, still it is striking that the Faculty of Medicine was the only faculty at the Universidad Central that admitted any female students at all until 1936, when Isabel Robalino enrolled in the first-year program in the Faculty of Law. Within the Faculty of Medicine, women were permitted first to study midwifery, then they were accepted into pharmacy (beginning in 1904, leading to four female graduates in 1909 but no more until 1929).[4] Women began to study nursing in 1917. Following Matilde Hidalgo's graduation as Ecuador's first female physician in 1921, it took almost fifteen years for the next woman, Reina Cadena, to graduate as the country's second doctora de medicina. In 1927, Lusitania Vivero graduated as Ecuador's first female dentist. In the academic year 1936–37, when the first woman registered in the Faculty of Law, there were twenty-five women studying in the Faculty of Medicine in the following fields: midwifery (two in year three), nursing (seven in year one, seven in year two), dentistry (one in the preparatory year, two in year three), and medicine (two in the preparatory year, one in year four, two in year five, one in year seven).[5] By that time, sixty-five women had graduated with midwifery degrees since 1890 (there were others before that date, and many more who undertook partial training), two as physicians, one as a dentist, six as pharmacists, and at least forty-three as nurses.[6]

While the Faculty of Medicine may have been the first to accept female students, midwifery students did not enter on the same footing as male students who registered in the faculty's other programs, such as medicine or dentistry. Most important, in order to study midwifery, it was not necessary at the turn of the century to have completed high school. In 1890, when an interim regulation governing the study of midwifery was passed by the Consejo General de Instrucción Pública (the national Council of Public Education) with the purpose of reorganizing midwifery training, it required that applicants should have some secondary education (although at the time there were no schools that provided for formal graduation as female *bachilleres*).[7] However, among the sixty-one students who began their studies in midwifery between 1890 and 1911, only one such student (in 1908) presented a high school diploma upon registering for the program. In 1899, Francisca de la Cruz had completed her studies with a grade of *sobresaliente* (outstanding) at Quito's Catholic Colegio de los Sagrados Corazones, when she would have been sixteen years old. When she registered in the midwifery program in 1908, she was at the advanced age of twenty-five and still unmarried; perhaps she sought a career after resigning herself to remaining single. If so, she seems to have met her goal: graduating in 1912, a quarter century later, she was still practicing in Quito in 1937 (then age fifty-four), and still apparently single, according to the practitioners' lists kept by the Sanidad. All other midwifery students who provided information about their educational background registered in the program on the basis of passing an exam set by the provincial Department of Education verifying their knowledge. This was the same exam taken to obtain credentials as a primary school teacher, granted based on the knowledge displayed rather than completion of formal studies.

This illustrates clearly the scarcity of educational opportunities available to Ecuadorian women at the time. As we know, even when the liberal government established in Quito the Instituto Nacional Mejía—its flagship institution of secular education—as a coeducational secondary school in 1897, it was only in 1903 that the first woman actually enrolled in this high school. Another option, study in one of the capital's three Catholic schools for girls (the most elite of which was the Sagrados Corazones), was limited to young women who could prove that they were from properly constituted homes—that is, who were themselves legitimate children and whose parents and grandparents had also been born in these circumstances—as well as those who could pay the relevant fees. A significant proportion of midwifery students would not have been able to satisfy these requirements. Another educational option in the early twentieth century was to attend the Instituto Normal Manuela Cañizares established by the liberals in 1901, but this institution formed female teaching professionals who went on to staff the nation's expanding system of secular schools, and it is unlikely that such students would have sought a different professional option in midwifery. Among midwifery students, it was only in the 1920s that three female registrants mentioned the schools in which they had studied, and only in 1928 that the first woman registered for midwifery with a formal high school diploma of bachiller: Quito-born Emma Franco had graduated with perfect grades from the Instituto Mejía earlier that year with a specialization in philosophy.

The 1890 regulation also specified that women should be at least twenty-one years of age to be admitted to the midwifery program. Yet again, we find that the reality did not match the rules, which highlights the importance of studying practice as well as policy. In fact, more than a third of the seventeen women who enrolled in their first year of studies between 1890 and 1899 were under twenty-one, including two sixteen-year-olds and one seventeen-year-old. While the average age at first registration did not differ significantly over time, the age range did differ somewhat (table 4.1). While in most time periods there were more students who began their studies between the ages of eighteen and twenty-two than in any other age group, in the 1900–11 period slightly more students entered aged twenty-three to twenty-seven than entered aged eighteen to twenty-two. This may indicate that, with the expansion of this field of study in that decade under the liberals, there was something of a backlog of women of a wider age range who had been waiting for an opportunity to train for professional work.

There is also a shift over time in the marital status of midwifery students. Among those who began their studies in the last decade of the nineteenth century, almost a third were identified as señora. In the following decade, the proportion of married women dropped to about a fifth, and the last married woman to register in the first year of the midwifery program did so in 1917. A small number of women did marry in the course of their studies (this differs from the case of nursing students, who were expected and required to be single). Nonetheless, among the fifty-four women in practice in 1932 who had registered their midwifery titles with the Servicio de Sanidad in Quito (as required by law), only eight were apparently married while two more were widows.[8] In general, over time the field evolved from one in which women of a somewhat wider age range initiated their studies, sometimes already married, and with little previous formal education, to a program in the 1940s in which students registered soon after graduating from high school (and most commonly having specialized in biological sciences at the secondary level) and always as single women.

Why might women seek training in this field? The records suggest that economic reasons were central to their search for decent forms of work. Many individual student files include petitions to have fees waived due to the student's lack of resources. For instance, the graduation fees of Manuela Ortega were waived in 1897 with the rationale that "her parents do not have property or fortune" and that she had undertaken her studies "in order to support her

Table 4.1. Midwifery Students: Age Range and Marital Status

| Year first enrolled | Total number of students | Age | | | | | "Señora" |
|---|---|---|---|---|---|---|---|
| | | Under 18 | 18–22 | 23–27 | Older than 27 | No age noted | |
| 1890–99 | 17 | 3 | 12 | 0 | 2 | 0 | 5 (29.4%) |
| 1900–11 | 44 | 1 | 18 | 19 | 3 | 3 | 9 (20.5%) |
| 1915–28 | 37 | 3 | 27 | 3 | 3 | 1 | 2 (5.4%) |
| 1933–34 | 2 | 0 | 1 | 0 | 1 | 0 | 0 |
| 1939–50 | 59 | 0 | 48 | 5 | 1 | 5 | 0 |

Source: Registration records of the Universidad Central's Faculty of Medicine, AGUC.

family."[9] Delfina Latorre (who graduated in 1898) presented a certificate from a high official of the Supreme Court verifying that she was "very honorable, discreet, and extremely poor, having distinguished herself by having helped her parents support the burdens of life." Her classmate Isabel María Racines similarly presented certificates that attested that she was "absolutely poor and an orphan" and that she had pursued her studies "in order to obtain a means of subsisting, suffering privations and sacrifices" in the process. In addition, for a few years in the first decade of the twentieth century the liberal government offered scholarships to allow some women to pursue this program of study, providing them with fee waivers and a small monthly stipend.[10]

The case of two young women from Ibarra (the capital of Imbabura province in the north) illustrates the transition from support from clergy to support from the state in the early years of the twentieth century. Archbishop Federico González Suárez certified in 1906 that he personally knew the sisters Zoila and Rosa Larrea and that they were very poor and deserving of financial support.[11] They may have also been orphans; although they were not identified as such in their registration records, the unusual omission of the names of their mother and father from those records suggests their absence. In any case the archbishop explained that it was at his urging that the Larrea sisters had gone to Quito to study midwifery, after a pastoral visit to the provincial capital Ibarra when he "discovered the considerable number of women who perished due to the not merely rudimentary, but even barbaric, manner in which certain maternity operations are practiced by empiric midwives." González Suárez himself initially supported the Larrea sisters financially, but when this was no longer possible, he sought state scholarships for them.

While many students appear to have had economic difficulties that may have led them to seek an opportunity to gain professional skills to support themselves, this begs the question of why they did not simply gain practical experience in this field rather than embarking on the arduous path of university training in Quito. What might have been the benefits of becoming a licensed *obstetriz* rather than an empiric *partera*? Part of the answer may lie in the signals that were being given by liberal governments that there might be an expansion of government jobs in these areas or other kinds of support for licensed practitioners. For instance, in the 1904–06 period, those students who received financial support for their studies were required on their graduation to take up practice in a location identified by the government; rather than a requirement, this might well have been perceived and experienced more as a promise of employment. Although there was not a formal program to hire midwives by the state at that time, and indeed this even predated the 1908 establishment of the Sanidad, midwives went on to work for municipalities and in some cases for the Junta de Beneficencia (later the Asistencia Pública) in provincial hospitals.[12]

There was also another form of government support that became increasingly important for many different kinds of medical practitioners. Under the Ley de Boticas of 1920 and its subsequent revisions, the Sanidad was tasked with professional defense: that is, with protecting the rights of licensed medical practitioners against those whose training was not recognized by Ecuador's universities and then, through their university credentials, by the state. While unlicensed practitioners could be tolerated and even given state permission to practice where no licensed practitioners existed, once a licensed practitioner set up practice in a population center, she had the right to insist that the Sanidad prohibit those without such credentials from continuing to practice, through a number of escalating punitive measures. Although this probably had very little effect in many rural or indigenous areas—mostly because few licensed practitioners would have settled there—the records of the Sanidad show that this was an important mechanism in more urban contexts, among midwives as well as pharmacists, dentists, and physicians.

Returning to the students' economic situation, beyond the general impression that permeates the records of the straitened economic circumstances experienced by female students, there is evidence that many of these women specifically lacked a male support figure able to maintain them financially, which was the gendered expectation in Ecuador whenever possible. In the last decade of the nineteenth century, almost a quarter of the women who registered to study midwifery were orphans or widows (table 4.2). The case of the one widow, Alejandrina Miranda, is especially poignant. In 1894, when she began her studies at the age of seventeen, she was faced with supporting her three legitimate children on her own following her husband's death, as she herself was also an orphan. After her first year of studies, she had to withdraw and

TABLE 4.2 Midwifery Students from Vulnerable Social Categories

| Year first enrolled | Total number of students | Illegitimate | Orphans | Widows | Total from vulnerable categories |
|---|---|---|---|---|---|
| 1890–99 | 17 | 0 | 4 (23.5%) | 1 (5.9%) | 4 (23.5%) (one was in two categories) |
| 1900–11 | 44 | 7 (16%) | 20 (45%) | 4 (9.1%) | 25 (57%) (six were in two or three categories) |
| 1915–28 | 37 | 0 | 13 (35%) | 0 | 13 (35%) |
| 1933–34 | 2 | 0 | 0 | 0 | 0 |
| 1939–50 | 59 | 9 (15.3%) | Not noted | 0 | 9 (15.3%) |

Source: Registration records of the Universidad Central's Faculty of Medicine, AGUC.

only returned to complete her second and third year in 1900–01 and 1901–02, graduating with perfect grades in 1902.[13]

In the first decade of the twentieth century, the number of women from what we can gloss as vulnerable social categories was even more significant. Over half of the first-year students (twenty-five of forty-four) were illegitimate daughters, orphans, or widows, and six of these women were members of more than one of those categories. There were no more widows among the students after 1910 (and no more married women at all after 1917), but there continued to be orphans and illegitimate daughters who made up significant proportions of the midwifery students. In Ecuador, children were considered to be orphaned when either or both of their parents died. Among the thirty-seven confirmed orphans who initiated studies of midwifery, twenty-three had lost their father, nine had lost both parents, and five had lost only their mother. This further underlines the important place that the absence of a male support figure in particular held in decisions to seek economic security through one's own work. While none of the three categories of vulnerability for which there is information can serve as a direct proxy for class, the absence of a male support figure could often cause downward social mobility, and being illegitimate in particular often declassed women—and even more so, their mothers.

The significance of these issues is further highlighted by a comparison of the social vulnerability of midwifery students with that of other female students in the Faculty of Medicine. There were no other fields in which widows studied, but there were illegitimate daughters and orphaned women studying for other paramedical or medical careers once those were opened to women. Table 4.3 summarizes this data for the five programs of study in the Faculty of Medicine that had female students. Although broad contrasts are clear, the raw numbers don't necessarily capture the social experience involved, since women in these categories were often clustered in specific time periods. For instance, midwifery students who were illegitimate were clustered exclusively in the periods 1900–11 (when enrollments expanded) and 1939–50 (after the School of Obstetrics was reopened as a separate academic unit within the Universidad Central), making up 15 to 16 percent of the student body in those decades. No doubt the experience at the beginning of the century was rather different than at midcentury; nonetheless, these women constituted a significant portion of their cohort, while the illegitimate women studying for other careers were often alone in their status.

Even there, the experience of the one illegitimate pharmacy student (who registered in 1905) was surely different from that of the one illegitimate dentistry student (who registered in her first year in 1942 but did not continue her studies). Of the four illegitimate women who pursued medical studies, one

TABLE 4.3. Illegitimate and Orphaned Women Studying for Medical Careers

| Program of study | Illegitimate women | Orphans |
|---|---|---|
| Midwifery | 10% (16 of 159) | 37% (37 of 100) |
| Nursing | 2.9% (11 of 375) | 2.7% (10 of 375) |
| Dentistry | 1.8% (1 of 57) | 3.5% (2 of 57) |
| Pharmacy | 5.6% (1 of 18) | 11.1% (2 of 18) |
| Medicine | 4.3% (4 of 93) | 2.2% (2 of 93) |

Source: Registration records of the Universidad Central's Faculty of Medicine, AGUC.

registered in 1937 and the remainder in the 1940s, although in the end only one of them succeeded in completing the program. Among orphans, the situation of midwifery students was even more striking, with thirty-seven confirmed orphans among the one hundred students who registered up through the 1930s, when this was being noted in the records. In contrast, there were ten students formally noted as orphans among nursing students between 1917 and 1950; only two among female medical students, both in the 1920s (one of whom was Matilde Hidalgo); two of the secular pharmacy students (both when the program first opened in 1904 and 1905, including Consuelo Rueda); and two female dentistry students, both in the early 1930s. Although the absolute numbers are not large, there nonetheless appears to be a disproportionate number of illegitimate daughters, and much more so of orphans, among women studying to be midwives.

Until the late 1920s, at the end of the third period, the registration records at the university also provide information about where students lived during their studies. As table 4.4 indicates, in the first period the majority of midwifery students lived with both parents, which may partly reflect the large number who were from Quito itself. Collectively they also do not seem to have been quite as vulnerable as the women who began their studies in the second period. Then the majority lived either alone (identified as "independent" in the records) or with their mothers. The number of women living alone is surprising, since this would have been very unusual for women in Quito at the time.

TABLE 4.4. Residential Arrangements of Midwifery Students

| Year first enrolled | Total with information | Independent | With both parents | With mother | With father | With others | With spouse |
|---|---|---|---|---|---|---|---|
| 1890–99 | 15 | 1 | 9 | 3 | 1 | 1 | 0 |
| 1900–12 | 30 | 9 | 4 | 9 | 1 | 5* | 2 |
| 1915–29 | 36 | 7 | 13 | 5 | 0 | 11** | 0 |

* includes two students who resided in convents.
** includes three students who boarded at the Maternidad.
Source: Registration records of the Universidad Central's Faculty of Medicine, AGUC.

Among the "independents," we find five widows and married women but also two orphans and another two women who do not fall into any of the vulnerable categories identified in the records. Those who lived with their mothers in that decade were almost exclusively orphans who had lost their fathers.

There were also a small number of women, especially among those who were not from Quito, who lived under the protection of (*bajo la dependencia de*) someone other than their parents; from their last names, they appear usually to have been extended family members. In two cases, midwifery students found lodgings in convents. In the third period, the largest two categories were made up of women who lived with both parents and those who lived with "others" (including three women who boarded at the Maternity Hospital). This may indicate, in the first case, perhaps a somewhat less vulnerable population; and in the second, the increasing numbers of women traveling to Quito from elsewhere in the country, to undertake advanced study.[14] Predictably, this became more common as travel was facilitated by improved transportation links. Interestingly, among those who came from elsewhere and lived with others was Julia González Delgado, who in 1920 lived with Matilde Hidalgo (then thirty-one and in her sixth year of studies in the medical program). González was born in Loja and undertook her first two years of study in Cuenca, much like Hidalgo who was also born in Loja and did her undergraduate medical degree in Cuenca before being accepted to the Universidad Central to study for the degree of *doctora de medicina*. Likely their families knew each other. This also suggests that Hidalgo's status as a physician in training made her an appropriate chaperone to a younger midwifery student, despite the fact that she was a single woman. Similarly, the university's registration records tell us that in 1930 twenty-one-year-old Blanca Rosa del Pino, a Riobamba-born student in the first year of the dentistry program, lived in Quito with Angela Torres, who at the time was twenty-seven years old, single, and in her fourth year of the pharmacy program. Although Torres was born in Guaranda, she had attended secondary school in Riobamba before traveling to Quito to study at the Universidad Central. These cases point to an emerging network of socially vulnerable professional women (for instance, both Hidalgo and Torres were orphans) offering concrete forms of mutual support.

One more interesting point emerges from the archival information about residence. Although there were sixteen married women who initiated their studies of midwifery between 1890 and 1917, only two of them were identified as living with their husbands. We know that five more of them were widowed, but nine still remain who were not living with their husbands. One possibility might be that these women traveled from other provinces to study, but the records show that this was the case for only three of the sixteen married women;

TABLE 4.5. Midwifery Students: Comparison of Entering Cohort and Graduates and Numbers from Vulnerable Categories

| Year first enrolled | Total number entering first year | Number who graduated | Number of students in vulnerable categories | Number of graduates from vulnerable categories |
|---|---|---|---|---|
| 1890–99 | 17 | 11 (64.7%) | 4 (23.5%) | 2 (50% of vulnerable group; 18.2% of total graduates) |
| 1900–11 | 44 | 27 (61.4%) | 25 (57%) | 12 (48% of vulnerable group; 44.4% of total graduates) |
| 1915–28 | 37 | 18 (48.6%) | 13 (35%) | 5 (38.5% of vulnerable group; 27.8% of total graduates) |
| 1933–34 | 2 | 0 | 0 | 0 |
| 1939–50 | 59 | Not available | 9 (15.3%) | Not available |

Source: Registration records of the Universidad Central's Faculty of Medicine, AGUC.

the remaining thirteen were all from Quito. While we cannot know why they were not living with their husbands, we might speculate that they were estranged. Although divorce was possible after 1902, it was still difficult both procedurally and socially.[15] If these women were indeed estranged from their husbands, they might appropriately be seen as adding to the group of socially vulnerable women entering this field of study.

Women experiencing specific kinds of social vulnerability—illegitimate daughters, orphans, and widows—seem to have been particularly interested in studying midwifery, likely to develop professional skills to be able to support themselves and their families. However, it was not easy for them to graduate (table 4.5). In no time period was the proportion of graduates from these categories equal to the proportion of registrants from these categories, and in no period did more than half of the women from vulnerable categories that enrolled in their first year actually graduate. Thus in 1890–99 they made up 23.5 percent of registrants but only 18.2 percent of graduates; in 1900–11 they made up 57 percent of registrants but only 44.4 percent of graduates; and from 1915–28 they made up 35 percent of registrants but only 27.8 percent of graduates. In other words, socially vulnerable women may have had particularly good reasons to pursue professional work, but perhaps their very lack of social support made it more difficult for them to complete their studies.

## Midwives at Work

Once they graduated and began to exercise their profession, licensed midwives sat in uneasy relation to two other categories of medical practitioners: unlicensed midwives (empirics or parteras) and physicians. As the letter from

Consuelo Rueda quoted at the beginning of this chapter suggests, professional midwives sought to displace unlicensed ones, but this was not easily achieved, especially in smaller population centers.[16] In addition, as the twentieth century progressed, professional midwives were increasingly in competition with male physicians as well. In the late nineteenth century, theoretical classes in obstetrics were provided to medical students at the Universidad Central, but without any opportunity for practical training. Only after the 1899 opening of Quito's Maternidad do we find in 1902 that sixth-year medical students began to attend the practical classes in obstetrics that were offered there by Juana Miranda, a licensed Ecuadorian midwife, who in 1891 became the only female professor on the payroll of the Universidad Central in her role as *profesora de obstetricia práctica* (she retired during the 1907–08 academic year at the age of sixty-five). In 1904, in order to graduate, medical students were required to have assisted at six deliveries; this was well beyond previous expectations but nonetheless compared rather poorly with the one hundred deliveries that female midwifery students attended prior to their graduation.

Upon Dr. Isidro Ayora's return from Germany, he was appointed director of the Maternidad in January 1910, and he set to work reforming the field of obstetrics in Ecuador both in terms of the practices at the Maternidad and the university curriculum in midwifery (for instance, the program of study for midwives was extended from three to four years later in 1910). Associated with this process of reform, in 1916 he threatened to resign as director of the Maternidad if a new female profesora de obstetricia práctica was appointed, rather than having a male physician offer practical classes to midwives and medical students alike. He won this battle, with the support of the Faculty of Medicine, despite the Junta de Beneficencia's insistence on its obligation to support women who had trained for a liberal profession. Ayora responded to this argument by pointing out that the primary purpose of the Maternidad was to offer an effective service to its patients:

> And to fulfill this objective above all else there is a need for competent personnel, that is, physicians and medical students who possess the knowledge and practical experience necessary for the scientific exercise of obstetrics, not the empirical kind, so fatal in its results.[17] A midwife, especially one of ours, is not capable of deciding what to do in a difficult case, much less treat it. . . . The protection of midwives that the Honorable Junta believes itself in the duty to pursue, should consist, as far as I am concerned, in making the Maternidad a true School of Obstetrics, where midwives learn to exercise their profession properly, and where they can come from time to time to forget the negligence and routine to which their professional exercise tends when it lacks medical

control. The Maternidad should be a model school for the midwives, and for that, it must be properly organized.[18]

This marked the end of the employment of a midwife in the Maternidad, through the end of our period of study.[19]

Simultaneous with this, Ayora promoted the initiation of the first nursing classes in the Maternidad, to train female professionals who would assist physicians rather than compete with them. As he put it, "Advanced nations such as the United States have suppressed the profession of midwifery; instead, they have created the profession of Nurse, to intervene in births as an assistant to the physician. Thus although it is true that one, perhaps lucrative, profession for women is eliminated, whose exercise involves a true danger for the public, it opens another one for them—that of nurse—that is not, like midwifery, a terrible weapon in inexpert hands."[20] The growing number of licensed nurses in Ecuador over the next few decades contrasts with the rather intermittent graduation of professional midwives—most markedly in the 1930s, when nursing studies intensified just as midwifery studies were almost entirely paralyzed, perhaps because women's activity in the latter sphere was increasingly invaded by physicians.

Evidence from 1947 indicates clearly the increasing competition from physicians in the area of maternity care in Quito. In a survey of medical establishments in Quito that year—none of which apparently employed any licensed midwives, although several public and private institutions did employ nurses— we find that in addition to the recently inaugurated Maternidad Isidro Ayora, with ninety-five beds, several other clinics offered obstetrical services.[21] The Clínica del Seguro with its ninety beds offered thirteen kinds of medical services to its affiliates, including obstetrics and gynecology. The Hospital Militar (266 beds) also had a maternity ward, presumably for the wives of military employees. At least as of 1935, the armed forces did not have a single woman among their 4,464 employees.[22] More strikingly, of the six private clinics that were then operating in Quito, four specialized in obstetrics and gynecology and one more offered these services along with general surgery and bone surgery. These clinics were the Clínica Pasteur (twenty-four beds), the Clínica Moderna (seventeen beds), the Clínica Quito (thirteen beds), the Clínica Román (ten beds), and the Clínica Narváez—which also offered bone surgery—with four rooms of two beds each (although in this case the second bed in each room was for the accommodation of companions or nurses rather than patients). Thus among private clinics in Quito, only the psychiatric Clínica Endara did not offer maternity services. Although there were certainly licensed midwives practicing in Quito at this time, evidently none of their clinics were considered formal enough to be included in this survey of medical establishments.[23]

Despite the clear evidence of increasing competition from physicians, licensed midwives were hired directly by the Ecuadorian state, through the Sanidad, when a new program of maternal-infant care was established in 1935. An important factor in the decision to hire midwives rather than physicians for this service was probably what was referred to as the "urbanismo" of physicians, who generally preferred to work in the country's largest cities. In 1938 of 610 physicians in the national territory, 390 (63.9 percent) were practicing in the three largest cities of Guayaquil (172, or 28.2 percent), Quito (151, 24.8 percent), and Cuenca (67, 11 percent), and a further 122 (20 percent) in all other provincial capitals combined (ranging from a high of 19 in Riobamba to a low of 3 physicians in Babahoyo); 82 more (13.4 percent) were distributed among 46 smaller population centers, including 1 physician in the Galápagos Islands but none in the Amazon region; and for the 16 remaining physicians no location was noted.[24] Additional factors influencing the hiring of midwives by the Sanidad were likely the lower salaries of midwives; possibly the perception that provincial, rural, and working-class women—in other words, most Ecuadorian women—would not be willing to have male physicians attend their deliveries; and perhaps, as elsewhere, physicians' general disinterest in taking over the time-consuming work of attending laboring women anywhere other than the main population centers where they may have experienced more intense competition for patients.[25]

The stated objective of establishing this outreach service was to oversee the well-being of Ecuadorian infants in three stages: prenatal, natal, and postnatal. The service was designed to be comprised of two employees: a professional midwife and a trained nurse (although budgetary constraints led to elimination of the nursing portion of the service in 1940). The midwife was charged with providing prenatal services, delivering babies, and offering immediate postnatal care. The nurse would then take over, monitoring infant health and providing advice to mothers during early childhood when children were most likely to add to the high figures of infant mortality. The Sanidad was to provide the medical implements and supplies necessary for this work, and these services were to be offered for free to the poor population. Midwives were permitted, however, to run a parallel private practice, charging a fee to those who could afford to pay for their services.[26] At the time, in many cases the provincial public health office was made up of a single room housed in another government office (for instance, the Sanidad delegate in Ambato used a room in the Gobernación, the offices of the provincial governor), so arrangements might be made for prenatal services to be offered in the local hospital. The home address of the midwife was also provided to members of the public, who were encouraged to contact her through the relevant office of the Sanidad or directly in her lodgings at any time of the day or night.

The initial program provided these services to the populations of provincial capitals throughout the highlands and to a limited number of county seats. First the urban residents of the provincial capital or county seat were to be attended, with the extension of services to outlying areas as possible and practical. In the few county seats included initially in this program, in some cases only one employee was named as an *inspectora visitadora sanitaria*, who did all of the work of maternal-infant protection as well as assisting in local campaigns to control infectious diseases. Consuelo Rueda was named to this post in Alausí, in the Chimborazo province. At the other extreme, the capital city of Quito, with a population of about one hundred thousand, was divided into three zones for this service, with a midwife and two nurses per zone. These employees had arrived at their posts by early June of 1935. In many cases they were not from the local area.

These female employees were conceived as being at the forefront of state projects of moral regulation over poor mothers in the provinces and in working-class neighborhoods in Quito. They were charged with providing instructions on and assistance with pregnancy, childbirth, and infant care, as well as other lessons in hygiene, during patients' visits to their workplaces or their own visits to local homes. In a sense this involved providing quite new services to the population; certainly the state had not previously made a serious attempt to intervene in such intimate practices anywhere other than in Ecuador's largest cities. However, it was also clear this was an explicit attempt to displace existing forms of knowledge and expertise. Indeed, when provincial delegates of the Sanidad advertised these new services to encourage people to take advantage of them, their persuasion often had a coercive tone. As the delegate in Tungurahua province in the central highlands pointed out in the flyer that he produced to promote this program, "with the availability of free services of a professional, there is no reason to expose yourself to the dangers of empirics, to whom we will apply the sanction established in Article 56.4 of the Public Health Police Code (Código de Policía Sanitaria), if they continue to illegally exercise the profession of midwifery."[27] These warnings extended not only to the empirics but also to those who consulted them. As the delegate in Imbabura province in the northern highlands stated in a similar flyer, after describing the need for these new employees due to the ignorance of mothers and poor hygiene of their homes: "You must not allow your children to die, without first exhausting every resource offered by medicine, thus demonstrating your love.

The death of a child due to the negligence of a mother is a crime that the Código de Policía Sanitaria, quite rightly, punishes very severely."[28]

In Quito, where there were many more services available to the public than in the countryside or provincial cities, the director general of the Sanidad instructed the *comisario de sanidad* (public health constable) in August 1936 as follows: "In order to prevent infant mortality, and there being no excuse given the number of services offered by the medical institutions as well as the Sanidad, you should proceed to judge and sanction any person who arrives at the respective office to apply for a birth or death certificate without having had professional medical attention."[29] In central areas like Quito there was a concerted effort to bring both birth and death under medical supervision, whether via state physicians and midwives or private physicians. In peripheral areas it was more difficult to insist upon this (despite the overblown claims of public health delegates in the flyers quoted earlier). For instance, the municipal council of Pelileo (in Tungurahua province) in 1946 passed a local bylaw regulating the services of the municipally funded midwife, specifying that no birth that had not been attended by the licensed midwife or a physician would be registered in the civil registry. However, as the regional director of public health in Quito pointed out when asked to approve this regulation, national legislation required all births to be registered, and until there were more medical professionals available, unassisted deliveries and those attended by empirics would still have to be registered. In those cases where professional services were readily available and people refused to use them, however, there, he argued, it would be appropriate to sanction the parents with all the severity that the law allowed.[30]

The uneven coverage of medical practitioners over space sometimes created problems for midwives quite directly. As Hortensia Cevallos—both a licensed midwife and trained nurse who was assigned to work in the county seat of Pujilí (in Cotopaxi province) in 1935—explained to the director of the Sanidad in Quito, the isolation of the town and general lack of medical services placed her in a situation in which she had access neither to a pharmacy nor to transportation for any complications that required medical treatment. Pujilí was two leagues' distant from the hospital in the provincial capital of Latacunga, and since there was not a physician any closer than that, if one of her patients were to die, she would surely be blamed by all of the "ignorant people of this place." She felt that her position was untenable and asked to be transferred to the county seat of Salcedo, closer to Latacunga. Besides, the local population had apparently made it clear to Cevallos that they had no need for a professional midwife, since they already had experienced parteras available locally, who had served them well for many years.[31] This kind of situation likely underlay the competition for posts in more accessible areas: ideally Quito but also some of the more central provincial capitals. Guaranda, for instance, was clearly not a plum posting. It was the capital of Bolívar province, to be sure, but it was a relatively isolated city situated between highlands and coast. There were so many problems in maintaining a state midwife there that in 1946 the Sanidad finally appointed a young local woman as a public health nurse on paid leave, so that she would receive her nurse's salary as a kind of scholarship while she pursued her midwifery studies in Quito for four years.[32]

The way in which provincial delegates of the Sanidad perceived the position of licensed midwives relative to empirics varied considerably. One place this can be seen is in the vital statistics forms that these officials had to submit to the regional public health office each month. Each birth in the jurisdiction had to be categorized in terms of the kind of professional attention it had received. The categories preprinted on the form were: (1) attended in the Maternidad; (2) attended at home by professionals; (3) attended by empirics; or (4) without assistance. While the second option would in principle apply to the work of licensed midwives, most provincial delegates seem to have had an implicit understanding that the word "professional" could only really be applied to physicians. In this context none of the preprinted options corresponded clearly to assistance from state midwives, and delegates had a variety of responses to this lack. Some crossed out Maternidad and typed in "attended for free" (Latacunga) or "Sanidad" (Ibarra, Latacunga), both of which referred to state-funded midwives. Various monthly forms from Riobamba (the capital of Chimborazo province) have "Sanidad" written in alternately on the line for "empirics" (crossed out) or for "professionals" (crossed out). Many delegates regularly left the line for empirics blank and insisted that the vast majority of births had lacked any assistance at all, presumably rather than admit that unlicensed midwives were conducting a brisk business in their jurisdiction. Indeed, on the February 1942 form for Pujilí county (in Cotopaxi province), it is clear that the figure entered for "empirics" was erased and this number added to a revised "without assistance" figure (although we do not know whether this correction was made in Pujilí or Latacunga; nor whether it was a simple error or was perceived as an inappropriate entry). In other forms the default category was clearly "empirics," with no births cited as without assistance, which was probably in most cases a more accurate reflection of the situation.

Table 4.6 summarizes the information provided on such forms for one month, where ultimately it is difficult to read how many births were attended by state midwives. Altogether, these forms indicate some ambivalence about where professional midwives fit within the range of existing services. While in general higher officials of the Sanidad showed support for the work of state midwives, at the provincial level feelings seem to have been rather more mixed.

TABLE 4.6. Type of Assistance Noted in Birth Registrations, Various North-Central Highlands Jurisdictions, September 1938

| Location | Maternity clinic | At home, by professionals | By empirics | Without assistance | Total |
|---|---|---|---|---|---|
| Tulcán (capital, Carchi) | 1 | 9 | 0 | 55 | 65 |
| El Angel (county, Carchi) | 0 | 0 | 14 | 0 | 14 |
| San Gabriel (county, Carchi) | 0 | 15 | 0 | 78 | 93 |
| Ibarra (capital, Imbabura) | 11* | 14 | 0 | 34 | 59 |
| Otavalo (county, Imbabura) | 0 | 8 | 0 | 62 | 70 |
| Latacunga (capital, Cotopaxi) | 6** | 1 | 21 | 62 | 90 |
| Ambato (capital, Tungurahua) | 29 | 28 | 48 | 0 | 105 |
| Riobamba (capital, Chimborazo) | 20 | 20 | 12* | 61 | 113 |

\* "Servicio de Sanidad"
\*\* "for free"
Source: Monthly summaries of birth registrations in various jurisdictions, LCR-Delegaciones Provinciales-II 1938, ASS/MNM.

Perhaps the one unmistakable conclusion that can be drawn is that these figures, once they are compiled at a higher level, simply cannot be used to interpret the numbers of births for each category, since the categories themselves seemed to mean rather different things in different local contexts (or even in a single place in different months). Although government registration of births was enhanced by such measures as the establishment of public health delegations in each provincial capital in 1926, who supported the work of civil registry offices by issuing birth and death certificates, it would be more accurate to characterize the information generated as claims about the state of birthing in each jurisdiction than objective records of the situation.

How far did the work of state midwives reach? According to the accounts of such midwives themselves, the number of births that were attended in a given month varied depending on demand and on the constraints on their time. Their reports show that a state midwife might attend up to thirty deliveries in a single month as well as between one hundred and two hundred (or even more) prenatal consultations, although the expectation was that they each assist at a minimum of ten deliveries.[33] In unusual cases a midwife might attend four deliveries in a single day. As Consuelo Rueda explained, when she was working as the state midwife in Ambato, capital of Tungurahua province, "For me there are no peaceful nights, no days of rest, no weekends, no holidays, no vacations. It would be nice if I were not so committed to my work, if it were a mechanical job of just doing a single thing; but the truth is that my work is simultaneously material, moral, and intellectual, and at any hour, in any circumstance, whether it is raining or not, day or night, I must run when I am called."[34] If one takes the September 1938 figures from Ambato presented in table 4.6, where admittedly it is unclear where the work of Consuelo Rueda might fit, nonetheless more than half of the births in the jurisdiction were attended by professionals of one kind or another. In the first months of 1930, in contrast, there had been twice as many births attended by empirics than by professionals in Ambato.[35] This does seem to imply a significant extension of services in at least some regions, while still recognizing (as the discussion of vital statistics reminds us) that many births continued to occur both beyond the reach of the Sanidad and more generally outside the view of the state.

In some cases the general public registered formal complaints about the state midwives. Most often these involved situations in which midwives charged for their services, they did not provide the necessary supplies, or they refused to attend a delivery. In sum, these complaints involved difficulties in accessing these free services rather than suggesting a rejection of them. There was a good deal of ambiguity regarding the first issue, since these state employees were authorized to charge fees to those who were capable of paying for their services, in the parallel private practices they were permitted to establish. They seldom received the necessary supplies from the (chronically underfunded) Sanidad, so that was a likely cause of the second problem; as a result, midwives might send a family member of a laboring woman to a local pharmacy to purchase supplies at the family's expense. In the third situation, it might be that the midwife was already out on a call and therefore could not be located by someone in need. These complaints tended to reflect concerns that people didn't have sufficient access to state midwives rather than suggesting that they did not want their services.

More prominent in the archival documentation than any tensions there may have been between the recipient population and these female practitioners, however, were the conflicts that erupted between more senior male functionaries of the Sanidad and these more junior female ones. In some cases public complaints provided a pretext for the disciplining of female public health employees. In several instances these women were accused by their male supervisors of quite serious moral flaws. This provides us with a glimpse of how unattached professional women were viewed, who were living in somewhat peripheral areas of the country—that is, in neither the hinterlands of the Amazon nor the largest cities but in county seats and provincial capitals in which they were often isolated from their social networks of support. The delegate in Tungurahua province in particular had the reputation for being a demanding taskmaster who expected the highest level of performance from his staff (as well as from his colleagues in other medical institutions, with whom he sometimes came into conflict). Over the first decade of this outreach service, a number of the midwives and nurses who worked for him ended up reporting to the regional director of the Sanidad in Quito, since they found it difficult to work under the direct supervision of the delegate (this wasn't the only province where this occurred, although it was most marked here). One of the first public health nurses in Tungurahua's capital of Ambato was accused by the delegate of "seeming to be dedicated more to prostitution than to fulfilling her noble mission."[36]

Consuelo Rueda, who was Ambato's state midwife from mid-1936 until March 1941, had a tense relationship with the delegate during most of her tenure, and at one point he speculated that her poor work might be due to her "habitual alcoholism."[37] However, the documents do not suggest that she was a poor employee, given that she worked for several years for the service, first in Alausí, then in Ambato, and from March 1941 to February 1942 in Machachi just south of Quito (after which she resigned to take a position working directly for the municipality of Machachi, for a better salary, as the municipal midwife). As Rueda herself pointed out in September 1940, in four and a half years in Ambato she had not had a single case of puerperal infection, much less a death under her care.[38] Indeed, the records of the Universidad Central show that she graduated at the top of her cohort in 1903, with perfect grades, and the evidence seems to point to her considerable competence.[39] Public complaints against her were limited to her occasional unavailability and to the fact that she did not provide all supplies. However, she defended herself against such complaints by insisting that people were perfectly satisfied with her services until they arrived at the provincial public health delegation to obtain a birth certificate and were subjected to an interrogation to discover whether she had provided all of the necessary supplies at no cost.

Like others in her position, Rueda seldom received the supplies that were supposed to be sent to her from the regional office in Quito. In some cases she was formally fined by the police for not being available to attend all patients who sought her services, leaving little of her salary for her living expenses. But as she explained, "it is impossible to attend to everyone, because often I am away on extended calls, and so of course, I am not at home when they come looking for my services."[40] Indeed, in the month to which she referred in this note, she had delivered nineteen babies (almost twice the minimum expectation) and had provided a large number of prenatal consultations. While the delegate in Ambato may have been a particularly difficult supervisor, there are other cases too in which accusations were made about these female employees, such as the longtime (unmarried) state midwife in the northern provincial capital Tulcán, who according to her supervisor lived in a "constant state of pregnancy."[41] The pattern that appears to emerge is that younger women were accused by their supervisors of sexual transgressions, while older women were accused of other flaws such as alcoholism.

Despite suffering what seems to have often been disrespectful treatment by their supervisors, these women carried on in their work. The documentation of the Sanidad suggests that they were motivated, at least in part, by the need to support their families. In numerous documents they referred to the need to support aging mothers and younger siblings or to support their own children (especially in the case of widows). A clear impression is given that there is no adult man in the family to provide support—there are no references to aging fathers, for instance. Nor do any of the state midwives appear to have been married at the time of their service, with a spouse to support them. As Señora Dolores Ayabaca, the state midwife in Guaranda, Bolívar province, explained to the regional director of the Sanidad in Quito in 1938, she and her nursing colleague, Rosa Martínez, were subjected to despotism and continual attempts to "stain our reputations" in the provincial office. In her case, it was only because of her pressing economic circumstances and in order to support her three children that she was willing to continue in her position.[42] Their economic and family situations placed many of these women in a vulnerable position, since they had few alternatives to working and they seldom had a network of support in the provincial capitals or county seats where they were appointed from Quito. This is fully consistent with what the archives of the Universidad Central revealed about the social profile, in general, of the women who opted to train for this career.

### Moral Issues and Midwifery

Throughout this period there was a great deal of attention paid to the morality of the women who studied or practiced midwifery. For instance, in the 1890 interim regulation governing the study of midwifery, it was specified that in order to take the final examination before graduation, the students were required to provide "legal proof of good conduct" (which came in the form of signed certifications from respectable men). In the decades of the 1890s and 1900s, too, women could apply to have tuition and graduation fees waived if their grades were high, their economic situation was difficult (as was so often the case), and their moral behavior was *intachable*, or irreproachable. In 1904 and 1905 the government signed contracts with some female students to pay them a small living allowance and their university fees while they studied midwifery, in exchange for three years of government service upon their graduation. However, a condition of their contracts was that they had to submit reports three times a year certifying both their grades and their moral conduct. Interestingly, Profesora de Obstetricia Práctica Juana Miranda had questioned this category of evaluation of her students as early as 1892, when she argued that she assumed that the category "conduct" meant not moral conduct but rather such faults as not paying sufficient attention or smoking in class.[43] Although there is no record of the answer to her query, the kinds of certificates submitted in the 1890s and 1900s cover such issues as frequency of church attendance and the modesty of women's behavior, so it appears that moral conduct was indeed what was being examined. The moral character of midwives who went on to work for the Sanidad was also called into question by their male supervisors at the provincial level.

While morality was consistently emphasized, it seems unlikely that midwifery students—dealing with some of the material consequences of sexual acts and with such intensely intimate bodily functions—would have been naive young women. From what we know about the backgrounds of at least some of them, they do seem to have been exposed to some of the realities—the difficulties—of women's lives. They strike one as women who did not have the opportunity to remain as naive as the social ideal; they do not appear to have been especially sheltered. This impression—that they don't fit easily with the more conservative stereotypes of virtuous women in highland Ecuador—is strengthened by the fact that prior education in a Catholic girls' school (and the social, economic, and cultural factors that might underlie that) was apparently not compatible with a decision to study midwifery. Although one early case of a midwifery student who had graduated from one of Quito's Catholic secondary schools is mentioned earlier, it is striking that this was only one of two such cases in all of the records reviewed. After midwifery training was intensified (again) with the establishment of the Escuela de Obstetricia in 1939, with only one exception—a young woman who had graduated from the Colegio Mariana de Jesús in Riobamba—the women who chose to enter this field of study had all graduated as *bachiller* in state secondary schools, such as what was by then Quito's flagship school for young women, the Colegio 24 de Mayo, or in the port, the Colegio Nacional Guayaquil.[44]

Despite clear statements such as Consuelo Rueda's opening remarks that aligned professional midwives with state objectives in these fields, these women often had a rather ambiguous position between unlicensed midwives and physicians and sometimes seemed to face in both directions at once. For instance, in early 1937 the provincial delegate of the Sanidad in Tungurahua accused Consuelo Rueda of having signed birth certificates for deliveries attended by one of Ambato's unlicensed parteras, Rosa de Gómez. Rueda admitted to the regional director of the Sanidad in Quito that she had done so, but explained that it was in response to "pleas and tears from those who thus save themselves from paying a fine and other difficulties." She had agreed to do this as a kind of interim measure, just "until the people become moralized and accustomed to the idea that without the certificate of a professional there will be no registration [of a birth in the civil registry], and thus they will seek out only professionals and not empirics."[45] Although the provincial delegate saw Rueda's actions as indications of personal immorality (as opposed to, say, a problem of professional ethics), his request that she be fired was not accepted.[46] It was a few months later that Rueda began to report directly to officials in Quito rather than to her nominal supervisor.

This dynamic in itself is revealing, since it suggests that government officials at one level were focusing on the usefulness of midwives (perhaps including their social backgrounds in this assessment), while those at another (geographically closer) site were focused more on what made them dangerous. On the former side of this divide, the midwives' pragmatic approach to maternal-infant protection may have ultimately made this program more effective, and the kinds of compromises they engaged in may indeed be more broadly representative of how frontline agents of government projects modify them in implementation. Interestingly, however, where this geographic difference was dissolved, the attitudes of officials in Quito might resemble those of their provincial counterparts. Thus some months after the initiation of this program, the director general of the Sanidad suggested (unsuccessfully) to the minister in charge of the public health portfolio that Quito's state midwives be replaced by male physicians and medical students who had specialized in obstetrics. As he put it: "The work of men, because they are better prepared, is more efficient."[47] In an unusual step the director referred to the state midwives in this note as *parteras* rather than as *obstetrices*, thus further emphasizing that their work did not meet his expectations. Later documents suggest that the main problem with the state midwives in Quito, from the perspective of the Sanidad, may have been that they were sufficiently busy with their parallel private practices that they were sometimes reluctant to take on free patients.

Both the mixed official feelings toward scientific midwives and the ways that such women sometimes pushed the limits of state projects indicate that these women were not passive conduits of state priorities. The fact that they both aimed and were expected to displace traditional parteras should not be taken to indicate a straightforward alliance with physicians or the state. That seems to be the assumption of the historian Ann Zulawski in her otherwise nuanced study of public health in Bolivia.[48] More strongly, the historian Kristin Ruggiero has referred to licensed midwives in late-nineteenth-century Buenos Aires as acting as "virtual 'gyneco-police'" or in a "quasi police" role, more aligned with male networks of power than women's networks of mutual support.[49] It is unclear whether the actual role of licensed midwives was different in Bolivia and Argentina, or whether the nature of the archival material drawn on here simply reveals to us more of the contradictory experiences and positioning of licensed midwives in the Ecuadorian context. The historian Steven Palmer, in contrast, begins to open up questions about the aspirations of these new professionals in early-twentieth-century Costa Rica.[50] No doubt he is right in suggesting that the young women recruited into these programs of study would have been more malleable than traditional midwives. Nonetheless, in Ecuador the difficulties scientific midwives encountered in their work relationships may have called into question for them the extent to which they were accepted as allies of physicians and perhaps in some circumstances partially realigned their allegiances.

The universe of medical practitioners offering obstetrical services in highland Ecuador was a shifting and complex one, even among those undertaking formal study: physicians and medical students participated as well as women with varying degrees of scientific training, which they might use to various ends.[51] One issue on which the records of the Universidad Central are silent is just how many of the women who initiated their obstetrical studies but did not graduate—forty-four of them (precisely 44 percent) from 1890 through the 1930s—nonetheless went on to practice their profession without being formally licensed to do so. In 1895, when it appeared that the practical classes for midwifery students might be suspended temporarily due to the reorganization of the university following that year's Liberal Revolution, Juana Miranda, profesora de obstetricia practica, argued precisely that if these classes were not reinitiated, it was logical to assume that her students would dedicate themselves to *empiricismo*.[52] We know that one particularly notorious midwife did just that, two decades later: Carmela Granja, a paternal orphan from the provincial city of Ambato, studied all four years of the midwifery curriculum at the Universidad Central from 1916 to 1919 but did not graduate. Popular memory in Quito attributes her failure to graduate to having been expelled from the university because it was discovered that she had begun to perform abortions while she was a student (however, the reasons she did not graduate could not be confirmed archivally). She went on to become Quito's most famous abortionist: she is rumored to have carried out some two thousand abortions during her professional life as well as providing general gynecological and obstetrical services.[53]

In 1929 public health authorities denounced the fact that Señora Carmela Granja, "without a degree, exercises not only the occupation of midwife, but also the medical profession, which is even more serious." Previously the Sanidad had fined her for her illegal exercise of the profession of midwifery, which was the only violation within their jurisdiction. A surprise raid on her premises in 1929 discovered: "first of all . . . three cauldrons of boiling water, prepared on electric elements at the center of the room, and ready for the washing; and in one of them sterilized obstetrical instruments were found, as well as a syringe on a kind of counter. Secondly, there is evidence that persons who live in this same house, not only act as midwives giving preparatory advice and medicine, but also detain people here to cause them to forcibly miscarry or abort, which can be observed and deduced by the baskets of food that are introduced from the street."[54]

The fact that instruments were sterilized, and that women were housed and fed here, suggests that this establishment was not quite as marginal as the authorities argued. Indeed, it compares favorably with descriptions of the care offered at the Maternidad. In 1942, in what he characterized as a patriotic effort to ensure improvement in the services provided there, the husband of a fee-paying patient at the Maternidad offered his observations of the conditions there to the president of the Junta de Asistencia Pública. While he credited the physicians with providing excellent care, he was much less impressed with the medical students:

> who even for a simple sentiment of charity should be more prudent and attend to the parturients individually and not collectively, as if the acts occurring in the Birthing Rooms were an exhibitionist spectacle, without understanding not only that the most exquisite delicacy should be shown, but also the primordial importance of surrounding the parturient with confidence and tranquility; even more so if it is not a poor woman who is there as a result of public charity, but a lady seeking the special services of a *pensionado*. . . . But unfortunately it is not thus: rather, the doors of the Birthing Rooms are opened without warning, by the interns or anyone else wandering the corridors—like servants or nurses—giving the impression that they merely aim to satisfy their curiosity.[55]

He added extensive critical commentaries on the lack of hygiene and shabbiness of the accommodations. Perhaps the chronic underfunding of state institutions had no parallel in Granja's practice: she may have been able to fund her busy illicit practice with patient fees more easily than state institutions were able to secure their own funding. It should also be noted that the description of her clinic suggests not a traditional midwife but someone working fully within the biomedical model. This did not preclude the use of herbal abortifacients in her practice. For instance, in September 1926 she was called to the offices of the Sanidad to answer for her illegal exercise of a profession; on the same day, all pharmacists and pharmacy owners in Quito were reminded by the Sanidad of the absolute prohibition against accepting any prescriptions signed by midwives that contained "rue, savin, mugwort, saffron, rye ergot and other similar substances known as abortifacients."[56]

Although there were repeated efforts to jail Carmela Granja for her "arbitrary actions," she deflected them by threatening to make public the list of all of the women whose pregnancies she had helped to abort. She apparently claimed that no elite family in Quito would escape scandal, if this list were made public.[57] Nonetheless, there is evidence that she was sent to the penitentiary sometime in the early 1930s for criminally inducing an abortion and again in 1938 when a young unmarried woman died as a result of an abortion that Granja performed.[58] That young woman's lover, interestingly, was a promising young physician who was himself forced to flee the country temporarily as a result of his involvement in seeking the abortion.[59] In 1941, when Carmela Granja was moved from the penitentiary to the Hospital San Juan de Dios's Camarote de Santa Marta—a combination municipal jail (where female prisoners served as laundresses for the hospital) and infirmary (where prostitutes with venereal diseases in a contagious state were interned)—it constituted the final straw that led the Hermana de la Caridad overseeing this wing to resign and the mother superior to refuse to assign another sister to this position. Although for years, indeed decades, the hospital director had been insisting that it was inappropriate to house such a facility within the hospital, detailing the very disruptive behavior of some of the female prisoners, it was the arrival of Carmela Granja that provoked a crisis in the management of this facility by the hermanas.[60] A paid laundry service was established at the hospital soon thereafter.

On her release from prison, Granja returned to her clinical practice, as the record of a further raid on her establishment in 1946 indicates. Public health inspectors discovered her in the company of an unmarried pregnant woman and with medical instruments in a pot of boiling water, but by the time the appropriate authorities arrived, she had hidden the instruments and her patient had fled.[61] Her insistence on pursuing her practice over several decades under such adverse conditions raises the question of whether she had a clear project of offering alternative health-care services to the women of Quito (rather than simply engaging in a lucrative business).[62] However, although we can read between the lines of official documents to trace some of the broad outlines of her career, any interpretation of her motivations based on those documents would be speculation.

While the moral behavior of any women in the public sphere was demonstrably under close scrutiny in this period, the main moral issue facing midwives may well have been abortion, as the case of Carmela Granja suggests.[63] Indeed, the director of public health, Alfonso Mosquera, was quite blunt about this in a communication to the police chief in 1929: "For a long time, the Dirección de Sanidad has been working hard to cleanse society of a fearsome evil which has the most disastrous consequences—that is, criminal abortion. On previous occasions, following suggestions from the Sanidad, the Police Intendency has already dealt with a woman named Carmela Granja, widely known as one of those who most practices criminal abortion. The Sanidad itself has pursued and sanctioned this person, within its sphere of authority; that is, judging her and fining her for the illegal exercise of a profession, since Granja does not have a degree."[64] His unprecedented reference to "la Granja" in the last phrase without using the honorific "Señora" stands out in this document and suggests the extent to which her actions marked her as a transgressor of what Mosquera considered to be fundamental social norms.

In the same document the director went on to report his suspicions that yet another midwife had criminally provoked an abortion, resulting in the hospitalization of her client.[65] In that case, however, the client was a married woman, suggesting that it was not only unmarried women needing to protect their honor who sought abortions. Married women, too, had few contraceptive resources available to avoid unwanted pregnancies. Indeed, an analysis of clinical histories of women who sought medical care in the Hospital San Juan de Dios between 1925 and 1965 demonstrated that between the onset of their reproductive lives and the age of fifty, on average the women sampled saw more than a third of their children die. Moreover,

> Certain women in the sample (and they are not isolated cases) had more than fifteen pregnancies, others suffered four, five, or six miscarriages, others still—or sometimes the same ones—arrived at the age of fifty having lost the majority of their children, dead because of infectious diseases, diarrhea, etc. A global analysis of the situation, necessary in order to achieve a certain level of generalization, often obscures the concrete reality of what it is, what it means to be a woman in eras and in societies where the social roles of each gender are heavily marked and determined by biological differences. Responsible for the lives and deaths of their children, while they had very few alternatives to plan births and to avoid diseases, women among the poorer sectors had to as-

sume this heavy burden—physically and psychologically—within the heart of the family, in addition to their domestic and extradomestic labors.[66]

The presumed association of midwives with abortion was again made explicit in the angry comments of a physician who had previously served as medical intern in Quito's Maternidad at the Second Ecuadorian Medical Congress in 1931: "The majority of criminal abortions, complete or incomplete, which arrive in our Maternidad, have been carried out by professional or amateur midwives, for whom the most profitable business is the practice of criminal abortions. For these reasons, I myself believe that the doors of the University should be closed to any woman who chooses to study midwifery."[67] Although it is unclear whether there is a direct connection, the doors of the university were indeed essentially closed to those who wished to study midwifery for most of the 1930s.

Given that so many of the women who studied midwifery were socially marginalized through their illegitimate birth or by losing a father or husband, it is possible that some of them might have been particularly sensitive to the difficulties associated with unwanted pregnancies. Whether or not in reality midwives were the main practitioners of illegal abortions, however, there was undoubtedly a perception on the part of physicians that such women were the main providers of these services.[68] Although there were no allegations that the specific midwives employed by the state provided criminal abortions, the fact that midwives by definition were suspect may well have had a strong influence over how physicians dealt with them, even when they were university-trained and licensed. This apparent distrust may have been intensified by the fact that unlike nurses, who generally were trained to work under supervision in hospital settings, midwives tended to work alone, carrying out their practice in people's homes or in their own offices or lodgings.

In the end, midwives were both the agents and objects of government projects. The overall campaign to address problems of infant mortality and maternal health—something that was regularized in the mid-1930s and continues today as a principal focus of the work of the Ecuadorian Ministry of Health—engaged midwives as frontline employees. As government employees, however, there was some distrust of them within local instances of the Sanidad, and they themselves became the objects of disciplining by their male supervisors. Part of this governing project indeed seems to have been directed at them. There were government projects to provide women with decent work in the early twentieth century, and the expansion of professional midwifery fit into that program. With the emergence of an increasingly active state in the 1920s, the government offered not just services but also employment to rather specifically situated people. In 1935 (just before the launching of the maternal-infant health outreach program), 95 percent of female employees of the Ministry of Government and Social Welfare—the third largest employer of women within the federal government, and where state midwives would be employed two months later—were unmarried (mostly single but also widowed or divorced).[69] It is difficult to know whether this means that only unmarried women sought work, or whether they were seen by the government as more worthy of a specific form of support: government employment. Certainly there are numerous suggestions in the archival documentation from the era that central government officials understood the state as having a paternalistic role as protector of women lacking other male supporters. However, the direct supervisors of some of these women did not appreciate the level of independence that they seem to have displayed, which would indeed have been required for them to become the well-qualified women that they were. Overall, the documents suggest the contradictory experience of government work for these women. It was both liberating, in providing them with a relatively stable form of employment (and we should not underestimate the importance of this), and constraining, in leading to an intensified level of monitoring of their work and behavior.

Nurses were seen as preferable to midwives in some of the materials on which this chapter is based, as Dr. Isidro Ayora's earlier statements make clear. Nonetheless, nurses, too, encountered difficulties as they attempted to promote a model of female professionalism and expertise that was almost entirely unknown to most Ecuadorians, including, it seems, some of the physicians and medical students alongside whom they trained and worked.

# The Transformation of Ecuadorian Nursing

I n 1942 the first cohort of Ecuadorian women enrolled in the newly estab-
lished Escuela Nacional de Enfermeras (ENE, National Nurses School), a
boarding school and training facility built adjacent to the Hospital Eugenio
Espejo in Quito and operated under the auspices of the Universidad Central.[1]
The school was funded by both the Ecuadorian government and international
institutions, including substantial financial contributions from the Servicio
Cooperativo Interamericano, a branch of the recently founded Institute for
Inter-American Affairs within the U.S. State Department. The Servicio funded
the construction of the building itself and provided technical staff—in the form
of U.S. nurses, known as *las Americanas*—to administer the Escuela for what
they expected to be its first five years of operation. The Rockefeller Foundation
also contributed. A private philanthropic foundation that previously led campaigns abroad against contagious diseases, the Rockefeller Foundation increasingly was involved in developing medical institutions and medical training. Its
contributions to the Escuela included payment of some salaries, technical advice, numerous donations of equipment and supplies, and provision of scholarships to Ecuadorian nurses to undertake advanced training in North America
so that they could return to Ecuador to teach at the school. While the Rockefeller Foundation was a private institution, the coordinator of Inter-American
Affairs himself—leader of the Institute for Inter-American Affairs—was Nelson A. Rockefeller from 1940 to 1944. In this position he was charged with ensuring the strategic defense of Latin America through work in the information,
economic, health, sanitation, agricultural, transportation, and cultural fields.

In this project the private foundation worked cooperatively with official U.S. government institutions.

The founding of the Escuela Nacional de Enfermeras formed one small part of a wide-ranging health and sanitation agreement signed by the U.S. and Ecuadorian governments in 1942 in the context of a comprehensive economic development and trade agreement, something quite new in United States–Ecuador relations.[2] This agreement was part of a larger project to develop a common front in Latin America against the Axis nations during World War II. In the Ecuadorian case this included, among other things, a Lend-Lease agreement that allowed the U.S. military to establish a base for their Pacific theater of war operations on Ecuador's Galapagos Islands and another in coastal Salinas; U.S. monopoly access to Ecuadorian rubber for the war effort; and Ecuadorian access to U.S. manufactured tires for its public transportation system; the breaking off of Ecuadorian diplomatic relations with Germany, Italy, and Japan (following the replacement the previous year of German Sedta by U.S. Panagra as provider of Ecuador's internal aviation service); provision of equipment and services from the Defenses Services Corporation (fully owned by the U.S. government) to the Ecuadorian armed forces, including boats, planes, munitions, training, and construction of barracks (the latter especially important to help consolidate army support for the embattled Ecuadorian president); and much-needed funding and assistance to rebuild Quito and Guayaquil's potable water systems. All of this occurred, too, in a context of internal political crisis related to the disastrous 1941 boundary war with Peru (in which Ecuador lost almost half its national territory, in the Amazon region) and rapid inflation. For internal political reasons any agreement involving military issues also had to include cooperation in the area of social development, given the economic crisis, political instability, and the fact that there was some sympathy among Ecuadorians for the Axis countries, particularly for the idea of a planned economy.

While these international and national political factors help to explain why there was funding and sufficient political will to found an institution such as the Escuela Nacional de Enfermeras, its establishment was also due to the vision of key Ecuadorian figures like pediatrician Dr. Carlos Andrade Marín, who at the time was minister of social welfare.[3] Nonetheless, the history and internal life of the Escuela cannot be reduced to either these international processes or the interventions of national medical and political leaders. This chapter focuses on the possibilities this dynamic created for a professionalization project for a group of Ecuadorian women, and the many challenges they faced. By 1952, at the end of the Escuela's first decade, a clear model had been consolidated of Ecuadorian nurses as both highly trained women with excellent technical skills and single women with a Christian devotion to their vocation who were required to display irreproachable moral conduct. The tension between the two dimensions of this model of professional womanhood, which seem to pull in different directions, can be seen as a response to sustained difficulties in promoting this female career in the social context of highland Ecuador in the mid-twentieth century. Despite the importance of the broader political context in the establishment of the school, the particular model of Ecuadorian nursing that emerged did so through a process of maneuvering through obstacles and difficulties that constrained the sphere of possibility of these new female professionals. To give proper attention to the Ecuadorian context in which this project was inserted, we begin with a consideration of early nursing in Ecuador.

### Precursors and Early Projects

In 1917, Ecuador's first nursing classes were established within the Maternidad, promoted by its director, Dr. Isidro Ayora. However, even before that there were two groups of women who, in rather different ways, could reasonably be seen as precursors to professional nurses in Ecuador. Indeed, the evidence suggests that both models influenced how trained nurses were perceived and treated. These women, who intervened in the hospital care of the sick, were on the one hand illiterate employees who were charged primarily with cleaning duties, both of patients and of hospital wards, and on the other hand members of the religious sisterhood the Hermanas de la Caridad (Sisters of Charity). While there is some clear continuity that can be traced between professional secular nurses and nursing nuns, it was the hospital servants, rather than the nuns, who were actually called *enfermeras* before the establishment of professional nursing, despite the large gap between this group and the new generation of nurses in terms of the work performed, training required, and professional aspirations.

In addition to being called enfermeras, hospital servants were also sometimes referred to by the outdated term *barchilonas*. They may have had their origin in the colonial period among women without resources who were taken in by the hospital as an act of charity. They were not technical staff; rather, these women were tasked with the "dirty work" on hospital wards and sometimes were simply referred to as servants. Even as the first half of the twentieth century progressed, there was a marked lack of specificity in the term *enfermera*. For instance, in 1938 the director of Quito's Hospital Civil San Juan de Dios had to request a formal change to the names of positions in the hospital, to reflect the fact that the new fiscal year's budget included categories that were not reflected in the existing names of positions at the hospital. Thus all of the men and women who had been working in the positions of *"velador(a),"* *"asistente de hombres,"* and *"asistente de mujeres"* were all renamed *"enfermero/as."*[4]

None of the employees named in that document had attended the nursing school that had begun in the Maternidad, which by that time had fifty-one formal graduates. A subsequent document that year similarly asked for formal approval to transfer a woman who had been working as assistant cook to fill a vacancy in the position of enfermera in one of the wards.[5] Although by the 1940s the word most often used for the positions filled by these employees was "*asistente*" (as in "assistant for the women's surgery ward"), increasingly these employees were referred to as "*asistente-enfermeras*" or "*auxiliares*," in an attempt to clarify the difference between these employees and the emerging group of graduated nurses. The latter were sometimes referred to as "*enfermeras tituladas*" (nurses with professional titles/diplomas) or after 1942 as "*enfermeras universitarias*." Courses began to be offered in the 1940s to formally train these asistentes as nursing aides, and other steps were taken to modernize their image, such as the 1946 provision of canvas shoes and two pairs of white socks to each such employee of the Hospital Civil San Juan de Dios.[6]

Despite a confusing continuity in name with the enfermeras in the hospital, it would be more accurate to identity the precursors of professional nurses as the nursing nuns who were so important elsewhere, too. Vowed women hold a special place in the history of medical establishments and medical care in Ecuador, centrally (but far from exclusively) in Quito's public hospital, the Hospital Civil San Juan de Dios. In the first half of the twentieth century, this was the oldest hospital still in operation in the Americas.[7] It had been founded in 1565 under the name of the Hospital de la Misericordia de Nuestro Señor Jesucristo. Initially, the hospital's mandate included not only care of the ill but also protection for the poor and for orphaned women without financial resources. It was funded by charitable donations. Its administration passed through the hands of several religious orders in the eighteenth and nineteenth centuries. Then in 1870, conservative president Gabriel García Moreno contracted the sisters of the order of San Vicente de Paul—the Hermanas or Hijas de la Caridad (the Sisters or Daughters of Charity)—as the hospital's administrators.

In France the religious community of the Sisters of Charity was organized by Vincent de Paul specifically to care for the ill, with a mandate to be the earthly expression of God's love and to "recognize in the afflicted poor the suffering face of Christ."[8] In contrast to cloistered nuns, the Sisters emerged as a community of vowed women who made up a nonenclosed sisterhood; rather than a contemplative life, work was central to their vocation.[9] The centrality of this work ethic may indeed be why the liberal state in Ecuador had relatively good relations with the Hermanas de la Caridad and continued to work closely with them after the 1895 Liberal Revolution at a time of significant church-state conflict in other realms and with other Catholic orders. Similarly, after the French Revolution among all of the Catholic religious communities, only the nursing sisterhoods in France were immediately recognized by the revolutionary state so that they could carry on with their duties under their contracts with municipal authorities.

On their arrival in Ecuador from France in 1870, the Hermanas de la Caridad took over the administration of the two most important Ecuadorian hospitals: in July that year the Hospital General de Guayaquil, and in December the Hospital San Juan de Dios in Quito. The relevant decree of the 1869 National Convention that placed Ecuadorian hospitals under their administration further specified that this included all of the hospitals of the republic with sufficient funds.[10] Thus over subsequent decades many additional institutions came under their administration, in provincial capitals and later also in county seats. Indeed, this became the dominant model of how Ecuadorian public medical institutions were administered for a century. This role as the contracted administrators of state health-care institutions differed from the experience of the Sisters of Charity in other national contexts, where the Sisters themselves fund-raised, established, and collectively owned, as well as administered, health-care facilities.[11]

A dual structure of authority existed within these hospitals, as the documentation of Quito's Hospital Civil San Juan de Dios demonstrates. Medical care itself was under the authority of the medical director of the hospital (until the mid-1920s still an unpaid—ad honorem—position), but the day-to-day functioning of the hospital was largely under the authority of the mother superior (*madre superiora*). She organized and oversaw the work of from twelve to seventeen Hermanas, depending on the era. The Hermanas in turn supervised the functioning of each ward, provisioned and oversaw the kitchen (which prepared food daily for some 250 to 300 patients and up to a hundred employees of various kinds), ran the hospital's apothecary, oversaw the Santa Marta wing and the work of its female inmates/patients in the hospital's laundry service, and lived in the institution to ensure round-the-clock care for its patients. The Hermanas were not employees of the hospital. Rather, a contract existed between the religious community and the government to provide administrative services to the hospital, and it was the religious order or *comunidad* that selected and assigned Hermanas to their specific positions within the hospital. In a review of archival documentation spanning three decades of hospital administration (1920–50), very few documents were encountered that suggested conflicts of jurisdiction or struggles of power between the hospital's medical administration and the sisterhood in general, or between the medical director and the Madre Superiora as individuals. There was apparently a relatively well-defined division of labor between physicians and Hermanas at the hospital.

The first formal classes in nursing were established in 1917 within the Maternidad, under the leadership of its director, Dr. Isidro Ayora.[12] A strong advocate for professional nursing, perhaps Ayora had developed his views of nursing during his period of advanced obstetrical study in Germany. In Ecuador at the time, professional secular nursing was an entirely unknown career. The nursing program initially involved two years of study, ostensibly under the auspices of the Universidad Central. However, the marginal status of the nursing classes is indicated by the fact that graduations were not noted in the university records until 1929 (in other words, even if students completed their studies, they were not considered university graduates). The curriculum was reformed in 1921 to include a probationary course of three months and then three years of study in an *internado* or boarding school that functioned within the Maternidad. Students would begin practical training with the patients in the Maternidad and go on to a practicum in the Hospital San Juan de Dios in their last year of study.[13]

According to a reformed 1921 internal regulation, within the Maternidad the instruction of nursing students would be offered by three people.[14] The director of the school (Ayora) gave classes in anatomy, physiology, pathology, therapy, and "*moral de la enfermera*" (which included appropriate "conduct with the patient, his family, the physician, other nurses, etc."). The *médico asistente* (a junior physician at the Maternidad) gave classes primarily involving demonstrations and practical exercises involving those same topics, in the anatomy amphitheater, the clinical laboratory, the operating rooms, and so on. And the enfermera would teach the students "everything relevant to domestic economy, attention to patients (tidying of the room, making beds, baths, etc.) and will also review with them basic topics of primary instruction (reading, writing, the metric system, etc.)." The students were charged with "paying special attention to being respectful to their superiors, very solicitous and discrete in their care of the patients, sincere in their relations with the other students, scrupulously clean in their person and lodgings, and, above all, irreproachable [*intachable*] in their conduct."[15]

To carry out this new structure of training, it was necessary to secure the services of a professional nurse to direct the students in the "details of the practice," services that were not available at the time in Ecuador. Thus in 1922, at Ayora's request, an Ecuadorian diplomat in Hamburg recruited a German nurse, Fraülein Frida Schwarz, to take up the position of nursing director of the Escuela de Enfermeras in Quito. According to the certificates she presented, she had begun her career as a nursing aide in Dassau in 1914, and there completed a nursing course. She went on to work in the inpatient clinic in the quarantine hospital in Dassau and then became head nurse in the surgical department in the Dassau hospital. By 1922 she was head nurse in the women's and children's ward in a Hamburg hospital as well as being involved in teaching religious novices. "Beyond that, she is a Señorita of high moral conditions, and her educational level is much superior to that of those who normally occupy such positions." She was at the time thirty-five years old, unmarried, and healthy.[16] She offered her services in exchange for first-class passage from Hamburg to Quito (and return passage after a four-year term); room, board, and laundry service; and a monthly salary of 160 sucres. The contract was signed in November 1922, on her arrival in Quito.

In 1922, Ayora commented that when eminent U.S. surgeons had recently toured South America on an official visit of the College of Surgeons, they mentioned in almost all of their reports the lack of nursing services in South America and vigorously recommended that this be remedied as quickly and effectively as possible. This, according to Ayora, was precisely the goal of Quito's nursing school. He summed up his hopes for the school in the following terms:

> We are convinced that one of the greatest necessities of the medical profession in Ecuador is that of forming good nurses, who will support intelligently the actions of the physician and offer to the ill professional care, of a technical nature, that cannot be offered by family, nor much less by people who are simply charitable but ignorant. It is the moral duty of physicians to encourage and support this new female profession, elevating it to its appropriate position to ensure that it is properly appreciated by the public, so that educated Señoritas from good social backgrounds will dedicate themselves to it. The field of action of the Nurse is enormously broad within the modern organization of Public Assistance: her services are used in Hospitals, Hospices, Orphanages, Milk Depots, Red Cross, Dispensaries, private Clinics and Doctors' Offices, Maternity Clinics, Childcare institutions, Quarantine Hospitals, etc., etc.[17]

In its early years the school was a work in progress, despite Ayora's concerted efforts to promote this new career. During the 1917–18 academic year, eleven young women registered in the first year of nursing study at the Maternidad; in all cases this required an authorizing order to the university secretariat from the rector of the university, since these women did not have the usual qualifications for university study.[18] The following year, seven of them went on to register for second year. In November 1918 ten Hermanas de la Caridad registered in year one and, presumably in recognition of their existing expertise, four of them were promoted to the second year of studies the following week (thus the second-year class in 1918–19 had seven secular women and four Hermanas). The remaining six Hermanas joined five secular women in the first-year class; no further Hermanas registered until 1931. Among secular students, annual registrations for first-year studies fluctuated: eleven registrations in 1917–18; five in 1918–19; none in 1919–20; one in 1920–21; five in 1921–22; none in 1922–23; five in 1923–24; and one in 1924–25. It is unclear where the first trained nurses worked, but we do know that some of the earliest secular students were able to obtain scholarships in the 1920s in the state-run nursing school in Panama, with the assistance of Colón E. Alfaro, the Ecuadorian consul in Panama and son of the former liberal president Eloy Alfaro.[19]

In 1925 the advent of the Revolución Juliana led to a number of reforms in public administration. Attention to health-related matters by the administration was no doubt enhanced by the rise of Isidro Ayora to national political prominence, first as minister of social welfare and then as president. Among other projects, concrete steps were taken to establish a modern hospital in Quito, the Hospital Eugenio Espejo. The nursing school was also reformed: the initial school that had operated under rather precarious conditions was replaced by a new school of nursing in 1927, which continued to operate its two-year program of studies in the Maternidad with additional practical training in the Hospital San Juan de Dios until the Hospital Eugenio Espejo was inaugurated in 1933. The 1927 reform constituted a revitalization of nursing studies, with twelve first-year students in October 1927, some of whom went on to comprise the first formal graduates—that is, graduates noted in the records of the university—in 1929.

One lesson that the early history of nursing training in Ecuador teaches us is that while nursing nuns were precursors to secular nurses, they were not superseded by them. Rather, they formed part of a joint cohort once more technical training became available in Quito. In preparation for the opening of the Hospital Eugenio Espejo in 1933, another wave of Hermanas undertook technical training in the nursing school, beginning in 1931 and graduating in 1933. Indeed, nineteen women graduated as nurses in October 1933, among whom two or three were secular.[20] The remaining graduates were all Hermanas de la Caridad. Following the opening of the new school in 1927, it produced thirty formal nursing graduates between 1929 and 1933; of those thirty, at least sixteen were Hermanas, all of them 1933 graduates. This suggests that nursing nuns were still considered the most appropriate administrators and staff for hospital facilities in the country. Outside of hospital work, however, secular trained nurses did begin to work in outreach activities for the Public Health Service (the Servicio de Sanidad) in the mid-1930s, and several also seem to have worked in the area of *higiene escolar*, providing some health monitoring of children within the school system. By the time the new nursing school was established in 1942, there were sixty formal graduates of this school that since 1933 had been operating out of the Hospital Eugenio Espejo.

## The Escuela Nacional de Enfermeras and the Rocky Road to Professional Nursing

Finally, at the late date of 1942, a modern nurses training facility, offering intensive studies in a boarding school context along with practical training at the adjacent hospital, was inaugurated in Ecuador with the enrollment of the first cohort of students at the new Escuela Nacional de Enfermeras. Although this model of professional nursing education and practice was well established elsewhere by this time, it was not easily adopted in Ecuador. In the account given below, a number of difficulties are interwoven: financial and administrative challenges, difficulties of carving out a distinct professional space for women within hospitals, and the ongoing project of defining what constituted an appropriate female professional of this kind.

### Administrative Challenges

The Escuela began to function on decidedly uncertain terms. The building was still under construction when the first students arrived in mid-1942 and through much of their first year of study (ultimately the physical premises of the school would be able to accommodate up to seventy-five students, twenty-five in each year of study, but the school was not always able to recruit or retain this number). The first prospectus for the school was only elaborated in May 1943, in preparation for recruiting the second cohort of students. The Executive Decree outlining government financial commitments to the school was only signed on January 7, 1944. Because the Junta Central de Asistencia Pública had already formulated its budget for that calendar year, however, it was unable to fulfill its obligations to pay utility bills or building repairs. In fact, during the school's first three years of functioning, the Junta paid no such expenses. The Escuela's decision-making mechanisms were also under construction. The school was governed by a *consejo ejecutivo* (executive council) chaired by the Universidad Central's dean of medicine and initially included a representative of the Junta Central de Asistencia Pública (Dr. Carlos Bustamante for many years) as well as the American nurses serving as *directora* and *subdirectora* of the school. However, in addition, the directors of the Hospital Eugenio Espejo and of the medical services of the *caja del seguro social* (social security system) also participated on the council, despite having no formal role under the Escuela's governing regulations. In 1947 a reorganization of the council brought additional representatives from the Servicio Cooperativo or the Sanidad, the Rockefeller Foundation, the general public, and the Madre Superiora of the Hospital Eugenio Espejo.

In addition to international funding and expertise that supported the school, Ecuadorian government institutions of various kinds and at various levels committed to providing support: the Universidad Central provided some administrative and teaching support; the Ministerio de Previsión Social and the Junta Central de Asistencia Pública provided financing for specific purposes; and various Ecuadorian institutions provided scholarships to nursing students (including municipalities as well as health-care institutions of various kinds). Under the scholarship system an institution would fund a local student's training for three years and that student would then return to work for the institution for three years upon graduation. The first cohort of students was funded by a range of institutions: the municipal governments of Ibarra, Ambato, Cuenca, Riobamba, Guaranda, and Otavalo (all but the last provincial capitals); the public health offices of Guayaquil, Esmeraldas, and Babahoyo; the Asistencia Pública of Latacunga and Cuenca; the *corporaciones de fomento* (development corporations) of Machala and Quito; the Red Cross; and other government social service agencies like the Hogares de Protección Social, Higiene Escolar, and the Caja del Seguro. Not all of these institutions paid their scholarship quotas on time; indeed, by the end of June 1943—eight months into the first cohort's studies—at least five of these institutions had made no payments at all. The school also had little or no ability to enforce the financial commitments of the Junta Central de Asistencia Pública.

The existence of full scholarships to fund study and living expenses in Quito for three years made it possible for a carefully selected group of young women from across the national territory to study for a professional career. We can imagine that each of them brought their own aspirations with them, and perhaps in another era some of them might have opted for a different career; however, only for nursing study was such a comprehensive scholarship system in place. Nonetheless, from the school's perspective, some aspects of the scholarship system were ill conceived from the start. The system seemed to suggest that the scholarships were to support individual students, while what the school needed was stable support for the institution itself. Scholarships were also intended to include financing for the initial equipment necessary to begin study (including uniforms, a watch, a thermometer, and so on) as well as funding of graduation expenses and the uniform and equipment necessary to begin professional practice. However, not all scholarships took into account these expenses, leaving the Escuela scrambling to ensure that both students and graduates were properly equipped.

Aspects of the scholarship system also posed some problems for students. Following the selection of students undertaken by the school directora and approved by the executive council, the favored candidates were themselves responsible for securing a scholarship, once the school had informed them of which institutions were offering scholarships that year.[21] Individual students thus had to negotiate with institutions and sign contracts for their scholarships, which among other provisions required them to work afterward for the institution, to present a financial guarantor, and if they did not complete their studies, to repay the scholarship monies disbursed. Some promising students had difficulties obtaining a sponsor. Among the first cohort that began studies in 1942, Señorita Flores had arranged sponsorship by a municipality in coastal Manabí. She was progressing well with her studies, but a new candidate then appeared with personal connections to members of the municipal council, leading the latter to decide several weeks into the term to switch their sponsorship (although it was too late for the second candidate to begin studies that year). Both the school administration and Flores spent months trying to secure a different sponsor for her education, since she was making excellent progress in her studies but she personally had "no resources but her willingness to study for this career."

One possibility was the Clínica Pasteur, a private clinic in Quito that had considered offering a scholarship to obtain a trained nurse. However, a "delicate problem" existed, since the clinic was administered by the Hermanas de la Caridad, who might object to having a secular nurse imposed on them after her graduation. Another possibility was the municipality of Quito, but they preferred to sponsor a local girl. Eventually the municipality of Esmeraldas stepped up to fund Flores's studies. Securing guarantors was also a problem for students of modest resources, and both Flores and her classmate Señorita Ochoa (another coastal student, sponsored by the municipality of Babahoyo) fell into this category. Both were excellent students but did not have anyone who could provide a guarantee of five thousand sucres.[22] Ochoa, for instance, was a maternal orphan, and her father had written a letter of thanks to the school's directora for favoring his daughter with a scholarship, explaining how welcome this was since he was a poor man with seven other children he was trying to raise and educate. When students were not progressing well, a further problem emerged: if they were unable to continue their studies, they would be required to repay the scholarship. School administrators attempted to ensure that students did not suffer financially if they had to suspend their studies, provided that this was due to something beyond their control (such as a health problem) rather than due to a lack of effort.

The first directoras of the Escuela were all American nurses working for U.S. government agencies. As such, they were required to go wherever they were posted by the U.S. government, which created marked instability in the administration of the school. The first directora, Miss Anne Cacciopo, was ordered by the U.S. government to return to the United States in March 1943. Cacciopo stated she would not accept another posting, the executive council added their voice of protest—including having the minister of social welfare lobby the American Embassy—but apparently Cacciopo was disappointed that the council did not intervene more strongly. She left on unhappy terms, refusing to provide the Escuela with a portrait so that they could honor her as the founding directora. Her subdirectora, Miss Kathleen Logan, was then appointed to the position of directora, and Miss Dorothy Foley (who had also been with the school since the beginning) was promoted to subdirectora. When Logan left at the end of that year, Foley became acting director, with the assistance of Miss Anne Middlemiss and Miss Isabel Needham. Foley was formally named directora in May 1944, at which point she was assisted by Middlemiss (now subdirectora), Miss Snell, and Mrs. Thomas and intermittently by Miss Froind and Miss Laffay. With the departure of most of these nurses in late 1945, Foley was assisted by Subdirectora Middlemiss and Miss Ruth Groves. When both Foley and Middlemiss left Ecuador in the spring of 1947, Miss Olive Nicklin took over as acting directora temporarily, with the assistance of Mrs. Ruth Ferguson, until Miss Pansy Virginia Murphy arrived. When Murphy left in April 1948, alluding to health problems that required her to return to the United States, Miss Genoveva Surette was named her replacement and continued in this role until June 1949 (when she too alluded to health problems causing her to resign). This brief account gives a sense of the dizzying rate at which the Americanas moved in and out of the directorship—a serious problem from the perspective of the executive council.

In recounting the origin of the directora Americana in 1949, Dr. Curtis of the Servicio Cooperativo characterized the arrangements with the school in the following way:

> Thanks to the Cooperative Program of Health and Sanitation agreed to by the governments of Ecuador and the United States, the Institute of Inter-American Affairs, when it founded the School, offered technical assistance in accord with its possibilities and the needs of the School, offering one, two, or three Americanas, who, from the foundation of the School to the present, in addition to cooperating with technical knowledge, have also assumed in part responsibility for the conduct and discipline of the teaching staff and students of the school, until there might be qualified Ecuadorian personnel available who could take over these functions.[23]

Although the initial agreements that established the school foresaw that in five years Ecuadorian staff would be available to take over its administration, it was only two years later, in 1949, that it was possible to appoint an Ecuadorian nurse as school director. Señorita Ligia Gomezjurado Narváez had been a member of the first group of graduates of the Escuela, whose exceptional performance earned her a Rockefeller Foundation scholarship to undertake postgraduate specialization in Canada and the United States. Born in Quito in 1918, Gomezjurado began her nursing studies with an exemplary level of preparation, having graduated with a *bachillerato* from Quito's première state secondary school for women, the Colegio 24 de Mayo. At the age of twenty-two, she then undertook some preparatory courses in the Universidad Central's medical program in 1940, and in the 1940–41 academic year she went on to first-year studies in medicine. She transferred in 1941 to the program in dentistry at the university.[24]

When the nursing school began to accept students in 1942, Gomezjurado enrolled in first-year study there and found her calling. Her mother (who had died during Gomezjurado's childhood, leaving her as the eldest daughter in a leadership position at home) was the cousin of prominent Quito physicians Aurelio and Alfonso Mosquera Narváez.[25] Aurelio served a term as rector of the Central University and rose to the position of national president in 1938, dying unexpectedly in office less than a year into his term; his younger brother Alfonso was a leading physician within the Servicio de Sanidad. On Gomezjurado's return from the United States in 1947 she began teaching at the school and was appointed subdirectora almost immediately. With the resignation of Surette in 1949, there was no debate or reservations about appointing Gomezjurado as directora, and she provided much needed stability at the school, continuing in this position for more than two decades (table 5.1). Without doubt, Gomezjurado personified precisely the kind of respectable, highly intelligent, well-educated, and very organized señorita that Ayora had always dreamed would become the model of professional nursing in Ecuador.

**TABLE 5.1. Early Directoras of the Escuela Nacional de Enfermeras**

| Name | Dates of Service |
| --- | --- |
| Miss Anne Cacciopo | November 1942–March 1943 |
| Miss Kathleen Logan | April 1943–December 1943 |
| Miss Dorothy Foley | January 1944–March 1947 |
| Miss Anne Middlemiss | April 1947 |
| Miss Olive Nicklin (acting) | May 1947–June 1947 |
| Miss Pansy Virginia Murphy | July 1947–April 1948 |
| Miss Genoveva Surette | May 1948–June 1949 |
| Señorita Ligia Gomezjurado Narváez | July 1949–1970 |

*Source*: Minutes books of the meetings of the Escuela's Concejo Ejecutivo, AENE.

Satisfying the institution's teaching needs was another chronic problem faced by the Escuela. From the school's founding in 1942, Doctora Fanny de Mora, who was not at that time exercising her profession as a physician, was hired on a full-time basis to teach many of the core medical courses in the curriculum (anatomy, physiology, bacteriology, and so on), while the Americanas offered the courses related directly to nursing. Fanny de Mora had graduated as doctora de medicina the previous year, only the fifth woman to graduate as a physician from the Universidad Central, a full two decades after pioneer Matilde Hidalgo had done so.[26] Given the cost of her full-time salary and the economic difficulties plaguing the school, the dean of medicine reminded the council in April 1943 that professors of the Faculty of Medicine were required to collaborate with the school and could be called on to teach in their areas of specialization as part of their duties to the university (where they had dual responsibilities for teaching in the classroom and supervising medical students at the public hospitals). While this appealed to the council, they had difficulties recruiting such professors. For instance, pediatrician Dr. Carlos Sánchez readily agreed to teach the nursing students, but only if he could do so on the same day he taught the medical students: in other words, the nursing students would have to receive their classes alongside the medical students. This was considered to be simply impossible, and not only because the kind of material covered should be different for each group.[27]

Only after further insistence by the dean did Sánchez finally agree, after a delay of several months, to offer separate classes to the nursing students. As the dean pointed out in general terms, however, "when we ask for something as a favor it isn't done properly, since some professors offer their services with very good will but for others this represents nothing but a burden."[28] Indeed, many of the medical professors seemed to see their duties at the school as a gentlemanly favor they were offering, rather than a responsibility, and slotted their teaching into spaces left after they had completed their classes for medical students, duties at the hospital, and often after they had attended patients in their private medical practices. They seemed unaware that the school had a formal curriculum, rather than the nursing students simply dabbling in different areas.[29] Indeed, the full curriculum included bacteriology, sixty hours of classes; chemistry, eighty hours; sociology, thirty hours; medicine, thirty hours; pathology, thirty hours; English, eighty hours; therapeutics, thirty hours; nutrition, twenty-five hours; psychology, thirty hours; surgery, sixteen hours; orthopedics, sixteen hours; contagious diseases, sixteen hours; pediatrics, thirty hours; urology, sixteen hours; psychiatry, thirty hours; obstetrics, twenty hours; gynecology, ten hours; dermatology, ten hours; social problems, sixteen hours; and otorhinolaryngology, twelve hours.[30] However, given the difficulties in scheduling classes, for instance, by July 1947 none of the following courses had yet been offered to the third-year students who were scheduled to graduate just three months later: nutrition, first aid, practicum in public health, practicum in pediatrics, otorhinolaryngology, dermatology, and advanced issues in psychology.[31] Later that year, Murphy insisted that she could not continue as directora if the situation with the professors was not resolved: she simply could not develop a timetable for classes based solely on the convenience of the physicians.[32] These chronic staffing problems were only resolved when the school began to offer hourly payments for each class taught, rather than the Faculty of Medicine including teaching at the Escuela as part of faculty members' general obligations to the university.[33]

The school's regulations also allowed it to retain the best graduates for its own teaching staff, which ran afoul of the aspirations of some institutions who had funded scholarships. Some of the graduates were retained in Quito to assist the Americanas and to oversee student practice as *supervisoras* on wards: of the first 1945 graduates, señoritas Adelina Sares, Piedad Ochoa, and Lucelina Mosquera were retained; in 1946 señoritas Judith Armas and Marina Diaz; in 1947 señoritas Tula Espinosa and Ligia Yépez. Others with appropriate performance and credentials were able to travel abroad on scholarship to undertake advanced training. Thus when the first cohort graduated, señoritas Ligia Gomezjurado, Victoria Grijalva, Olga Granja, and Filomena Lituma all traveled to North America to undertake advanced training, with the intention of returning to the school to teach rather than serving the institutions that had provided their initial scholarships. When the first three returned in the middle of 1947, the directora aspired to having them named "*profesoras universitarias de enfermería*" to distinguish them from less qualified instructors, but the university only consented to name them adjunct professors.

Granja left again in April 1948 for Panama for additional advanced study. Some of those initially retained internally subsequently also had the opportunity for study abroad. After two years working at the school, Judith Armas was awarded a scholarship for advanced study in the United States; after a period teaching at the school following her return, she received yet another scholarship and left again for the United States in November 1952. She went on to become a consultant for the Oficina Sanitaria Panamericana.[34] In 1949 two nurses returned from studies in the United States: Lucelina Mosquera had specialized in surgical nursing, and Colombia Galvis was an expert in ward administration. Tula Espinosa left at the end of 1949 to work for Shell, and Guillermina Murillo (a 1949 graduate) was retained to work at the school as her replacement. Murillo then went to the United States with a Rockefeller scholarship in mid-1952 to specialize in surgical nursing. In addition, in 1950 postgraduate studies in public health were undertaken in Chile by 1949 graduates Teresa Verduga and Mercedes Romero, thanks to scholarships from the Oficina Sanitaria Panamericana.

In 1949–50, for the first time, the Escuela had a fully Ecuadorian teaching staff rather than relying on Americanas.[35] However, the school was chronically short of supervisoras and instructors, partly due to the flow of trained nurses out of the country as well as to the nursing services of private companies such as Shell Oil in Ecuador or to staff new facilities such as the recently inaugurated Maternidad Isidro Ayora. Ligia Gomezjurado and the executive council were also concerned in general about the constant problem of emigration to seek better salaries. The only solution, they thought, would be the establishment of an association to defend nurses' rights—not just salaries but also hours of work and other working conditions.[36] Certainly, the graduates of the school seemed to have numerous opportunities open to them, including advanced study abroad.

### Professional Competition

Despite the growing recognition in some circles of the expertise of the school's graduates toward the end of the 1940s, there was ongoing concern about the proliferation of short courses being offered with some element of nursing training, given the general public's continuing lack of understanding of what professional nursing implied. For instance, in May 1943 Quito's daily newspaper *El comercio* announced a course offered by the Escuela de Enfermeras de la Provincia de El Oro. Not only was there no nursing school in the southern coastal province of El Oro but the course was only a few weeks long. At the time the Red Cross was also offering a nursing course of a few months' duration. The council of the Escuela pointed out to Cruz Roja president Dr. Benjamín Wandemberg that first the Cruz Roja did not have a nursing school, and second the course's students should be clearly identified as auxiliary nurses or nursing aides rather than as nurses. A certificate could be awarded upon completion but not a diploma of any kind. The Universidad Central itself had also begun to offer, through its newly established cultural extension program, a short course of a similar nature. The council began to wonder if they should be calling ENE students by a different name, given the proliferation of courses in nursing that the public had difficulty distinguishing from the university education offered by the Escuela.[37] These problems were still of concern to the school council in 1952. There were numerous short courses (*cursillos*) being offered in nursing, after which their participants called themselves nurses. However, as Gomezjurado pointed out, to become a nurse, you needed six years of secondary school, three years of nursing school, and a degree from the Universidad Central. The council requested, yet again, that the names of such courses be changed from "rapid courses in nursing" to "courses for nursing aides" or "first aid courses."[38]

Although the Escuela was concerned about the confusion caused by the proliferation of short nursing courses, *enfermeras universitarias* were in more serious competition with two other groups of recognized nurses with whom they had strained relations. It was predictable that there would be tension between Hermanas de la Caridad and the new Escuela early on. Among the first group of students admitted to the school in 1942 for the five-month probationary preclinical period were three Hermanas. They were among the very few students who were not accepted to continue in the program because of their low grades in the preparatory courses.[39] It turned out that they had no secondary education, unlike their classmates, who all had a minimum of four years of secondary school and in several cases also had *bachilleratos*. The Hermanas had been selected to receive this training by the religious community itself, rather than by the Escuela. It was conceded that the governing council of the Faculty of Medicine had erred in allowing the Hermanas to register in the program, knowing from the beginning that they would never be able to achieve professional degrees but rather simply aspired to be better prepared to serve their humanitarian function. This reveals some confusion within the Faculty of Medicine itself about the mission of the Escuela when it was first established. The religious order was urged to undertake a more rigorous selection process so that better-prepared Hermanas could be nominated as students the next time: they should meet the same qualifications for admission as any other student. In addition, they should be prepared to dedicate all of their time to their studies rather than continuing to carry out multiple other duties. However, given additional conflicts between the order and the Escuela, in the end no further Hermanas applied to attend the school. Instead, they sought to establish their own Catholic nursing school.[40]

Indeed, problems had started early, when an experienced sister, Sor Margarita, had been enlisted to offer the first cohort of nursing students their chemistry classes during the preclinical period. By January 1943, when the students should have already completed experiment number 10, the chemistry teaching laboratory had never been used.[41] The Escuela's council was at pains to replace Sor Margarita without offending sensibilities, appreciating that she had only offered to teach as an act of solidarity with the new school and recognizing that she was very busy with her other commitments (at the time she was Madre Superiora of the Hospital Civil San Juan de Dios). The Escuela tried offering her an honorary appointment in recognition of her support but having someone else teach the classes; while they first thought of appointing a fifth-year female student in the pharmacy program, they opted instead for a doctor of pharmacy,

Dr. Alberto Di Capua. Perhaps the choice of a (male) professional rather than a (female) student made it all too clear that Sor Margarita was being fully replaced. The Escuela's best attempts at diplomacy failed.

This led to the withdrawal of another important form of collaboration: Sor Emilia, who had been overseeing the student residence, was removed from the Escuela by the religious order in May 1943. Although a few months earlier there had been six Hermanas assisting in various ways at the school, by the end of May there were only two remaining (and in later years there are no references to Hermanas working within the school). It was clear to the school administrators that this general withdrawal of support could be attributed to the fact that the three preclinical students had not been approved for formal studies. The withdrawal of Sor Emilia, in turn, led to concern that some parents might remove their daughters from the school, since a guarantee of appropriate supervision had been removed. This underlines how unusual it was to consider sending a daughter to Quito for professional training in a boarding context. While one might send a daughter from the provinces to secondary school in Quito, proper supervision would normally be ensured by lodging them with trusted extended family members. In the end it was agreed that a secular employee would take over these duties. The emphasis on the teaching staff living onsite—a model that was consolidated under the directorship of Gomezjurado—was a result of these ongoing concerns.

Conflicts also occurred with the nursing graduates of the *antigua escuela*, the school formerly operating under the university's auspices, which suspended admissions upon the establishment of the new nursing school. When all of the existing students completed their studies in 1944, the old school was closed despite a public petition to the Consejo Universitario that it be permitted to remain open. It was at this time, too, that the ENE's council heard rumors that the president of the republic had been informed that the training offered at the ENE was inadequate; he was quickly invited to visit the school so they could remedy that impression. Moreover, there had been ongoing criticisms of the school because it was administered by foreigners, with the suggestion that the truly "national" school of nursing was the one that had been operating in the Hospital Eugenio Espejo.[42] An opportunity to prove the value of the school came at the end of 1944, when the students responded effectively to an outbreak of poliomyelitis in Quito. Indeed, third-year student Colombia Galvis fell ill during this outbreak. A fundraising campaign was successfully conducted to send her to the United States for treatment, and she proceeded from there to obtain a scholarship to complete specialist training in the treatment of poliomyelitis.[43] She returned to the school in mid-1946 to complete her few remaining months of study and was released from her obligation to practice for her sponsoring institution since, because of her illness, she was better suited to a teaching position.[44] Nonetheless, by early 1948 she was working as head nurse at the new Clínica de la Caja del Seguro (CCS), although she later returned to teach at the school.[45]

In addition to general issues of the status of the new and old schools, strain also existed in the interactions between graduates of the old school and the students and teachers of the new school. When the first students began study at the ENE in 1942, they necessarily fell under the supervision of *graduadas* of the old school when they began their practice in hospital wards. This created difficulties given the different training involved. Indeed, in general there were difficulties associated with training the students in the Hospital Eugenio Espejo, since there were factions within the hospital that were antagonistic to the school, including both the former graduadas and the Hermanas. It was hoped that if the students could practice instead in the Clínica de la Caja del Seguro once it was opened, some of these problems might be avoided.[46] Unlike the Hospital Espejo, the equipment and procedures in the new clinic were expected to be "just like in an American hospital." However, when the CCS opened, there were rumors that its director of nursing might be Señora Anne Cacciopo de Cevallos (married by then to an Ecuadorian husband), and many of the graduates of the ENE that had gone on to work there were precisely those most sympathetic to her.[47]

The school feared potential difficulties since the supervisoras would be more likely to follow the orders of Señora de Cevallos than those of the school (indicating further divisions and rivalries even among the school's graduates). In March 1947 it was agreed that students could begin practice at the CCS, as long as they were supervised by Escuela supervisoras and not considered employees of the Caja. Throughout the decade, however, there continued to be tensions with the graduadas of the old school of nursing, who felt they suffered discrimination in employment conditions. Gomezjurado conceded that it was not their fault that they were from the old school, which was admittedly the best school available previously. However, in her view the difference in their background preparation, methods of work, and their sloppy appearance led physicians to treat them differently from the graduates of the new school. Some were working in the CCS, especially those who had been able to take some advanced training outside the country, but Gomezjurado felt that it was mostly in the Sanidad that they were well accepted, where they were engaged more often in outreach activities involving domestic visits or campaigns against contagious diseases than in hospital work.[48]

### Defining an Arena for (and the Character of) Professional Nursing

Some of the people whom nursing leaders hoped would support them did not always fulfill expectations, revealing some of the difficulties of achieving recognition of this field as a professional one. Miss Pansy Virginia Murphy was taken aback in 1948 when she met personally with the director of the Junta Central de Asistencia Pública, who not only denied that the asistencia had any obligation to fund the school but also stated baldly that in his opinion nurses were overpaid in Ecuador.[49] Physicians, too, indicated a less-than-serious attitude toward nursing education when they neglected their teaching duties at the school. A number of specific incidents with physicians help us to understand some of the pressures on nursing students and on the larger institutional project to forge a new model of professional women.

After the school's first year of functioning, disgruntled directora Kathleen Logan offered her resignation. As the dean of the Faculty of Medicine summed up her concerns to the other members of the Concejo Ejecutivo: "It seems that in the Hospital wards where the students are practicing, there is sabotage against the education and practice of the students; the Madres de la Caridad are hostile to the Escuela for no good reason. Besides, in terms of equipment, the majority of the supplies that the Escuela provided for the practice of the students have disappeared." Logan herself articulated a rather different problem, however. In the seven months in which the school had been offering services on the wards, not once had she received any positive feedback: "All we have had are complaints, not once have we received an encouraging word about the work we carry out in the Hospital."[50] To address this lack, the council invited the chief physicians of the various wards in which students were training (the doctors Salgado, Arauz, Sánchez, and Estupiñán) to attend the next council meeting to offer their comments on the nursing services.

When they did so on December 6, 1943, much discussion focused on the lack of appropriate equipment on the wards for nursing practice, such as thermometers that broke easily and were expensive to replace.[51] Similarly, extensive discussion revolved around the fact that when physicians arrived on their rounds, sometimes the nursing students had not completed recording the temperature of patients. In exasperation, Logan commented that apparently the physicians had not noticed that the system of taking temperatures by the students was entirely different from the practice of the barchilonas, who either just pretended they had taken the temperature or "put the thermometer in the mouth of each patient without disinfecting it; what we are doing is completely different." The physicians rushed to assure her that, of course, they had noticed an enormous difference in the care offered in the wards. Indeed, given the quality of care, Arauz emphasized his desire that the nursing students practice at night and on holidays, since during the day the patients could be cared for by physicians, by medical students, and by the Hermanas de la Caridad. At night, on the other hand, patients "are under the care of the barchilonas, rough folk who know nothing nor have the obligation to know anything about what to do with a patient; so the night service is a disaster." Sánchez added that it would be especially important to have nursing students on duty on holidays, "because these are the days when there are many complications. It is necessary to indicate to the barchilonas, for instance, that they take better care of the items and equipment on the wards, to avoid theft by members of the public." The council agreed that once there were three classes of students, it would be possible to increase the shifts and night service could be extended once sufficient supervisoras could be obtained to oversee the students' work.

Logan further commented that the tasks being given to the students were very monotonous, that many of the patients were essentially healthy, and that she would like to extend practice to the operating room. Ward 3 had few operations and few patients in general. However, this ward had been chosen for a reason: many of the patients were *pensionistas* (fee-paying) and were thus more likely to accept nursing care. In Ward 1 (surgery), for instance, "patients are not accustomed to this kind of treatment and wouldn't put up with being bathed, while the patients in Ward 3 are pensionistas and thus more rational, they are already accustomed to cleanliness." The students had been assigned to Ward 3 with the idea that there they would have access to both clinical and surgery patients, and as affiliates of the Caja del Seguro (who received treatment in the hospital before the opening of the Caja's own clinic), those patients were more "rational and know how to appreciate the attention they receive from the nurses, and when they are released they will comment positively on the students of this School." However, Bustamante agreed with Logan that perhaps it had been an error to assign the students to Ward 3, since its patients were noticeably different from other patients in the hospital.

> On the other hand, I can assure you that in the surgery wards patients are also used to being bathed—of course, only when the Hospital has running water—and we have never had to deal with resistance of any kind. Besides, the students have to become accustomed to dealing with this kind of patient, with *indios, cholos*, because such is our population. What is happening is that we have 25 students practicing in two wards [Ward 3 and the pediatric area, Ward 6] with 140 patients and what has to be recognized is that they have

little nursing work and instead a great deal of servants' work; the coming year when we have 50 students, it is indispensable that the second-year students begin to practice in the operating room.

After some questions from the physicians about whether the nursing students were really prepared for surgery practice—Logan assured them that there would be no problem whatsoever in this regard—the directora was authorized to gradually extend the students' practice as she saw fit. A crucial additional concern was expressed, though: if student nurses began practical training in the operating room, this would bring these female students into contact with the male medical students. As one surgeon suggested, "to protect the prestige of the school, it will be necessary to instruct the medical students that they must maintain a perfect comportment with the nursing students, that they must not take the liberty of engaging in any kind of teasing." The physicians agreed that if any medical student was overly familiar with the nursing students, the latter should immediately make this known to the physician in charge of the relevant service. Despite this frank discussion with the physicians (although their flowery assurances frequently expressed a condescending tone), Logan left Ecuador soon thereafter, making good on her resignation from the directorship.[52]

This conversation highlights two problems in particular that constrained the radius of practice of the students: concerns about potential interactions with male medical students (which became a chronic problem) and concerns about what kind of patients the nursing students treated. It was not by chance that the first nursing classes had been established in the Maternidad, where students would deal with female patients. Nor that their initial practical training after 1942 was on the children's ward, where they apparently spent quite a lot of time practicing bathing infants and young children. Bathing and treating adult men—that is, naked and semiclad men—was a very different matter. The more "rational" fee-paying patients were considered more likely both to understand the benefits of cleanliness and to understand the meaning of such intimate treatment by young women who were neither Hermanas nor barchilonas.

Interwoven with the difficulty of gaining access to sufficient (and appropriate) patients for teaching purposes was the shortage of the necessary equipment on hospital wards. When the first cohort was to begin work on wards in the spring of 1943, numerous items were needed to facilitate their practical training: sheets, mattresses, blankets, a stretcher to transport patients, and so on.[53] Each student had a thermometer and a syringe, supplied by the school; but on the wards they found that there was no cotton, no alcohol, no gauze, none of the basic materials that they needed to treat patients. It was unclear who should supply this—the hospital, it was largely agreed, but its storerooms were under-provisioned. Problems in Ward 3A (the pensionistas) continued in 1949. Many of the ward's patients paid fees for their surgery on the assumption that they would receive better service. Two or three patients at a time might arrive, be bathed by the nursing students and treated for intestinal parasites, have their surgery, and then they would transfer to other wards where they did not have to pay fees. In other words, the students never had an opportunity for postoperative practice.[54] The following year Dr. Tello, the new director of the Hospital Espejo, solicited increased services from the nursing students. He agreed that Ward 3A did not offer enough patients for the nursing students and suggested they extend their services to other wards.

> I have sometimes seen a whole group of students trailing along behind a physician, others holding folders or washing windows, two or three bathing a child, when the principal task of the students should be to attend patients: giving them medicine, attending a wound, applying casts, etc. I know that the students must be trained in all kinds of activities, but I think they have had enough practice with feeding children, bathing them, etc. . . . I don't mean to say they are not working—they are always working—but seldom with patients. I think it would be very important to have them working in other wards where patients are currently being clumsily attended by servants.[55]

While the sphere of practice of the students was a chronic concern, with the school continually trying to find additional placements for them in which they could learn useful skills, Gomezjurado was insistent that the school's priority was to ensure that the students had an opportunity to learn modern nursing techniques, not to fulfill the needs of the hospital. The other wards (and most medical institutions) still did not have the appropriate equipment for students to be trained in modern nursing practice. Nursing students increasingly practiced in newer, more technically sophisticated facilities, a number of which opened in the late 1940s and early 1950s in Quito: the Clínica de la Caja del Seguro, the new Maternidad Ayora, and the Baca-Ortiz Children's Hospital. These were also places where the Escuela's graduates increasingly found work (as well as with the Compañía Shell and some other private facilities). The Hospital Civil San Juan de Dios, in contrast, still had no professional nursing staff in 1949; older institutions (and those in more peripheral areas) continued to work under the established model of nursing and administration by the Hermanas de la Caridad.

Although the nurses were being trained within a modern professional model, many of the people they came into contact with in their practice were clearly not used to thinking of them in this way. Some additional conflicts with physicians are instructive in this regard. Despite his assurances at the council meeting in December 1943 that he appreciated the services offered by the nursing students, a significant conflict erupted between Dr. Augusto Estupiñán and the nursing school and its students in March 1945. The physician had decided not only that the students were not helpful in his ward, but he had accused them of causing injuries to his patients. Moreover, he had made these accusations in front of the medical students. When he had calmed down, Estupiñán commented privately that he could accept the students back as long as they observed appropriate discipline and principally that they "obey him, as the physician."[56] However, Miss Anne Middlemiss pointed out that the students could not be expected to respect someone like Estupiñán, who made them look bad for no reason and kept changing his instructions; she was the first to admit that, knowing that Estupiñán was involved, she was unwilling to impose any additional rules on the students.

Miss Dorothy Foley proceeded to remove the student nurses from the children's wards the following month, simply explaining that although the goal of this work was to teach the nursing students, there was little work provided to them in these wards and the tasks assigned could just as easily be carried out by the unskilled hospital's female servants. There were two medical chiefs of the pediatric ward (which was divided into girls' and boys' wards): the well-known pediatrician Dr. Carlos R. Sánchez and the surgeon Dr. Augusto Estupiñán. Given her failed attempts to resolve this situation, Foley indicated her intention not only to withdraw the students, but she also threatened to remove from the ward all of the equipment that belonged to the nursing school (medical implements, bedding, and so on; in the end this equipment was left there, however). She indicated to the director of the Asistencia Pública that incidents had been occurring for two years in this ward (essentially since the inauguration of the Escuela).[57] One possible solution was to separate the infant surgery patients from the other patients, but this was impossible because it would requiring mixing boys and girls in the same ward.[58]

The director of the hospital reminded the council that Estupiñán himself had solicited the services of the students, so conflicts of this kind were simply the result of his difficult character. A resolution of the conflict was brokered by the dean of medicine, in response to the protests of the Junta Central de Asistencia Pública about the withdrawal of the student nurses, following a negotiation among the dean and the directors of the Asistencia, the hospital, and the Escuela. The director was of the opinion that with this, Estupiñán would be taught a "severe lesson" and no doubt he would apologize and they could be sure that in the future he would act in a more gentlemanly way. In communicating this resolution to Estupiñán, the dean diplomatically pointed out that he was concerned to ensure the efficient fulfillment of both the medical courses in infant surgery under the responsibility of Estupiñán and the teaching mission of the nursing school. The resolution—all expressed in the spirit of ensuring the harmonious work of the various institutions involved in the hospital (which likely did not reduce the sting)—was that effective immediately Sánchez, professor of pediatrics, would be the sole physician-in-chief of the pediatric ward; that all patients related to infant surgery would be moved to the surgery wards, where Estupiñán could carry out his teaching mission; that the Asistencia Pública would do its best to make any necessary renovations to the surgery wards to accommodate the children; and that the nursing students would return to their work in the pediatric ward as soon as these changes were made.[59]

In March 1946, Sánchez requested that this work be reinitiated, promising that both he and the hospital director would guarantee the good behavior of Estupiñán.[60] However, in June, Middlemiss explained that due to the reduced number of students in the school (some of whom were on vacation), it was not possible to reestablish this service in the children's wards; perhaps this would be possible the following year.[61] In April 1947, Estupiñán himself formally petitioned to have the student nurses return to both Wards 6 (pediatric) and 1A (surgery) to assist him; however, Middlemiss explained that the students were already assisting him in the operating room and that his wards lacked both appropriate equipment and sufficient supervisoras for student practice.[62] She elaborated that in any case, the practice they had carried out previously in that ward was limited to bathing the children, and besides, they had left there four thousand sucres' worth of equipment and supplies that had deteriorated so badly that they would need to be replaced (which was impossible because of the lack of resources) before practice could be recommenced.

Although this suggests the difficulty at least one physician had in adapting to the new image of the professional nurse, it might be a mistake to assume that his attitude was representative of all physicians. Estupiñán had a reputation for being rather difficult. Another incident may be more revealing of the common difficulties faced by nurses. In 1948 a conflict occurred between graduated supervisora Tula Espinosa and her student nurses on one side, and the medical staff of the operating room on the other.[63] The purpose of the nursing students' practice in surgery—as articulated in 1944, when this was first being established—was (a) to teach them how to prepare for the operation, including sterilizing the instruments; (b) to assist in the operating room by passing to the surgeon whatever he needed under sterile conditions; and (c) to assist with surgical instrumentation (a service previously provided by medical students but not as well as it was thought a nurse could).[64] The dean of the Faculty of Medicine, Dr. Carlos Pólit—who in that capacity also served as chair of the nursing school's executive council—was chief of surgery at the hospital.

According to Espinosa, the nurses were simply fulfilling their obligations in the area in which they were in charge in the operating room: that is, in overseeing and ensuring an aseptic environment. What had happened was that "the operating room was ready, with all of the sterilized material, when Dr. Gutiérrez entered without a cap or mask; as he was dressing, he contaminated the apron with his bare hands, then he contaminated the gloves, which is strictly prohibited. . . . As the supervising nurse I did the same as I had seen the American nurses do in similar circumstances, pointing out the contamination—suggestions that in their case have always been accepted by the surgeons, but in my case the response was negative, perhaps because I am Ecuadorian." The surgeon then began to criticize the instrumentation prepared by the students, which had been selected not by them but by the Hermanas. At the last minute he requested a different scalpel, which could not be provided because the Hermana with access to the instruments was absent. This contributed to Pólit's explosive reaction; he began to insult Espinosa and the students, along the lines of, "Who is in charge here, who is responsible for this? It is an embarrassment for the nursing school to have employees like this, you've shown us what you are, I want all of your names!"

Espinosa concluded:

> The students have been accused of having pretensions and of considering themselves to be like physicians, because they make small suggestions about asepsis to the surgeons and the medical students, after having been trained to do precisely this: the person in charge of asepsis is the nurse. It is unclear what the attitude of the students should be, since if they are pleasant and courteous, there are physicians who confuse this with flirting and take liberties with the students, leading them to change their attitude. Then they are accused of being pretentious and despotic. I request that the Concejo resolve this matter, indicating to us the norms of conduct we should follow in the future.[65]

When this was discussed in the council meeting of July 29, 1948, the dean commented that the students had behaved in an infantile way, bursting into tears.[66] He had thought that the school had proper supervisoras, but it was obvious that the graduadas still needed to be under the direct supervision of the directora and subdirectora. Subdirectora Gomezjurado responded that some of the physicians, and almost all of the medical students, regularly violated the basic rules of asepsis, continually contaminating material that was sterilized in preparation for surgery—and that whenever the supervisoras or students commented on this, the reaction was excessive.

While the dean conceded that this might be so, ultimately he believed that the nurses should simply be more understanding of the stresses the surgeons experienced: "It is necessary to inculcate in both the supervisoras and the students a greater spirit of abnegation and tolerance, because the mental state of the surgeon changes entirely during an operation and some violent reactions are the result of the nervous tension he experiences in moments in which the life of a patient is in his hands. . . . A lack of cooperation on the part of the Nurse goes directly against the patient's interest, since if an operation is poorly conducted, the patient's recuperation can be seriously delayed." In other words, how nurses treated surgeons—most importantly, not questioning their actions and therefore adding to their stress—was more important to the success of an operation than whether a proper aseptic environment had been maintained![67]

A rather different kind of problem emerged with a physician the following year—although it echoes the concerns expressed by Espinosa—when it was discovered that over half of the third-year cohort were in danger of failing to graduate because they had received very low grades from the physician teaching the course in orthopedics.[68] Signed statements were collected from a number of students who explained that the conflict was due to the immorality of the physician: he had asked for a kiss, or tried to hold their hands, or made inappropriate jokes to various students. Having observed this physician for several years in the hospital, the doctors on the council explained that the professor lacked not morality but culture (that is, manners, delicacy). Indeed, one of the student statements (from an excellent student who went on to teach at the school) recounted that the professor had made jokes along the lines of: "if a student has a physician for a boyfriend, I will give her 100 in the course; if she dates a medical student, I'll give her 80; if she dates a policeman, 20; and if she doesn't have a boyfriend at all, I'll give her 0 for her ineptitude." These were extraordinarily inappropriate jokes, given cultural norms about proper intergender relations as well as the struggles of nurses to be recognized as professionals. The professor finally admitted that he had indeed made jokes of this kind, although he claimed not to have otherwise abused his position. The physicians on the council argued that having the course taken away from him would be punishment enough, since it would imply that he had not properly fulfilled his duties; any more explicit action would potentially create a scandal that would damage the reputation of the school itself. The administrators of the nursing school were in a quandary—with so little time before graduation, and with this a required course, how could the third-year students be rescued from this situation? An elegant solution was arrived at: an Ecuadorian physician who had just returned from advanced training in Spain would be asked to offer an intensive "mini-course" to the students to allow them to complete the material just in time for graduation, and his assessment of their work would replace that of the dismissed professor. All of the students easily passed the new exam following these additional classes.

This incident lays bare some of the ambiguities surrounding the nursing professionalization project: in short, this professor-physician treated the nursing students as sexual beings available to the men with whom they came into contact during their training, rather than as asexual female professionals. This goes to the heart of some of the difficulties nursing students faced, who were set apart from the Hermanas de la Caridad by the quality of their technical training but confronted difficulties as single women that the Hermanas did not. The Hermanas' own professional space was achieved through annihilation of their personalities as symbolized, for instance, through giving up their names. As the nursing historian Siobhan Nelson has argued, the triumvirate of attributes that characterized religious women included asexuality, conservatism, and submissiveness; paradoxically, this was precisely what allowed them to pioneer certain forms of relatively autonomous work.[69]

What is perhaps most surprising of all about this situation is that the physician who returned to save the day was none other than Estupiñán, who had left for Spain for a year in September 1948. It was unusual for such an experienced physician to receive a scholarship for advanced study abroad, but this may have been because of his experience with orthopedic surgery—a field whose importance had been highlighted by the polio epidemic. In November 1952 he was appointed as the representative of the Junta Central de Asistencia Pública in the executive council. On assuming this position, he commented: "I am very happy to accept my appointment, since I feel very close to the school due to the long time that I have worked alongside it; since its foundation with Miss Cacciopo I have offered all of my energies to support the school. During however long my position here lasts, I will do everything in my power to support the school."[70] His change of attitude seems almost inexplicable. However, an explanation is readily available: it appears that the increased stability of the school under Gomezjurado's irreproachable direction, her Ecuadorian citizenship, and her model of virtuous female vocation in general won over early opponents of the school. Certainly Estupiñán became a staunch ally and supporter of the school.

While the establishment of the Escuela seemed to signify a kind of decoupling from the tradition of nursing nuns, some continuity nonetheless existed. Indeed, this sense of continuity was intensified under the directorship of Ligia Gomezjurado, who was in a position to understand the Ecuadorian context much better than her predecessors. Like nuns, nursing students lived together in a female community and were expected to be single, dedicating themselves fully to their nursing vocation. At the Escuela Nacional de Enfermeras they learned not only technical skills but were also forged as moral young female professionals. Both written and oral accounts indicate that there was a mystical flavor to this training that presented nursing as a spiritual calling. This can be seen, for instance, in the comments of Directora Gomezjurado at the 1952 festivities celebrating the tenth anniversary of the Escuela's founding. As she put it, "The ideal pursued by the Nurse is to alleviate human suffering, wherever there is a tear, a complaint, an injury, there is the place for the Nurse. Where there is suffering, the white legions will advance; but one should not think that all is pain, the satisfaction of fulfilling one's duty is the great delight that fills the soul of the Christian Nurse, because charity, humanity, comprehension, this is the Divine mandate, the apostolate of Faith, Hope and Charity."[71]

Señorita Filomena Lituma, a graduate of and sometime teacher at the Escuela, spoke in representation of all of the school's graduates (who numbered 118 by that time), commenting that these nurses served in all parts of the national territory, offering their "scientific knowledge and pure souls." She credited Gomezjurado as an inspiration to all, and as an example to which Ecuadorian nurses should aspire. "*Compañeras de Labor*! You have experienced wonderful and unforgettable moments, nourishing your spirits with the wise advice and self-sacrificing example of our self-denying [*abnegada*], virtuous and intelligent Directora, who has made of her life a mystic of service at the gospel of the infirm and needy."[72] Students who attended the Escuela during Gomezjurado's two decades of leadership commented in interviews about how central moral issues were in their formation as female professionals. "Our school was secular, part of the Universidad Central, liberal, secular, but no, in reality it was very Catholic, very conservative. We even had a chaplain as if it were a convent, it was convent-like. At that time the Catholic school already existed, and I think that they were less convent-like than we were."[73] As another recalled: "One of the principal arteries in the school of Ligia Gomezjurado was ethics and morality, what she called professional adaptations. . . . The teaching of ethics and morality was a requirement to be able to graduate then. A requirement sine qua non of respect, devotion, respect for the human being, devotion, even faith in God, belief in God, to apply Christian principles in the management and care of the patient."[74]

Beyond the considerable financial and administrative difficulties faced in establishing and maintaining the nursing school, a central problem its leaders confronted was defining just what constituted an appropriate kind of female professional. What characteristics and social background made an Ecuadorian nurse in the 1940s, in a context where notions of professional nursing were not widely understood or accepted? The selection process aimed to find young women with the right academic preparation and promise, but also the right vocation to become nurses given the multiple challenges involved in working with patients, medical students, and physicians and completing important technical tasks accurately. Educational requirements were initially four years or more of secondary or normal school, or holding a diploma as a commercial accountant. Given the small number of students in the preclinical period in October 1946, it was agreed that the school could also accept young women who had graduated from technical or secretarial schools.[75] Indeed, one of the eleven students entering that year had a diploma as a seamstress from a technical school, rather than an academic background. Following the appointment of Gomezjurado as directora, the years of few applicants ended. In 1949 so many *bachilleres* and *normalistas* applied that the school did not consider any students with lesser qualifications.[76]

Although the situation with scholarships appeared bleak in mid-1950, the Servicio Cooperativo stepped forward to itself finance twelve scholarships, allowing the school to accept twenty students (one of whom was a pensionista, a paying student) in October 1950. That year there were seventy applicants, allowing for a good selection. In 1951, too, there were seventy candidates, all bachilleres and normalistas, competing for twenty-one student spaces (including three pensionistas, two from Colombia and one from Ecuador). And again in May 1952 the large number of bachilleres and normalistas among the applicants led the council to disregard those with lesser qualifications.[77] Building on this progress, in 1952 the admission criteria were formally changed to require a bachillerato. This represented a significant advance from the situation a decade earlier, when the school first began: the first group of students included seven bachilleres, seven students with six years, five with five years, and eight with four years of secondary education. The case of the three Hermanas with no secondary school who hoped to form part of that first class shows some of the early ambiguities around the school's mission. The decline in enrollment in the middle of that decade had also been rectified by the time Gomezjurado took over; rather, she appears to have herself rectified it through her actions as subdirectora and then directora.

In addition to educational qualifications, appropriate personality as well as moral character was needed for nursing. For instance, in 1944 a student from Guayaquil was in danger of not advancing after the preclinical period, for the following reasons outlined by the dean of medicine: "As a student she is very good and intelligent, however the state of her health and psyche is bad; she has neuritis in one of her eyes for which there is no remedy, but besides this, her nervous state is altered, she changes character easily, and sometimes does strange things. . . . For all of these reasons, I don't think she can continue at the school, because if a nurse loses her composure, she might commit a serious error."[78] Mrs. Thomas had spoken with the student, who had tried to improve her conduct, but it had become clear in that meeting that she had a problem at home. "It's true," confirmed the dean, "there must be a serious situation at home, because this young woman enrolled in the school against the wishes of her parents, who reacted violently."[79] Thomas pointed out that it would not be right to send her home with the possibility that her family might not accept her back. The Escuela agreed to accept her conditionally and monitor her conduct and state of mind.

Indeed, she went on to register for second year, but two very serious violations that year ended her potential career as a nurse. In June 1945, at the end of her vacation period, she left Guayaquil on the train to Quito, proceeded to disembark in Riobamba for three days, and arrived at the school several days late. When she arrived and realized that the school had contacted her family inquiring as to her whereabouts, she falsified a telegram to her family, supposedly from the directora, apologizing for the error in the previous telegram and stating that indeed she had arrived on time. When she was called in to explain her actions to the council, she admitted both to having stayed without permission or supervision in Riobamba and to having impersonated the directora in the telegram. She was expelled from the school.[80] As the dean explained in a meeting with the school's entire student body, "as a man, I can be flexible, I am not interested in knowing what she did [in Riobamba] or with whom, but what does concern me is protecting the dignity of the Escuela." He elaborated:

As long as you are the dignified women that you are, you guarantee the prestige of the Escuela. But I want to remind you that any little fault, any error as insignificant as it might seem, is very serious when it occurs in a women's institution. It may seem minor, but hostile elements will always judge it harshly. You are currently facing crude opposition. The Hermanas de la Caridad will be the first to judge you; as soon as they see something, they jump to criticize. At the moment the Hermanas are interested in establishing another School of Nursing, but the Faculty has rejected their project. For this reason I ask you to ensure that all of your acts express the healthiest discipline, the healthiest correctness, to thus avoid any unfavorable commentaries.[81]

In evaluating the second-year students in July 1944, the council also confronted the problem of what makes a good nurse.[82] All those who went on to their third year would form the first graduating class of the school. There were three students in particular whose work in theoretical classes was satisfactory but who were not doing sufficiently well in their practical courses. True, they weren't doing so badly as to fail, but it was feared that they would never make good nurses. The dean suggested that it wouldn't be fair to fail them—it wasn't their fault that they did not have a vocation for nursing. Dr. Bustamante was adamant, however:

> The Escuela was established to form nurses and must graduate good nurses. It would be an embarrassment for the Escuela to graduate someone incapable of carrying out the sensitive work of a nurse; it would cause damage to the student, to the Escuela, and to the institution that funded her education. Let's suppose that after she graduates she is put in charge of a provincial hospital where there will be no one to help her or show her how things should be done.[83] She herself will have to confront all of the challenges that present themselves, and if she is not well prepared she will be a failure.

One student hadn't fallen into obvious mistakes only because she always chose the easiest tasks to complete—she never challenged herself. Another was otherwise good at her practice but had problems when conflicts erupted with her classmates. Another "has no security in what she is doing, she doesn't understand why she is performing certain procedures, or why she is giving a certain medication, and whenever she commits an error and is rebuked, she does not tell the truth." One of the problem students was from another provincial capital and the other two were from smaller towns in the highlands—they may have all had additional stresses on them in Quito. Bustamante's opinion was that a student might be permitted to lose points in almost any other subject of study, but not in nursing practice. The solution that the council came up with was to create an additional basis for evaluating all students—vocational aptitude—that would be assessed by the Escuela's administrative staff as a matter of subjective judgment. For the current assessment this would replace the existing criteria of conduct within the Escuela, which would be folded into the assessment of vocational aptitude. In the end, two of these students did go on to graduate; the other got married and therefore had to withdraw from the Escuela in any case.

In defining the profile of a future nurse, the Escuela prospectus became increasingly detailed as unanticipated problems arose. First, students were required to be single.[84] In 1948 it was discovered that a preclinical student, although unmarried, was nonetheless the mother of a three-year-old child. The requirements were then modified to read "single, without children," and this student was asked to leave. It was then discovered that one of the second-year students also had a child; since she had already advanced with her studies, in her case it was deemed too late to ask her to leave.[85] In September 1948 a divorced woman sought admission; it was specified in the discussion of her application that she was unable to have children, which was apparently a relevant issue in the view of the council.[86] This application was considered "from various angles—social, moral, disciplinary, and ethical—and after much discussion and based in part on the Reglamento sobre Conducta, which was modified in the sense that the Escuela would seek references regarding past behavior, conditions, lifestyle, etc. of the candidates, in this case it was determined that this would not be a good candidate for the Escuela," something that was agreed unanimously by the council. Like the invention of the criteria of vocational aptitude, this too demonstrates how the criteria for admission and evaluation were moving targets. In this case, an applicant was measured against a standard created to deal precisely with her application. As a result, the school prospectus itself was then further modified to read "single, without children, not divorced."

More ambiguous was the application of an Afro-Ecuadorian woman from the coastal province of Esmeraldas to the school.[87] Gomezjurado feared that the applicant might have social difficulties with some of her classmates; she was also concerned that accepting this student might undermine the school's prestige. However, the physicians on the council were adamant that her racial background should not be considered an impediment, since even in the United States African-Americans could study different medical careers, and the Universidad Central itself had already graduated three male Afro-Ecuadorian physicians. In a seemingly irrelevant comment—but apparently in an attempt to say something positive about the abilities of the country's Afro-descendant population—one of the physicians reminded the other council members that there was an Afro-Ecuadorian woman in Quito's Normal School who had joined the basketball team and was "much appreciated by her classmates and the public." The nursing applicant was partially funded by the Asistencia Pública of Esmeraldas and partly self-funded, suggesting that she had some resources that might help to counterbalance her skin color.

In a rather different example, in May 1952 a woman with four years of midwifery study wished to enter directly into the second year of nursing school.[88] While the Americana who continued to serve on the council as technical consultant spoke well of the applicant and her qualifications, Gomezjurado opposed this: "It is necessary not only to consider the scientific dimension, but also the moral and disciplinary ones; I know that this Señorita does not have good conduct, in which case it would be impossible to accept her even with an entrance exam. Besides, all of the students must begin together and pass through the same experiences." A physician on the council stated that as professor of pathology in the midwifery program, he "knew very well their deficiencies: they are not required to be bachilleres and so they are always failing and having to repeat years." Another member of the council objected "from a practical point of view; since she is a midwife she has her means of livelihood and she does not need another one." Another affirmed that in the university it was not permitted to skip years of study. And Gomezjurado stated that she knew for a fact that this student wasn't really interested in nursing, but instead saw this as a stepping-stone toward an opportunity to leave the country. When they reviewed the minutes at the next meeting, the council corrected the erroneous statement that midwifery students did not require bachilleratos—indeed, the midwifery school had insisted on high school diplomas for admission well before the nursing school had been in a position to do so—but the council did not change their decision on the applicant.

Moral behavior, broadly defined, was also central to the characterization of a proper nurse. In 1947, with the departure of Directoras Foley and Middlemiss—who had provided a certain amount of stability to the administration—a crisis in discipline occurred in the Escuela, leading to an unprecedented written reprimand from the Junta Central de Asistencia Pública to the acting directora, Miss Nicklin. She had arrived in a difficult moment, since the Instituto de Asuntos Interamericanos had never before withdrawn all of the experienced Americanas at the same time. Indeed, Nicklin had come to Ecuador as a representative of the U.S. Children's Bureau, to develop a similar office of child welfare in Quito, but she had been unexpectedly asked to direct the school following the departure of the former administrative staff, just until the new directora arrived from the United States. Regardless of the reason, though, the dean of medicine affirmed: "The School is going through a period of crisis in terms of discipline and morality."[89] In addition to the rebelliousness of the students in the wards—who were disregarding the authority of the supervisoras—discipline within the school walls was also deficient. Students wandered the halls in their dressing gowns, made a ruckus in the dining room, continued to make noise after 8:30 at night—all things that had never before been permitted. Dr. Bustamante added:

The students are permitted to leave the school frequently; too often I come across them in the street, and always in company. I know of one student whose parents ordered that she not leave the school unless she was accompanied by one of the supervisoras, but nonetheless she went out and did not return until 9:00 at night, and the Junta Central de Asistencia Pública has had to respond to her family's complaints. And when the students do go out in public, they are never properly dressed. Even in the wards, they don't wear their full uniforms and present an unpleasant sight with sweaters of all different colors. The students simply are not being properly controlled as they used to be; they spend their time conversing with the medical students within the Hospital, and these conversations have gone so far as to convert themselves into frankly immoral acts carried out on Hospital property, these students have been found in truly immoral postures and acts.[90]

Miss Parker, who was supposed to be overseeing the internal discipline of the establishment at night, simply stayed in her room in the midst of all of these irregularities; Nicklin had already decided to sleep at the school to attempt to rectify the situation.

The arrival of Miss Pansy Virginia Murphy at the end of June 1947 marked a return to discipline in the school. Dr. Charles Miller, the new director of the Servicio Cooperativo Interamericano in Quito, explained bluntly that the Servicio would only continue its support of the school if the Americanas were guaranteed the full cooperation of the council, taking the criticisms of discipline as criticisms of Nicklin. The dean explained that discipline was of fundamental importance, "since we have to take into account the fact that in Ecuador, parents are skittish [quisquillosos] and want to ensure that their daughters conduct themselves in the most correct way, and under the maximum of care. . . . On many occasions students have not enrolled precisely because their parents have not had sufficient knowledge of or confidence in the care or supervision their daughters would receive."[91] Moreover, the Concejo Ejecutivo was expanded at this point, to include representatives of the Servicio Cooperativo (Dr. José Gómez de la Torre, a senior physician in the Sanidad), the Rockefeller Foundation (Dr. Carlos Andrade Marín, who had previously served on the council as director of the medical services of the Caja del Seguro), the Madre Superiora of the Hospital Eugenio Espejo, and a "representative of the public" who rarely attended meetings over the following five years. These changes aimed to ensure both the regular functioning of the school and its reputation.

Among the administrative reforms that Murphy immediately instituted were the creation of an inventory of the school's equipment, establishment of a proper archive for the school's documentation and records, and the practice of providing memoranda to the council before each meeting with the points that she wished them to discuss (essentially she herself set meeting agendas). School discipline in turn was enhanced by her reduction of the free time available to students; the return of the Ecuadorian graduates who had undertaken specialist training in the United States, two of whom agreed to live on the premises (including Ligia Gomezjurado); and the separation from the school of four students for unacceptable behavior or academic performance. Possibly precisely because of the changed leadership style, the three graduadas who had been working for the school, supervising the students who were practicing in the Clínica de la Caja del Seguro, resigned their positions to work directly for the

CCS. While they could be replaced as supervisoras by the graduadas who had returned from the United States, Murphy did not want the students to practice any longer at the Caja under the influence of the former supervisoras, so the students' practice was shifted to the Sanidad.[92] Despite her marked concern with reestablishing discipline, however, Murphy expressed surprise that she was expected to actually grade students on their conduct; she had had better luck using a system of penalties for specific infractions. As she put it: "For me, it is impossible to grade conduct, this is the first time that I have seen such a thing in a school for adults, this is for kindergarten children; we assess conduct each time we evaluate the efficiency of their work."[93] However, given all of the critical eyes watching the school and the disciplinary crisis a few months earlier, the executive council considered this an important form of control over students' behavior.

Oral histories as well as written sources emphasize the strict discipline under which these young women lived—frequently referred to as an "almost military style of discipline"—and the extent to which their behavior was monitored.[94] The "military" tone was attributed in part to the fact that some of the American nurses who first organized the Escuela were literally affiliated with the U.S. military or its allied services. There was also a strict hierarchy observed within the school, such that as students progressed from year to year they also moved up in rank; when first-year students arrived at the school, they were expected to step aside when more senior students passed them in the corridors.[95] Thus they were inculcated with a sense of hierarchy early on, which was reinforced when they began their hospital work. Indeed, the course on ethics included such rules as that the nurse must always greet the physician as a gesture of respect.[96] And another central message of that course as taught by Ligia Gomezjurado was that nurses must always obey physicians: "You must meekly and blindly obey the orders of the physicians," the students were told.[97] Moreover, students followed very strict ("almost military") schedules of work, study, meals, and sleep, which led some students to hide under their covers after lights-out to catch up on their studying.[98]

The figure of the professional woman that was developed at the school was one that included relatively short hair, little make-up, and few accessories or jewelry. She also must have an absolutely tidy and clean general appearance.

> At first it cost us effort to accept the discipline, the hours of study, of eating, having to pass inspection in a line-up before going to the hospital, the inspection that we had to undergo of personal cleanliness, of overall presentation, of the state of our uniforms, if something needed to be mended or not, if something was out of place. If all of that at first seemed tiresome and bothersome,

it served us well. It served us as professors to be able to project a certain image for our students, and also to know how to project an image, a hard-fought image in the work environment, in the hospital, in health posts, etc. . . . The fact that we had discipline internally, in all aspects of everyday life, also was reflected in the external: in the external because what you saw was a very tidy nurse, a nurse who fulfilled all of her obligations, and who knew why she was doing what she was doing.[99]

Part of the students' training was indeed how to behave: "We were taught how to be [respectable] people. How to sit at the table, how to interact with people, how to maintain personal cleanliness, how to greet people, where, when, how. I think in this way, we were all brought up to the same level, regardless of having come from different socioeconomic backgrounds."[100] Moreover, nurses were expected to keep their emotions in check, to leave them behind when they entered their work space. Georgina de Carrillo, who went on in 1971 to succeed Gomezjurado as directora, commented that as a student, the first time there was a death at the hospital during her shift, the supervisora overheard her comment that it was frightening. The latter immediately took her to the morgue and left her there with the cadaver so that she could get used to dealing with death.[101]

Honorable conduct was also necessary because as nurses they might handle valuable items belonging to patients as well as valuable equipment belonging to the hospital and school, not to mention holding the lives of patients in their hands.[102] Ligia Gomezjurado was very aware that she was inventing a new profession and a new kind of woman, an invention that relied on absolute correctness and morality: "That is why the internal regulations themselves of the school said that students could not date medical students, could not flirt, could not laugh, couldn't do anything, in other words appropriate behavior was defined so rigidly because she was constructing an image within a social space that was absolutely moralistic, and absolutely . . . deep down, that blocked and resisted the entrance of women."[103] Much of the school's first years of functioning, explored in this chapter, can be seen as a kind of prehistory to the Gomezjurado period of much greater stability and clarity about the mission of the school. When Gomezjurado took over leadership of the school and the profession, she had already developed some clear notions of appropriate behavior for professional nurses. Her aspirations for professional nurses can be found in a new regulation for the graduadas on the school's staff, which was one of her first projects on assuming the directorship. What was considered appropriate behavior in defense not only of a nurse's reputation but also the reputation of the profession and the school? The regulation offers insight not only into Gomezjurado's modeling of appropriate behavior but also some of the perceived sources of unruliness that had been affecting the school. These provisions further consolidated a moralizing professional project, something that had been more ambiguous under previous directoras.

## Norms of Conduct for *Supervisoras Profesoras*

These norms of conduct were written by Ligia Gomezjurado Narváez and approved by the Concejo Ejecutivo on June 30, 1949.[104]

### Responsibilities of the *Graduada*

- Supervise and control the students in your assigned ward.
- Schedule shifts and distribute tasks among the students in your ward.
- Communicate any problem that arises in your ward first to the directora, before informing the Hermanas de la Caridad or the hospital director.
- Monitor the schedule for changes in your hours of work.
- Always comply with your scheduled shift, eight hours per day according to the schedule; but please do not be annoyed if you sometimes must work a little longer, since a good nurse has to make sacrifices for the well-being of others and the exaltation of the profession.
- Do not change your hours of work without consulting first with the directora.
- Do not leave your ward during your shift in order to visit other wards or to return to the school unnecessarily.
- Make notes and observations regarding the work and aptitude of each student in the notebooks provided for that purpose in the nursing office, so that this forms a record of the efficiency of the students.
- Prepare in advance the classes that you are assigned to teach as well as attending classes of the relevant physician.
- Be untiring in expanding your knowledge; never believe that you already know too much.

### Other Responsibilities

- You should neither entertain students in your room nor visit students. Between the graduadas and the students a prudent distance should be maintained; don't be overly familiar with them, remember that you are a graduada and a role model for the students.
- Treat all students equally, without favoritism or injustice. When you must reprimand someone, do so without fearing recriminations against you.
- Do not communicate to students any disagreeable incidents that occur within the school; this undermines discipline.

- Do not communicate administrative matters or issues involving the graduadas to the students; these should remain confidential among the teachers.
- You are not permitted to receive visitors in the school or the hospital during your working hours. No visitors in the school after 8:30 p.m.
- Each *enfermera* graduada is permitted to go out until midnight twice a week. When you do so, please advise the residence supervisor or the sub-directora so that the door is not double-locked.
- The recreation room is for the use of students; if you wish to use it, please do so when students are not present.
- Meal times are:
  Breakfast from 6:30 to 8:00, depending on your shift
  Lunch from 12:00 to 1:00
  Dinner from 6:00 to 7:00
- Moderate your voice in the hallways, washrooms, and in your own rooms; avoid singing or whistling; control your gestures and way of walking; be feminine at all times.
- Be loyal to the school, its leaders, your coworkers, and the students; do not gossip behind their backs; if you have a suggestion for someone, make it to her directly. Show character.
- Cooperate always with anyone who needs your help. Conserve harmony with the graduadas and others who work with you. Be tolerant of other opinions.
- Do not administer medication without a doctor's orders. The medicine in the school infirmary is exclusively for the students, not for hospital patients. Be thrifty in the use of medication.
- Be severe in your morality to protect the good name of the profession, the institution, and to be a good example to your students. Respect yourself and you will be respected.
- Use your complete uniform when you are working, and try to display an attractive appearance in street clothes. In uniform your appearance should be very neat (fingernails trimmed and very clean, hair pulled back, shoes well maintained, no jewelry, buttons complete, no pins, etc.).
- Do not smoke in the dining room or hallways; do it only in your own room and never in uniform.
- Have a joyful spirit; always be optimistic and happy.
- Control your emotions; don't offer a spectacle to observers.
- At the end of each day examine your actions, and if you identify any deficiencies, try to correct them the next day.
- If you encounter difficulties at work that lead to you resign, notify the dir-

ectora at least a month in advance; then in your resignation don't mention weaknesses of others, couch it in courteous terms. If you leave your position in a hostile form, your good reputation will be destroyed. Always leave your work well organized, leaving the directora or your replacement well informed about its status.

• Always comply with the regulations of the school.

These rules are made to protect the well-being of the school and the good name of the graduadas.

Just like the world of obstetrical services, the universe of nursing services in Ecuador in the middle third of the twentieth century was also a complex and shifting one in which the new professional trained nurses' expertise and behavior was judged alongside barchilonas, nursing nuns, and the graduates of the nursing school that had previously existed in Quito. While various officials and physicians contributing to the administrative correspondence of the Hospital Civil San Juan de Dios were quite careful to avoid the term *barchilona* even from relatively early in the 1920s, it is striking how freely the physicians and nurses engaged in discussions within the Concejo Ejecutivo of the Escuela Nacional de Enfermeras used this term to refer to subaltern employees of hospitals. This marks a persistent effort to distance the work of the graduated nurses and nursing students from that model of care, which apparently continued to influence how nurses were perceived and treated.

The role of nurses as not only highly trained technical staff but also young women whose technical skills were applied in work with semiclad and sometimes naked bodies was a difficult balance to maintain in the conservative social environment of Quito even in the 1940s, leading to a constant emphasis within the school on dignified, respectable, and at the same time feminine behavior. There was clearly a pull toward working in environments with female or young patients, leaving the care of adult men more often—although not exclusively—in the hands of the Hermanas de la Caridad. According to an oral history account of the era, "in the Caja de Pensiones and other public offices the work spaces of men and women were separate, because it was believed that this was morally correct."[105] The overlapping of men's and women's work spaces in hospitals was thus still unusual, and despite the clear hierarchies within the hospital, nurses tried to eke out their own spheres of action and authority. In this time period in Quito, the figure of *la chulla quiteña* was a prominent one: in the 1940s and 1950s the feminine form of the term *chulla* referred to unmarried women of the emerging middle sectors who just might be sexually available.[106] The prominence of this negative image may have constituted partly a response and rejection on the part of elite society to some of the social changes associated with the populism of the 1930s and 1940s. There are many traces in the archives of attempts to distance nurses and nursing students from any such image. Nonetheless, some of the women who came to the Escuela from the provinces or even from local neighborhoods in Quito probably experienced in shifting degrees both the pressures and possibilities their new freedoms posed.

A nurse whose enrollment in the Escuela coincided with Gomezjurado's appointment as directora pointed out: "Despite the fact that I arrived at the school some years after it opened, still the level of prestige of nursing was very low. . . . So I think that the kind of rigidity, of discipline, had the objective of placing the nurse in the position that she deserved, so that she would both act and be recognized as professional in every way. And I think it was successful."[107] The archival materials support that interpretation: Ligia Gomezjurado was a central figure in establishing, through a process of trial and error and of learning from past conflicts and mistakes, a palatable model of a female nursing professional appropriate to the Ecuadorian highland context as it existed at midcentury. By 1970 this model had exhausted itself, and when political events led to the university's closure, reform, and then reopening in 1971, the new directora, Georgina de Carrillo, took the school in a different direction. The boarding school was eliminated to allow for an exponential increase in nursing enrollments to begin to meet the needs of a country experiencing an oil boom, where at least some of the new resources were used to expand medical services.[108] By 1980 a decade had been added to the average life expectancy in Ecuador and infant mortality had been reduced by 40 percent.[109] The model of a very meticulous selection and careful cultivation of a small number of nurses gave way to new ways of thinking about the key role of nurses in expanding medical service coverage throughout the national territory. Although this departed in significant ways from the model cultivated for over two decades at the school, perhaps this was possible precisely because of the achievements of Ligia Gomezjurado and her students in persuading state actors and the general public of what Ecuadorian nurses could offer to a project of comprehensive social development.

# Conclusion

A central dimension of state formation is what historical sociologist Philip Corrigan has called "the materiality of moral regulation and the moralization of material reality."[1] This book explores both, examining some of the concrete ways that women's moral behavior was regulated in a range of different social arenas as well as how women's efforts to deal with some of the material constraints they faced were perceived and addressed in moral terms. In each chapter state projects are scrutinized. What lent such projects considerable legitimacy was not so much their ability to impose behaviors, but rather the ways that they *enabled* certain kinds of actions or possibilities for differently situated Ecuadorian women. They enabled poor women to find (particular kinds of) solutions to their need to feed and educate their children, or to find free medical attention or sterilized milk for those children. They enabled some women who went so far as to register themselves with the venereal prophylaxis service to find a solution to their economic difficulties in prostitution (sometimes temporarily), providing them with medical treatment for sexually transmitted diseases. They enabled quite different kinds of women to seek new educational opportunities and to professionalize themselves as midwives and nurses, which might lead to state employment. There were ways in which all of these programs acknowledged, furthered, and sometimes even dignified women's aspirations and situations, at the same time as they disallowed or undermined other dimensions of women's behavior and identity.

The chapters range widely over women's lives, state practices, and health issues in highland Ecuador—especially, but not exclusively, in the capital city of Quito—in the first half of the twentieth century. Nonetheless, some issues weave their way through several chapters, and one of the prominent themes is sexuality. While sexuality was repressed (for women), it was also everywhere— a prominent window through which women's behavior was judged and a primary way in which their role was understood. Its prevalence can be seen, too, in the number of male secondary school students who were sexually active from their adolescence, often with the many women who prostituted themselves regularly or occasionally to make ends meet. It can also be seen in the behavior of medical students: in a kind of voyeurism or salaciousness they could not seem to help exhibiting with pregnant women in the Maternidad, or when they hung around the offices of the Servicio de Profilaxis Venérea hoping to get to know some of its clients (registered prostitutes).

Nurses, too, found it difficult to forge a new professional space in which they would not be treated primarily as sexual beings; it is no wonder that nursing leaders concluded that only a nunlike persona could help nurses project an appropriate image within the hospital. Unattached women who took up positions in the Public Health Service's outreach program of maternal-infant health might also be accused of sexual transgressions by their supervisors. A registered prostitute in Guayaquil recounted in 1951 that she had tried to make a living in other ways, including working "like a man" cutting and moving rock in the municipal quarry, but once her male coworkers discovered that her name was in the registry, they made her life impossible. This incident led the director of venereal prophylaxis in Guayaquil to conclude that women were only ever considered as sexual objects by men, who were interested in possessing them (and if they failed, hated them), but who had no interest in understanding them.[2] Emphasizing their sexuality in these ways, in contexts where women did not themselves foreground it, was a way that men exercised power over women.

A related theme that appears frequently in these pages is morality, including in the obvious double standards of morality that judged women harshly for missteps that were commonly accepted for men: indeed, men's sexuality was seen as a natural, instinctual urge, in a way that women's rarely was. Perhaps more interesting is the very different ways that morality was seen as problematic for midwives and for nurses. The main moral issue for midwives seems to have been abortion, and it was suspected that they were likely to identify too much with the conundrums of their female clients (or simply seek the fees they could earn for an illegal service) rather than to keep in mind their obligations as medical professionals. They worked alone in people's homes or in their own private practices by necessity, since they were frozen out of work in larger medical institutions such as the Maternidad as well as from teaching positions in the midwifery program in the Universidad Central for many years. But this also meant that they undertook their work for the most part without regular supervision by other professionals, which seems to have intensified physicians' mistrust. For nurses the moral issues were rather different: a strict moral rectitude on their part (and again we see the double standard here) was needed given that they worked alongside physicians and medical students in mixed-sex workplaces, something still very unusual in the 1940s. They also carried out their duties working with naked and semiclad bodies, including those of adult men—something unheard of for respectable women.

Structural working conditions had other implications for midwives and nurses. If we look at their history and professional status over the larger trajectory of the twentieth century, there are important differences between the experiences of midwives and nurses. Midwives began as true pioneers of higher education for women, and throughout the 1940s, for instance, it was necessary to have a completed *bachillerato* (high school diploma) to register in this four-year degree program at the Universidad Central. The training of nurses began later, and they often entered their studies with less prior educational preparation. Only in the 1950s was the Escuela Nacional de Enfermeras able to recruit consistently women with bachilleratos. However, some of those women had opportunities to travel abroad for specialist training as their potential contribution within the health-care system was more recognized in international contexts than at home—and that training then vaulted them into positions of authority when they returned. Moreover, the very model of training in a boarding school context, under the supervision of other women, seems to have created an esprit de corps among nurses that was difficult to generate among the more isolated midwives. This was sustained as nurses worked alongside not only physicians and medical students but other nurses, too, in medical institutions. The particular ways in which their professionalism was belittled and their work was marginalized was much more likely to be experienced collectively, unlike midwives, who experienced such undermining more often on an individual basis. It is not by chance that it was nurses who became leaders in defending working conditions and salaries in Ecuador in the last decade of the twentieth century—not only for themselves but more broadly for a range of paramedical practitioners in public health-care institutions.[3]

Midwives have been less successful in organizing to protect and promote their professional space, including in pressuring the state to create positions for midwives in the staff complements and budgets of public medical institutions. Still, nurses and midwives interviewed seemed to agree that for both professions there are often more interesting opportunities outside the context of large urban institutions.[4] For nurses, in the more varied and creative work they might be called upon to do in rural health posts, where they have more latitude to organize the overall work processes of such clinics; and for midwives, in provincial contexts where they are more likely to be able to establish busy and remunerative private practices than in urban areas where they are in greater competition with physicians. Medical anthropologist Elizabeth Roberts's ethnographic research on assisted reproduction in Ecuador reveals another dimension of the marginalization of midwifery: today some urban Ecuadorian women's preference for highly medicalized forms of childbirth is expressed through the elevation of the Caesarean section scar to a status symbol.[5]

Another recurring theme is the problem of illegitimacy, which physicians thought could bring along with it all kinds of additional medical and social problems. When they discussed these issues publicly, as in Dr. Antonio Bastidas's lecture to medical students in 1932, empathy with illegitimate children was combined with a distancing that seemed to make illegitimacy a problem requiring physicians' and future physicians' support, understanding, and social action. It was not presented as something with which they might be intimately familiar. However, illegitimacy was widespread in Ecuador and might indeed touch the lives not only of the popular classes but also of medical professionals themselves. Such was the case of the physician who had to flee the country as the result of his involvement in seeking an abortion for his lover, which resulted in her death. And the medical director of the Servicio de Profilaxis Venérea in the early 1920s had an illegitimate son. A female medical student and single mother supported her illegitimate son with her work as an intern at the Hospital Civil San Juan de Dios in 1949. A nursing student managed to gain enrollment in the Escuela Nacional de Enfermeras—and thus a way to support herself and her family in the future—despite having had a child out of wedlock a year or two prior to that.

Of the women who registered to study midwifery in the Universidad Central—the first field of study opened to them—in the two decades of greatest expansion of enrollments some 15 to 16 percent of midwifery students were illegitimate daughters. More striking still are the figures of women like María Luisa Gómez de la Torre and Rosa Stacey who, regardless of their illegitimate birth—or perhaps precisely because of the ways that birth inevitably placed them at the margins of respectable society—became trailblazers of social and educational change in a restrictive environment, with an impact not only in their own lives but also for many cohorts of young women whom they taught. The legal status of "illegitimate"—defining different rights for illegitimate versus legitimate children—was only eliminated in the 1967 Civil Code, redefining relatedness in terms of the biological fact of birth and not the legal status of the parents' relationship.[6] Until that date, illegitimate birth was registered on birth certificates and identity cards and noted in formal records such as the enrollment books of the Universidad Central (a boon to historical scholars but to illegitimate children a constant reminder of their irregular status). Given demographer John Saunders's finding that a third of Ecuadorians born in 1955 were of illegitimate birth, this condition was far more common than either dominant representations of family life in Ecuador, or scholarly analyses of Ecuadorian society, have recognized.

The prevalence of illegitimacy in Ecuador—even in the more socially conservative highlands and even among middle- and upper-class sectors—merits additional research, and not only to explore more systematically the country's demography. From the perspective of understanding how social change occurs, it seems that there was something about being marginalized but not fully disadvantaged (and of course not all illegitimate children fell into that category) that predisposed people to take risks and to strike out in new directions. While having a more economically secure social position might have offered greater resources to do this, those circumstances did not especially lend themselves to being daring. Indeed, for women in particular, a more comfortable and respectable social position might also lead to restrictions on their ability to engage in public life, except in narrowly defined ways. In the end, perhaps there is nothing surprising about this conclusion. Four decades ago, the anthropologist Eric Wolf came to a similar position in his exploration of what sector of the peasantry was more likely to rebel: neither the poorest peasants who couldn't afford to take the risk nor the wealthiest peasants who had a stake in the status quo, but rather the middle peasantry.[7]

Like those middle peasants studied by Wolf, the women whose lives are explored in this book had a social position that was not only middling but also contradictory, pulling them in different directions simultaneously. Although their actions did not constitute a collective social movement as occurred with peasant revolutions, they were undoubtedly involved in processes of social transformation. And while they did not participate in visibly dramatic mobilizations, their lives were characterized by a considerable degree of personal drama. In addition to the illegitimate daughters and women with illegitimate children who populate this book, noteworthy in general were the large numbers of unattached women, who by 1950 constituted a quarter of all urban women over age thirty in Ecuador (and more if we add widowed women to those who were single). Being unmarried might involve a wide range of lived experiences, from abandonment and economic misery for some to a sense of freedom for others. This book begins to explore some of those social circumstances, seeking to provide a narrative about Ecuadorian history in which more women can recognize themselves.[8]

While nursing and midwifery offered opportunities for professional advancement—very hard-fought opportunities—the women who were in a position to pursue those opportunities were very specifically situated. They were literate and were increasingly drawn from the ranks of liberal (meaning in part, more secular) urban families whose daughters attended state secondary institutions. They were not necessarily wealthy families, to be sure, but they were also not among the destitute urban (or much less, rural) poor. Where we can distinguish the voices of popular-sector women, it is clear that the options available to them were very different from the women able to achieve some modicum of social mobility through education and professional work. It would be interesting to explore whether for some women from smaller population centers and relatively humble homes, joining the Hermanas de la Caridad (the Sisters of Charity) might have been a more realistic option. The archival records hint that more Hermanas than secular nursing students were drawn from smaller towns in the early years of professional nursing training; more targeted research would be needed to understand the processes of recruitment and the social profile of the Ecuadorian women who became Hermanas. Of course, that alternative would not have been available to women who were not born into legitimately constituted families.

The Ecuadorian state projects explored throughout this book were pursued in the context of a range of different transnational processes. In all cases the designers of regulations or the founders of institutions were in dialogue with the ways such things were done elsewhere. Sometimes external influences were very direct, as when the Servicio Cooperativo Interamericano and the Rockefeller Foundation helped to found the Escuela Nacional de Enfermeras, even providing American nurses to design curriculum and administer the institution and then sending early Ecuadorian graduates abroad for advanced training. In other cases, such relations were less direct, when representatives of foreign governments requested information on infant mortality or child welfare institutions or when questionnaires were sent by international associations regarding venereal prophylaxis programs, and Ecuadorian public health experts used the opportunity to further an exchange of ideas over additional matters of mutual interest. The Gota de Leche, too, was modeled on similar institutions elsewhere, and of course the Red Cross was an international organization. Nonetheless, an institution such as the Gota de Leche also took a very Ecuadorian form, founded and run by the elite wives of modernizing dairy farmers. While physicians read widely about health conditions and social policy elsewhere, they used that information to interpret an Ecuadorian reality, in Ecuadorian ways.

One of the goals of this book has been to portray a range of women's experiences that are not widely known in Ecuador. However, it also shows that there was significant diversity within the category "Ecuadorian women" or even "women of the north-central highlands" or even "urban women of the middle sectors." Among "Catholic women" themselves, there was a range of forms of participation in public activity: charitable work such as that carried out by the Señoras de la Caridad, philanthropic work such as that of the elite women who formed the Sociedad de La Gota de Leche, work in institutions of Beneficencia undertaken by the Hermanas de la Caridad, not to mention the heavily Catholic tone of Ecuadorian professional nursing. Indeed, many of the women who pioneered new forms of professional work were themselves practicing Catholics, like the majority of their fellow Ecuadorians—except perhaps in eras when the Catholic Church made it difficult to reconcile these two identities given its harsh treatment of women who opted for the only kind of advanced education that might provide future opportunities to support themselves independently, in secular secondary schools. Ecuadorian society underwent a significant process of secularization in the first half of the twentieth century, on the foundation of the separation of church and state pushed through by liberal governments at the beginning of the century, in which the expansion of state-run education played a central role. By the 1930s—given Ecuadorians' relatively short life expectancy—the vast majority of the population had been born since the 1895 Liberal Revolution.[9] Nonetheless, some of the ambivalent ways that professional nursing at midcentury engaged Catholicism attests to the ongoing influence of religion in Quito, in ways that were particularly significant for women's roles.

Just as the category "women" is highly diverse, the state, too, appears in various guises in this book. All of the chapters analyze state projects; however, such projects involved significant disagreements over design, goals, and implementation, often even within a single state institution. This suggests that we need to be careful about what a "state" project toward "women" might mean: both categories were highly differentiated internally, and state institutions themselves included and engaged women who might be positioned in a range of ways in relation to those projects, including serving as their often ambivalent agents. In some ways the Ecuadorian state seemed to be acting on society in these projects. That is, state institutions sometimes seemed to offer opportunities to women in the face of constraints placed on them by "society." This was articulated especially clearly by liberal policy makers in the early decades of the century when they presented themselves as forging new spaces for women to support themselves honorably and defend their virtue, articulated precisely against conservative social values and the Catholic Church. However, the narrative of this book also shows the extent to which "state" and "society" were intermingled. The state agents who populate this book were not faceless bureaucrats following administrative mandates issuing from a single source; they were complex figures immersed in broader social relations. In some situations they had considerable leeway to exercise their own judgment about how to act, and their views of what to do were surely formed as much in their private lives and personal histories as in their public roles.

When one begins to inquire into the activities of state actors, it becomes increasingly difficult to see the state as a monolithic entity with a single set of interests. The state is an assemblage of different institutions and agencies that recruit a range of kinds of agents who embody different experiences, aspirations, and perspectives. State programs may contradict each other, and state agencies and their agents themselves may come into conflict. It may be that it is the room for maneuver generated by such disjunctures that creates a world of shifting possibilities for people with different positioning vis-à-vis social programs. Perhaps this is also how states normally function, despite efforts by state actors to make states and their projects appear coherent and rational.[10]

# NOTES

## Chapter 1. Gendered Experiences and State Formation in Highland Ecuador

1. Philip Abrams, *Historical Sociology* (Ithaca: Cornell University Press, 1982), 227.

2. Abrams, *Historical Sociology*, 240.

3. Among many useful theoretical discussions of structure and agency, some of those most relevant to the concerns of this book can be found in Abrams, *Historical Sociology*; Philip Corrigan and Derek Sayer, *The Great Arch: English State Formation as Cultural Revolution* (London: Basil Blackwell, 1985); and William Roseberry, *Anthropologies and Histories: Essays in Culture, History, and Political Economy* (New Brunswick: Rutgers University Press, 1989).

4. For biographical materials about the two women discussed here, see Jenny Estrada, *Una mujer total: Matilde Hidalgo de Prócel (biografía)* (Guayaquil: Imprenta de la Universidad de Guayaquil, 1980), and Raquel Rodas, *Nosotras que del amor hicimos . . .* (Quito: Fraga, 1992). The lives of Matilde Hidalgo and María Luisa Gómez de la Torre are also discussed in the context of a rather different argument in A. Kim Clark, "Feminismos estéticos y antiestéticos en el Ecuador de principios del siglo XX: Un análisis de género y generaciones," *Procesos* (Quito) 22 (2005): 85–105.

5. This information is drawn from the enrollment records of the Faculty of Medicine at the Central University, "Matrículas de la Facultad de Medicina, Farmacia, Odontología, Obstetricia, 15 de octubre de 1912 a 18 de junio de 1930," Archivo General de la Universidad Central (AGUC).

6. Indeed, in his 1910 annual report to the nation, an earlier minister of the interior himself had pointed this out and urged the congress to amend the Law of Elections to make it consistent with the spirit of the constitution, granting women the right to vote. See Octavio Díaz, *Informe que a la nación presenta el ministro de lo interior, policía, beneficencia, obras públicas, etc. en el año 1910* (Quito: Imprenta y Encuadernación Nacionales, 1910), xi–xii.

7. Uruguay followed soon thereafter, granting women the right to vote in national elections in 1932. In Chile women were permitted to vote first in municipal elections,

effective in 1934. However, neither Chilean nor Argentinean women could vote in national elections until after the Second World War. See Asunción Lavrin, *Women, Feminism, and Social Change in Argentina, Chile, and Uruguay, 1890–1940* (Lincoln: University of Nebraska Press, 1995). In Ecuador a literacy requirement continued to be linked to voting rights for both men and women until the 1979 constitution established compulsory universal suffrage.

8. In 1933 women made up 12 percent of the registered voters in Ecuador, at a time when the electorate was only 3.1 percent of the total national population. By 1968 the percentage of female registered voters had increased to 39 percent of the voting population, with just under 20 percent of the population comprising that electorate. See Juan Maiguashca and Liisa North, "Orígenes y significado del velasquismo: Lucha de clases y participación política en el Ecuador, 1920–1972," in *La cuestión regional y el poder,* edited by Rafael Quintero (Quito: Corporación Editora Nacional, 1991), 133.

9. Jorge Gómez, *Las misiones pedagógicas alemanas y la educación en el Ecuador* (Quito: Abya Yala and Proyecto EBI-MEC-GTZ, 1993).

10. From the 1920s this began to be publicly demonstrated in the choreographed gymnastics exercises that women from secular schools began to perform for audiences. Students from private schools of all kinds, most of which were Catholic schools, were required to take their final examinations at state schools. When they did so in physical education, female students from Catholic schools did not even have appropriate uniforms for athletic activities, much less any practice at undertaking them. See Ana María Goetschel, *Educación de las mujeres, maestras y esferas públicas: Quito en la primera mitad del siglo XX* (Quito: FLACSO/Abya Yala, 2007).

11. As late as 1951, the archbishop of Quito reminded Catholics that it was prohibited to send their children to non-Catholic schools. Lilo Linke, *Ecuador: Country of Contrasts* (London: Royal Institute of International Affairs, 1954), 97.

12. Leonardo J. Muñoz, *Testimonio de lucha: Memorias sobre la historia del socialismo en el Ecuador* (Quito: Corporación Editora Nacional, 1988).

13. On the Revolución Gloriosa, see Carlos de la Torre, *La seducción velasquista* (Quito: Libri Mundi, 1993).

14. On María Luisa Gómez de la Torre's work in indigenous education, see Raquel Rodas, *Crónica de un sueño: Las escuelas indígenas de Dolores Cacuango* (Quito: Proyecto EBI-MEC-GTZ, 1989); and more broadly on the alliances between urban leftists and peasant activists, see Marc Becker, *Indians and Leftists in the Making of Ecuador's Indian Movements* (Durham: Duke University Press, 2007).

15. There are many excellent studies of the emergence of CONAIE, including these works in English: Becker, *Indians and Leftists*; José Antonio Lucero, *Struggles of Voice: The Politics of Indigenous Representation in the Andes* (Pittsburgh: University of Pittsburgh Press, 2008); and Amalia Pallares, *From Peasant Struggles to Indian Resistance: The Ecuadorian Andes in the Late Twentieth Century* (Norman: University of Oklahoma Press, 2002).

16. Interview with Rosa's niece, Aurelia Stacey, Quito, 28 June 2006.

17. Thanks to Rosa's great nieces, Alicia and Ximena Andrade Stacey, for review-

ing these comments about Rosa Stacey and for sharing this family story (personal communication, Quito, 16 May 2010).

18. Wilson Miño Grijalva, *Eduardo Larrea Stacey: Visionario y precursor de un nuevo Ecuador* (Quito: Banco Central, 2006), 37.

19. Goetschel, *Educación de las mujeres*, 153.

20. See the interview with Rosario Mena de Barrera in María Cuvi Sánchez, ed., *Quito casa adentro: Narrado por mujeres* (Quito: FONSAL, 2009), 70–123.

21. Interview with Mireya Salgado de Fernández in Cuvi Sánchez, *Quito casa adentro*, 28.

22. Cuvi Sánchez, *Quito casa adentro*, 19. The other four medical students were Isidro Ayora, Ricardo Villavicencio, Mario de la Torre, and Luis Dávila.

23. Adriana Valeria Coronel, "A Revolution in Stages: Subaltern Politics, Nation-State Formation, and the Origins of Social Rights in Ecuador, 1834–1943" (PhD diss., New York University, 2011).

24. On the struggles of peasants see, for instance, A. Kim Clark and Marc Becker, eds., *Highland Indians and the State in Modern Ecuador* (Pittsburgh: University of Pittsburgh Press, 2007).

25. Linda Alexander Rodríguez, *The Search for Public Policy: Regional Politics and Government Finances in Ecuador, 1830–1940* (Berkeley: University of California Press, 1985), continues to be a useful source for this time period. See also Cecilia Durán, *Irrupción del sector burócrata en el estado ecuatoriano, 1925–1944* (Quito: Abya Yala and PUCE, 2000), and Juan Paz y Miño Cepeda, *Revolución Juliana: Nación, ejército, y bancocracia*, second edition (Quito: Abya Yala, 2000).

26. Pablo Arturo Suárez, A. López, and Cornelio Donoso, "Estudio numérico y económico-social de la población de Quito," *Boletín del Departamento Médico Social* 1, no. 1 (1937): 7–11.

27. Juan Maiguashca, "Los sectores subalternos en los años 30 y el aparecimiento del velasquismo," in *Las crises en el Ecuador: Los treinta y ochenta*, edited by Rosemary Thorp (Quito: Corporación Editora Nacional, 1991), 79–94; Carlos Marchán Romero, "La crisis de los años treinta: Diferenciación social de sus efectos económicos," in *Las crises en el Ecuador*, 31–60; and Maiguashca and North, "Orígenes y significado del velasquismo."

28. See, for instance, Goetschel, *Educación de las mujeres*, chapter 1; and Erin O'Connor, *Gender, Indian, Nation: The Contradictions of Making Ecuador, 1830–1925* (Tucson: University of Arizona Press, 2007), chapter 3.

29. See especially Derek Williams, "Assembling the 'Empire of Morality': State Building Strategies in Catholic Ecuador, 1861–1875," *Journal of Historical Sociology* 14, no. 2 (2001): 149–74; and more generally, see Marie-Danielle Demélas and Yves Saint-Geours, *Jerusalén y Babilonia: Religión y política en el Ecuador, 1780–1880* (Quito: Corporación Editora Nacional y Instituto Francés de Estudios Andinos, 1988).

30. Mensaje de Eloy Alfaro a los diputados, sesión ordinario de 13 de Junio de 1897, in Eloy Alfaro, *Diario de debates* (1897): 1734–35.

31. Ibid.

32. Presidential Decree of 19 December 1895, reproduced in Jenny Estrada, *Mujeres de Guayaquil* (Guayaquil: Banco Central and Archivo Histórico del Guayas, 1984), 324.

33. José Peralta, *Informe del ministro de instrucción pública al congreso ordinario de 1900* (Quito: Imprenta de la Universidad Central, 1900), 12.

34. The arguments summarized in this and the following paragraph are developed in detail in A. Kim Clark, *The Redemptive Work: Railway and Nation in Liberal Ecuador, 1895–1930* (Wilmington: Scholarly Resources, 1998), chapters 3 and 4.

35. Rafael Quintero and Erika Silva, *Ecuador: Una nación en ciernes*, vol. 1 (Quito: FLACSO and Abya Yala, 1991).

36. See Clark, *Redemptive Work*, chapter 3, for a discussion of some prominent state-church conflicts during the first half of the liberal period; and Enrique Ayala Mora, ed., *Federico González Suárez y la polémica sobre el estado laico* (Quito: Banco Central and Corporación Editora Nacional, 1978).

37. See chapter 4 of O'Connor, *Gender, Indian, Nation*, for more information about debates around and effects of some of the legal changes discussed here, as well as Martha Moscoso, "Discurso religioso y discurso estatal: La mujer sumisa," in *Y el amor no era todo . . . Mujeres, imágenes y conflictos*, edited by Martha Moscoso (Quito: Abya Yala and DGIS, 1996), 21–57.

38. See the presidential decree of 4 July 1895, in Rafael Gómez de la Torre, *Informe concerniente a las secciones de instrucción pública, justicia y beneficencia que presenta el ministro de gobierno a la convención nacional de 1896–1897* (Quito: Imprenta Nacional, 1897). This same decree permitted Palmieri to register in medical studies at the Universidad de Guayaquil; however, Raquel Rodas has commented that Palmieri withdrew from those studies after being sexually harassed by one of the professors (see Raquel Rodas, "De los inicios de la República a la Revolución Juliana," in *Historia del voto femenino en el Ecuador,* edited by Raquel Rodas Morales [Quito: CONAMU, 2009], 70).

39. See, for instance, Enrique Ayala Mora, *Historia de la revolución liberal ecuatoriana* (Quito: Corporación Editora Nacional, 1994), 293.

40. Compañía Guía del Ecuador, *El Ecuador: Guía comercial, agrícola e industrial de la república* (Guayaquil: Talleres de Artes Gráficos de E. Rodenas, 1909), 563–67, 1199–1201.

41. Information on women's enrollment in the Universidad Central comes from the registration records of the Faculty of Medicine (AGUC), supplemented with the lists of students registered in each program published regularly in the *Anales de la Universidad Central*.

42. Luis A. Martínez, *Memoria del secretario de instrucción pública, correos y telégrafos, etc. al congreso ordinario de 1905* (Quito: Tipografía de la Escuela de Artes y Oficios, 2005), xxiv–v.

43. The following quotations on this issue all come from Dr. Enrique Gallegos Anda to the director of the Junta de Beneficencia, Quito, 31 January 1925, LCR (Libro

de Comunicaciones Recibidas) 1925, Archivo de la Asistencia Pública/Museo Nacional de Medicina (AAP/MNM).

44. Caja de Pensiones, *Segundo Censo de Afiliados, realizado el 30 de Abril de 1935* (Quito: Publisher, 1936). For a history of Ecuador's social security system, see Jorge Núñez et al., *Historia del Seguro Social Ecuatoriano* (Quito: Instituto Ecuatoriano de Seguridad Social, 1984).

45. Nómina de empleados, Hospital Civil San Juan de Dios, October 1949, Archivo del Hospital Civil San Juan de Dios/Museo Nacional de Medicina (AHCSJD/MNM).

46. The information about this student's progress through the medical program comes from the enrollment records of the Faculty of Medicine at the Universidad Central (AGUC).

47. The female students who were permitted to study pharmacy in the first decade of the twentieth century, for instance, neither began studies with the same credentials as male students nor graduated with the same degrees. University authorities noted later that when they said that female students finished as "licenciadas," they did not mean that they completed their licentiate degrees as men did but rather that they were licensed to practice the basic tasks of pharmacists (although not more complex operations).

48. On the career of Dra. Elvira Rawson de Dellepiane, see Lavrin, *Women, Feminism, and Social Change,* 127–29.

49. Susan K. Besse, *Restructuring Patriarchy: The Modernization of Gender Inequality in Brazil, 1914–1940* (Chapel Hill: University of North Carolina Press, 1996), 147–48.

50. Quintero and Silva, *Ecuador,* chapter 9.

51. Rodas, "De los inicios de la República," 106–10, 121.

52. Piedad Larrea Borja, "Biografía de la mujer en el Ecuador: Romanticismo y siglo XX," *El espectador* (Quito) 1 (1943): 3.

53. Goetschel, *Educación de las mujeres*; Martha Moscoso, "Imagen de la mujer y la familia a inicios del siglo XX," *Procesos* 8 (1996): 67–82; O'Connor, *Gender, Indian, Nation*; Ana María Goetschel, "Las paradojas del liberalismo y las mujeres: Coyuntura 1907–1909," in *Celebraciones centenarias y negociaciones por la nación ecuatoriana,* edited by Valeria Coronel and Mercedes Prieto (Quito: FLACSO and Ministerio de Cultura, 2010), 209–40.

54. Many examples are reproduced in Ana María Goetschel et al., *De memorias: Imágenes públicas de las mujeres ecuatorianas de comienzos y fines del siglo veinte* (Quito: FONSAL and FLACSO, 2007).

55. Michel Foucault, *The History of Sexuality,* vol. 1, *An Introduction* (New York: Vintage Books, 1980), 139.

56. See Michel Foucault, "Governmentality," in *The Foucault Effect: Studies in Governmentality,* edited by Graham Burchell, Colin Gordon, and Peter Miller (Chicago: University of Chicago Press, 1991), 87–104; among many other elaborations on his work, see Mitchell Dean, "'Demonic Societies': Liberalism, Biopolitics, and

Sovereignty," in *States of Imagination: Ethnographic Explorations of the Postcolonial State*, edited by Thomas Blom Hansen and Finn Stepputat (Durham: Duke University Press, 2001), 41–64; and for Ecuador, see Eduardo Kingman Garcés, *La ciudad y los otros, Quito 1860–1940: Higienismo, ornato y policía* (Quito: FLACSO and Universidad Rovira e Virgili, 2006).

57. Recently scholars have begun to examine these internalizations in contexts of "neoliberal governmentality." For Latin America, Verónica Schild's work stands out: see, for instance, her "Neoliberalism's New Gendered Market Citizens: The 'Civilizing' Dimension of Social Programs in Chile," *Citizenship Studies* 4, no. 3 (2000): 275–305; and her "Empowering Consumer Citizens or Governing Poor Female Subjects? The Institutionalization of 'Self-Development' in the Chilean Social Policy Field," *Journal of Consumer Culture* 7, no. 2 (2007): 179–203.

58. Paulo Drinot, *The Allure of Labor: Workers, Race, and the Making of the Peruvian State* (Durham: Duke University Press, 2011), 11.

59. Lynn Morgan and Elizabeth Roberts, "Rights and Reproduction in Latin America," *Anthropology News* (March 2009): 12.

60. A groundbreaking study of the profound cultural effects of state formation is Corrigan and Sayer's *Great Arch*.

61. Gilbert Joseph and Daniel Nugent, eds., *Everyday Forms of State Formation: Revolution and the Negotiation of Rule in Mexico* (Durham: Duke University Press, 1994), brings together early examples of this perspective applied to a Latin American case. Several of the chapters in Hansen and Stepputat's *States of Imagination* pursue a similar approach in exploring how state power operates and is engaged in everyday contexts in a variety of ethnographic and historical cases.

62. James Ferguson and Akhil Gupta, "Spatializing States: Toward an Ethnography of Neoliberal Governmentality," *American Ethnologist* 29, no. 4 (2002): 981–1002. For a useful perspective from geography, see Joe Painter, "Prosaic Geographies of Stateness," *Political Geography* 25 (2006): 752–74.

63. Christopher Krupa, "State by Proxy: Privatized Government in the Andes," *Comparative Studies in Society and History* 52, no. 2 (2010): 319–50.

64. David Nugent, "State and Shadow State in Northern Peru circa 1900: Illegal Political Networks and the Problem of State Boundaries," in *States and Illegal Practices*, edited by Josiah McC. Heyman (New York: Berg, 1999), 63–98; and Akhil Gupta, "Blurred Boundaries: The Discourse of Corruption, the Culture of Politics, and the Imagined State," *American Ethnologist* 22, no. 2 (1995): 375–402.

65. For a pioneering study of the intersection of honor, gender, and class in Latin America, see Verena Martínez-Alier, *Marriage, Class, and Color in Nineteenth-Century Cuba* (Cambridge: Cambridge University Press, 1974); more recently, see Carol A. Smith, "Race-Class-Gender Ideology in Guatemala: Modern and Anti-Modern Forms," *Comparative Studies in Society and History* 37, no. 4 (1995): 723–49; and Tanja Christiansen, *Disobedience, Slander, Seduction, and Assault: Women and Men in Cajamarca, Peru, 1862–1900* (Austin: University of Texas Press, 2004).

66. Sueann Caulfield, Sarah C. Chambers, and Lara Putnam, eds., *Honor, Status, and Law in Modern Latin America* (Durham: Duke University Press, 2005).

67. Chad Thomas Black, *The Limits of Gender Domination: Women, the Law, and Political Crisis in Quito, 1765–1830* (Albuquerque: University of New Mexico Press, 2010).

68. J. V. D. Saunders, *The People of Ecuador: A Demographic Analysis* (Gainesville: University of Florida Press, 1961), 28.

69. Saunders, *People of Ecuador,* 29. The relative lack of men in Quito may help explain why women made up 32 percent of the factory labor force in the city, much higher than in other parts of the country; also see Pablo Arturo Suárez, *Contribución al estudio de las realidades entre las clases obreras y campesinas* (Quito: Imprenta de la Universidad Central, 1934), 25–26.

70. Saunders, *People of Ecuador,* 53–54.

71. Pierre Bourdieu, "The Forms of Capital," in *The Handbook of Theory and Research for the Sociology of Education,* edited by John Richardson (New York: Greenwood Press, 1986), 243.

72. In 1936 domestic servants made up 21.1 percent (7,464 people) of Quito's economically active population; see Suárez, López, and Donoso, "Estudio numérico y económico-social." A majority of these domestic servants would have been women.

73. Ann Stoler, *Along the Archival Grain: Epistemic Anxieties and Colonial Common Sense* (Princeton: Princeton University Press, 2009), 32.

74. Mercedes Prieto, *Liberalismo y temor: Imaginando los sujetos indígenas en el Ecuador postcolonial, 1895–1950* (Quito: FLACSO, 2004).

75. Becker, *Indians and Leftists.*

76. O'Connor, *Gender, Indian, Nation.*

77. Esben Leifsen, "Moralities and Politics of Belonging: Governing Female Reproduction in Twentieth Century Quito," PhD diss., University of Oslo, 2006, 225.

78. In 1950 both urban and rural women had lower literacy rates than men in those regions. Having benefited from the expansion of primary education, younger men and women (ages ten through fourteen in 1950) were almost equal in literacy in each zone: 87.7 percent of urban males, 85.3 percent of urban females, 50.5 percent of rural males, and 47.8 percent of rural females were literate. However, among those age sixty-five and over in 1950, literacy rates were 80.1 percent of urban males, 62.7 percent of urban females, 39.4 percent of rural males, and only 17.6 percent of rural females. Saunders, *People of Ecuador,* chapter 8.

79. Compare Marisol de la Cadena, "'Women Are More Indian': Ethnicity and Gender in a Community near Cuzco," in *Ethnicity, Markets, and Migration in the Andes,* edited by Brooke Larson and Olivia Harris (Durham: Duke University Press, 1995), 329–48; and Smith, "Race-Class-Gender Ideology."

80. See Mercedes Prieto's recent research on these issues: "Las trampas del silencio: Estado y mujeres indígenas en Ecuador, 1925–1975," presented at the conference Off-Centered States: State Formation and Deformation in the Andes, Quito, May 2010;

and "Rosa Lema y la misión cultural ecuatoriana indígena a Estados Unidos: Turismo, artesanías y desarrollo," in *Galo Plaza y su época*, edited by Carlos de la Torre and Mireya Salgado (Quito: FLACSO and Fundación Galo Plaza Lasso, 2008), 157–91.

## Chapter 2. Gender, Class, and State in Child Protection Programs in Quito

1. For an extended Latin American case study, see Donna Guy's *Women Build the Welfare State: Performing Charity and Creating Rights in Argentina, 1880–1955* (Durham: Duke University Press, 2009), which has influenced the analysis presented here. The various chapters collected in Seth Koven and Sonya Michel, eds., *Mothers of a New World: Maternalist Politics and the Origins of Welfare States* (New York: Routledge, 1993), explore women's participation in child welfare activities in a range of European, U.S., and Australian historical conjunctures. For studies that aim to capture more of children's experience, see Tobias Hecht, ed., *Minor Omissions: Children in Latin American History* (Madison: University of Wisconsin Press, 2002).

2. Esben Leifsen's research on child circulation, popular practices, and state action in Quito focuses especially on the period following the 1938 Child Code; see Leifsen's "Moralities and Politics of Belonging: Governing Female Reproduction in Twentieth Century Quito," PhD diss., University of Oslo, 2006. A preliminary analysis of the contours of public discussions of child welfare in the early twentieth century can be found in A. Kim Clark, "Género, raza y nación: La protección a la infancia en el Ecuador, 1910–1945," in *Palabras del silencio: Las mujeres latinoamericanas y su historia*, edited by Martha Moscoso (Quito: Abya-Yala, DGIS-Holanda, and UNICEF, 1995), 219–56.

3. See Abelardo Moncayo, *Informe del ministro de lo interior y policía, beneficencia, etc. al congreso ordinario de 1898* (Quito: Imprenta Nacional, 1898), 19. Guayaquil's prosperous commercial economy based on a busy import-export trade provided more disposable income for philanthropic activities than highlands agriculture. For a fascinating analysis of the Guayaquil Junta de Beneficencia, see Patricia de la Torre, *Lo privado y local en el estado ecuatoriano: La Junta de Beneficencia de Guayaquil* (Quito: Abya Yala, 1999).

4. Two additional sources of financing for Beneficencia programs were: (1) line items in the national budget, and (2) various donations or bequests earmarked by the donors for specific projects.

5. Octavio Díaz, minister of the interior, to the president of the Junta de Beneficencia, Quito, 25 October 1910, AAP/MNM.

6. Abelardo Moncayo, *Informe del ministro de lo interior y policía, beneficencia, etc. al congreso de 1899* (Quito: Imprenta Nacional, 1899), 16.

7. See Modesto A. Peñaherrera, *Informe que Modesto A. Peñaherrera, ministro de lo interior, municipalidades, policía, obras públicas, etc., presenta a la nación en 1916* (Quito: Imprenta y Encuadernación Nacionales, 1916), cx; and León Becerra, "Informe del director general de sanidad pública," appendix to Peñaherrera, *Informe . . . 1916*, 546.

8. Ann Blum's *Domestic Economies: Family, Work, and Welfare in Mexico City,*

*1884–1943* (Lincoln: University of Nebraska Press, 2010) influenced the interpretation presented here of the Ecuadorian archival materials, although her close analysis of admission and release records at Mexico City's foundling home unfortunately could not be matched for Quito's orphanages.

9. Sor María, visitadora, to the president of the Junta de Beneficencia, Quito, 26 July 1901, Archivo de la Asistencia Pública/Museo Nacional de Medicina (AAP/MNM). The figure appears to include both orphans and abandoned children.

10. "Informes sobre protección maternal y puericultura en el Ecuador, para la Asociación Internacional de Higiene Infantil de Washington," appendix to the subdirector de sanidad to the minister of sanidad, Quito, 18 October 1922, Archivo del Servicio de Sanidad/Museo Nacional de Medicina (ASS/MNM).

11. Dr. Luis M. de la Torre, physician of the Casa San Vicente to the director of asistencia pública, Quito, 2 April 1928, AAP/MNM.

12. Manuel Jijón Larrea, inspector of San Carlos, to the president of the Junta de Beneficencia, Quito, 30 July 1903, AAP/MNM.

13. Sor María Eudocia, superiora of La Providencia, to the president of the Junta de Beneficencia, Quito, 10 May 1909, AAP/MNM.

14. "Informes sobre protección maternal y puericultura en el Ecuador, para la Asociación Internacional de Higiene Infantil de Washington," appendix to the subdirector of sanidad to the minister of sanidad, Quito, 18 October 1922, ASS/MNM.

15. Sor Josefina to the president of the Junta de Beneficencia, Quito, undated 1915, AAP/MNM.

16. Lino Cárdenas to the president of the Junta de Beneficencia, Quito, 6 June 1912, AAP/MNM.

17. Superiora del Buen Pastor to the governor of Pichincha province, Quito, 21 January 1918, AAP/MNM.

18. José L. Román, provincial director of education, to the director general of Beneficencia, Quito, 15 June 1920, AAP/MNM.

19. See, for instance, Miguel Ortiz to the president of the Junta de Beneficencia, Quito, 7 November 1911; and Modesto A. Peñaherrera, minister of the interior, to the president of the Junta de Beneficencia, Quito, 20 November 1915, both AAP/MNM.

20. Contract signed in Quito, 31 July 1919, AAP/MNM.

21. Contract signed by Temistocles Terán, director of the Junta Central de Beneficencia, Quito, 30 September 1922, AAP/MNM.

22. Contract between Señorita Carmen Tobar and the Junta Central de Beneficencia, Quito, 7 August 1924, AAP/MNM.

23. Petition from Obdulia Chiriboga de Araujo to the director of the Junta de Beneficencia, Quito, 15 November 1920, AAP/MNM.

24. Contract between Angel F. Araujo and Obdulia Chiriboga de Araujo and the Junta Central de Beneficencia, Quito, 2 June 1923, AAP/MNM.

25. President of the Tribunal de Menores de Pichincha to the director of the Junta Central de Asistencia Pública, Quito, 20 April 1945, LCR 1945-I, AAP/MNM. See also Leifsen, "Moralities and Politics of Belonging," 181.

26. The debates over and provisions in the 1948 adoption law are discussed in Leifsen, "Moralities and Politics of Belonging."

27. Sixto M. Durán, provincial intendente general of police, to the director of the Junta Central de Beneficencia, Quito, 22 September 1920, AAP/MNM.

28. Petition from Virginia V. v. de Pinto to the director of the Junta Central de Beneficencia, Quito, first half of 1922 (undated), LCR-1922-I, AAP/MNM.

29. Lola Crespo de Ortiz Bilbao, *Mi vida tal como la conté a uno de mis hijos* (Quito: Corporación Editora Nacional, 2003), 55–56. For analyses of a range of practices of child circulation in various Latin American contexts, see, for Quito, Leifsen, "Moralities and Politics of Belonging"; for Mexico City, Blum, *Domestic Economies*, and Blum, "Cleaning the Revolutionary Household: Domestic Servants and Public Welfare in Mexico City, 1900–1935," *Journal of Women's History* 15, no. 4 (2004): 67–90; and for Peru, Jessaca Leinaweaver, *The Circulation of Children: Kinship, Adoption, and Morality in Andean Peru* (Durham: Duke University Press, 2008).

30. Petition from Rosa M. Valdez de Corral and Jose M. Francisco Corral to the president of the Junta de Beneficencia, Quito, 2 February 1917, AAP/MNM.

31. Luis Rosalino Cruz to the Junta de Beneficencia, Quito, 30 September 1927, LCR 1927-II, AAP/MNM.

32. Petition from Carlos Ochoa to the Junta Central de Asistencia Pública, Quito, 5 October 1927, AAP/MNM.

33. Petition from Genoveva Ortega to the Junta Central de Asistencia Pública, Quito, 10 October 1927, AAP/MNM.

34. See, for instance, Lino Cárdenas to the president of the Junta de Beneficencia, Quito, 6 June 1912, AAP/MNM.

35. Carlos R. Sánchez, "Protección a la infancia," *Anales de la Universidad Central* 246 (1923): 62.

36. José L. Román to the president of the Junta de Beneficencia, Quito, 5 October 1911, AAP/MNM. By 1914, Román was provincial director of education for Pichincha.

37. Lino Cárdenas to the president of the Junta de Beneficencia, Quito, 6 June 1912, AAP/MNM.

38. Petition from Rosa Zumba to the president of the Junta de Beneficencia, Quito, end of 1915, AAP/MNM.

39. Petition from Margarita Valencia de Valencia to the director of the Junta Central de Beneficencia, Quito, second half of 1923 (undated), LCR-1923-II, AAP/MNM.

40. José María Vera to the president of the Junta Central de Beneficencia, Quito, 2 May 1922, AAP/MNM.

41. Miguel Ortiz to the president of the Junta de Beneficencia, Quito, 7 November 1911, AAP/MNM.

42. Petition from Emperatriz Escobar de Ruiz to the president of the Junta de Asistencia Pública, Quito, 23 August 1937, LCR 1937-II, AAP/MNM.

43. J. M. Quiñones, comisario de orden y seguridad, to the president of the Junta de Beneficencia, Quito, 3 May 1906, AAP/MNM.

44. Ann Zulawski offers an excellent analysis of the medicalization of inappropriate behavior as mental health problems in her *Unequal Cures: Public Health and Political Change in Bolivia, 1900–1950* (Durham: Duke University Press, 2007), chapter 5.

45. Director of the hospicio and manicomio to the chief of the inspección de farmacias y profesiones médicas, Quito, 12 November 1947, LCR (Jefatura de Farmacias y Profesiones Médicas) 1947-I, ASS/MNM.

46. Kristin Ruggiero, "Wives on 'Deposit': Internment and the Preservation of Husbands' Honor in Late Nineteenth-Century Buenos Aires," *Journal of Family History* 17, no. 3 (1992): 253–70.

47. María H. del Hierro to the president of the Junta de Beneficencia, Quito, undated (between 1906 and 1909), AAP/MNM.

48. Petition from Rosario Vaca v. de Aguirre to the president of the Junta de Beneficencia, Quito, 5 November 1921, AAP/MNM.

49. Rosario Baca v. de Aguirre to the president of the Junta de Beneficencia, Quito, 22 December 1923, AAP/MNM.

50. Sor M. Magdalena, superiora of the Orfelinato de San Vicente de Paul, to the director of the Junta Central de Asistencia Pública, Quito, 13 February 1936, LCR 1936-I, AAP/MNM.

51. Sor M. Magdalena, superiora of the Orfelinato de San Vicente de Paul, to the director of the Junta Central de Asistencia Pública, Quito, 14 May 1936, LCR 1936-I, AAP/MNM.

52. Of all of the documents that evoke the Dickensian world of orphaned and abandoned children in Quito, perhaps none does so more than the 1922 response of the police chief to a reminder that before sending children on to orphanages, police officials should first obtain an admission slip from the Beneficencia. This was impossible for very young infants, he explained, because they might be found at any time of the day or night and needed immediate lactation or they would perish. "There have been occasions when infants have been found at unearthly hours and it has been impossible to attend to them if there are not by chance *mujeres contraventoras* [arrested women] in the cells of the Police station, and the infants have perished" (Sixto M. Durán, provincial intendente general de policía, to the director of the Junta Central de Beneficencia, Quito, 18 August 1922, AAP/MNM). The image of hungry abandoned infants being nursed by women held temporarily in the jail suggests that these women may have been prostitutes. However, given the general lack of access to contraceptive resources, many or most sexually active women experienced ongoing cycles of pregnancy and breast-feeding throughout their reproductive lives that might allow them to feed such infants on a moment's notice.

53. "Informes sobre protección maternal y puericultura en el Ecuador, para la Asociación Internacional de Higiene Infantil de Washington," appendix to the subdirector of sanidad to the minister of sanidad, Quito, 18 October 1922, ASS/MNM.

54. Ann Blum has pointed to the relationship between public welfare institutions for the children of poor women and the preferences of employers for domestic

servants without distractions from their own children in her "Cleaning the Revolutionary Household."

55. José María Suárez M., president of the Sociedad Protectora de la Infancia, to the director of the Junta Central de Asistencia Pública, Quito, 21 September 1931, LCR 1931-II, AAP/MNM.

56. Carlos A. Miño, subdirector of sanidad, to the president of the Junta de Beneficencia, 9 February 1914, LCR 1914, AAP/MNM.

57. Guillermo Bustos, "Quito en la transición: Actores colectivos e identidades culturales urbanas (1920–1950)," in *Quito a través de la historia* (Quito: Municipio de Quito, 1992), 163–88.

58. Modesto A. Peñaherrera, *Informe que Modesto A. Peñaherrera, ministro de lo interior, municipalidades, policía, obras públicas, etc., presenta a la nación en 1913* (Quito: Imprenta y Encuadernación Nacionales, 1913), xxxiii.

59. Antonio J. Bastidas, *Contribución al estudio de la protección infantil en el Ecuador y demografía nacional* (Quito: Imprenta Municipal, 1924), 51.

60. L. Estuardo Prado, "La protección de la infancia en el Ecuador," *Revista del Centro de Estudiantes de Medicina* 13–14 (third series, 1930): 15. In 1927, Prado had been the medical intern at the Gota de Leche.

61. Michel Foucault, "Governmentality," in *The Foucault Effect: Studies in Governmentality*, edited by Graham Burchell, Colin Gordon, and Peter Miller (Chicago: University of Chicago Press, 1991), 87–104. For an example of an ethnographic application of this concept to a child welfare project, see Akhil Gupta, "Governing Population: The Integrated Child Development Services Program in India," in *States of Imagination: Ethnographic Explorations of the Postcolonial State*, edited by Thomas Blom Hansen and Finn Stepputat (Durham: Duke University Press, 2001), 65–96.

62. See Eduardo Kingman Garcés, *La ciudad y los otros, Quito 1860–1940: Higienismo, ornato y policía* (Quito: FLACSO and Universidad Rovira e Virgili, 2006).

63. See Bruce Curtis, *The Politics of Population: State Formation, Statistics, and the Census of Canada, 1840–1875* (Toronto: University of Toronto Press, 2001), chapter 1.

64. For Chile, see Jadwiga Pieper Mooney, *The Politics of Motherhood: Maternity and Women's Rights in Twentieth-Century Chile* (Pittsburgh: University of Pittsburgh Press, 2009); for Costa Rica and Cold War fertility-control policies, see María Carranza, "'In the Name of Forests': Highlights of the History of Family Planning in Costa Rica," *Canadian Journal of Latin American and Caribbean Studies* 35, no. 69 (2010): 119–54.

65. Carlos R. Sánchez, "La importancia del estudio de puericultura en la enseñanza escolar," *Anales de la Universidad Central* 41, no. 265 (1928): 18.

66. Luis G. Dávila, "La Gota de Leche: Lo que se puede aguardar en Quito de esta obra de protección infantil," *Anales de la Universidad Central* 31, no. 247 (1923): 199–254, 200.

67. Sánchez, "Protección a la infancia," 64.

68. Gonzalo Córdova, *Informe del ministro de lo interior y policía, obras públicas, etc. al congreso ordinario de 1903* (Quito: Imprenta Nacional, 1903), 23–24.

69. For analyses of the social arguments embedded in the 1950 census, see A. Kim Clark, "Race, 'Culture' and Mestizaje: The Statistical Construction of the Ecuadorian Nation, 1930–1950," *Journal of Historical Sociology* 11, no. 2 (1998): 185–211; and Mercedes Prieto, *Liberalismo y temor: Imaginando los sujetos indígenas en el Ecuador postcolonial, 1895–1950* (Quito: FLACSO, 2004), chapter 5.

70. León Becerra, "Informe de la Dirección del Servicio de Sanidad Pública del Ecuador," appendix to Modesto A. Peñaherrera, *Informe que Modesto A. Peñaherrera, ministro de lo interior, municipalidades, policía, obras públicas, etc., presenta a la nación en 1914* (Quito: Imprenta y Encuadernación Nacionales, 1914), 434.

71. Carlos Miño, "Informe de la Subdirección de Sanidad de la provincia de Pichincha al ministro de sanidad y al director del Servicio de Sanidad Pública," appendix to Peñaherrera, *Informe que . . . 1914*, 442.

72. Delegate of sanidad to Charles Baker, Quito, 11 September 1913, LCE 1913, ASS/MNM.

73. Acting governor of Pichincha (jefe político Rafael Grijalva Polanco) to delegate of sanidad for Pichincha, Quito, 24 September 1913, LCR 1913, ASS/MNM.

74. Carlos A. Miño, subdirector of sanidad for Pichincha, to the president of the Junta de Beneficencia, 9 February 1914, LCR 1914-I, AAP/MNM.

75. Miño, "Informe de la Subdirección de Sanidad," 445.

76. A. Villamar to the president of the Junta de Beneficencia, Quito, 6 May 1915, AAP/MNM.

77. Semestral report of Carlos García Drouet, director of the dispensario, to the president of the Junta de Beneficencia, Quito, 11 July 1917, AAP/MNM.

78. Dr. Carlos García Drouet to the director of the Junta de Beneficencia, Quito, 17 February 1920, AAP/MNM.

79. Sánchez had previously been one of the assistant physicians at the dispensario and went on to serve as director and médico ad honorem of the clinic until 1937 (thus working a full two decades there), combining these duties with his role as chief physician of the pediatric ward at the Hospital Eugenio Espejo following its 1933 inauguration. He also had teaching duties as professor of pediatrics at the Universidad Central.

80. Dr. Carlos R. Sánchez to the director of the Junta Central de Beneficencia, Quito, 1 February 1924, AAP/MNM.

81. Secretary and chief of statistics at the Subdirección de Sanidad de Pichincha to the encargado of the Dirección de Sanidad in Guayaquil, Quito, 15 May 1923, LCE-1923 ASS/MNM.

82. Carlos Andrade Marín, *La protección a la infancia en el Ecuador* (Quito, 1929), 76.

83. Salvador Allende, *La realidad médico-social chilena*, second edition (1939; reprint, Santiago: Editorial Cuarto Propio, 1999), 110.

84. See, for instance, Antonio J. Bastidas, *La ilegitimidad, factor de letalidad infantil* (Quito: Imprenta de la Universidad Central, 1932).

85. President of the Sociedad de La Gota de Leche to the director of Beneficencia, Quito, 14 June 1920, APP/MNM.

86. "Informes sobre protección maternal y puericultura en el Ecuador, para la Asociación Internacional de Higiene Infantil de Washington," appendix to the subdirector of sanidad to the minister of sanidad, Quito, 18 October 1922, ASS/MNM.

87. Luz María Freile de Zaldumbide, president of the Sociedad de La Gota de Leche, to the president of the Junta Central de Beneficencia, Quito, 27 November 1920, AAP/MNM.

88. On the SNA and the Ley de Fomento Agrícola, see Clark, *Redemptive Work*, chapter 5; for a broader analysis of the SNA, see Carlos Arcos, "El espíritu de progreso: Los hacendados en el Ecuador del 900," *Cultura* 19 (1984): 107–34.

89. This funding was also potentially available to similar institutions in the provinces, but only in 1934 were the first steps taken to establish a Gota de Leche in the provincial capital Ambato, for instance, an initiative of the women's auxiliary to the Tungurahua provincial branch of the Cruz Roja Ecuatoriana, which received some funding from the Junta Central de Asistencia Pública. See Señora Blanca Martínez de Tinajero, president of the Asociación de Damas de la Cruz Roja de Tungurahua, to the director of asistencia pública, Ambato, 13 August 1934 and 5 October 1934, LCR 1934-II, AAP/MNM.

90. President of the Sociedad de San Vicente de Paul to the director of the Junta Central de Asistencia Pública, Quito, 4 September 1931, LCR 1931-II, AAP/MNM. Note that this account of the society's history and activities was typed partially on pages of letterhead of the Sociedad de las Señoras de la Caridad and partially on the stationery of the Conferencia de San Vicente de Paul, a material indication of the linked operations of these two associations.

91. Gioconda Herrera, "El congreso católico de mujeres en 1909 y la regeneración de la nación," in *Celebraciones centenarias y negociaciones por la nación ecuatoriana*, edited by Valeria Coronel and Mercedes Prieto (Quito: FLACSO and Ministerio de Cultura, 2010), 241–63.

92. The first Ecuadorian Red Cross association was established in 1910 in Guayaquil by a group of the port's physicians in the context of a border conflict with Peru. In the second half of 1922, the national Cruz Roja Ecuatoriana (CRE) was formally established as an affiliate of the international League of Red Cross Associations partly through the efforts of Luis Robalino Dávila, the Ecuadorian consul in Switzerland. Because Robalino's diplomatic activities made it difficult for him to personally direct the CRE, he was succeeded in the CRE presidency in 1924 by Dr. Isidro Ayora.

93. Cruz Roja solicitation to Dr. Luis G. Dávila, 27 November 1925, LCR-1925-II, ASS/MNM.

94. Leifsen has argued that a guiding focus on children's rights only became dominant in Ecuador after the country ratified the 1989 U.N. Convention of the Rights of the Child (in 1990), with a rewriting of the Child Code in 1992 that implemented the basic principles of the rights of the child. This was partly the result of the interventions of children's rights activists who had gained prominence in the 1980s (a decade that also saw a proliferation of NGOs working in Ecuador in various fields) in

the context of some public scandals involving irregularities in adoption processes (see Leifsen, "Moralities and Politics of Belonging," chapter 8).

95. Miño was likely referring not only to European or North American centers but also to Guayaquil, where private philanthropy had a stronger tradition than in Quito (perhaps in part due to the greater disposable income generated by coastal export production compared to highland production for the domestic market).

96. Carlos A. Miño, subdirector of sanidad, to the director of the Junta de Beneficencia Nacional, Quito, 2 December 1920, AAP/MNM.

97. Director of the Junta Central de Beneficencia to the subdirector of sanidad, Quito, 7 December 1920, ASS/MNM.

98. Subdirector of sanidad to the president of the Sociedad Gota de Leche, Quito, 13 December 1920, ASS/MNM.

99. Rector of the Universidad Central to the president of the Junta Central de Beneficencia, Quito, 13 December 1920, AAP/MNM.

100. "Informes sobre protección maternal y puericultura en el Ecuador, para la Asociación Internacional de Higiene Infantil de Washington," appendix to the subdirector de sanidad to the minister of sanidad, Quito, 18 October 1922, ASS/MNM. Following his 1916 graduation as a physician from the Universidad Central, Bastidas traveled to Paris to undertake specialist studies in pediatrics until 1919. After working for a few years as the appointed physician of the rather precarious in-patient facilities for children at the Hospital Civil, he worked for a time for the sanidad and was subsequently appointed profesor de medicina legal at the Universidad Central.

101. María Lasso de Eastman, vice president of the Sociedad de La Gota de Leche, to the jefe de asistencia pública del Distrito Norte de Sanidad, Quito, 10 October 1925, LCR-1925-II, ASS/MNM. Ayora was at the time on the brink of being named minister of social welfare; he was also serving as the president of the Cruz Roja Ecuatoriana as well as director for some fifteen years by then of Quito's Maternidad. Pablo Arturo Suárez, in turn, would be named the new director general of sanidad in mid-1926, when the institution's main office was moved to Quito. Señora Lasso succeeded to the presidency of the Gota soon after she sent this letter.

102. María Lasso de Eastman, president of the Sociedad de La Gota de Leche, to the director of sanidad del Distrito Norte, 20 November 1925, LCR-1925-II, ASS/MNM.

103. Director of the Distrito Norte del Servicio de Sanidad Pública to the president of the Sociedad de La Gota de Leche, Quito, 28 November 1925, LCE-1925, ASS/MNM.

104. President of the Sociedad de La Gota de Leche to the director del Distrito Norte del Servicio de Sanidad Pública, Quito, 2 December 1925, LCR-1925-II, ASS/ MNM.

105. José María Suárez M., president of the Sociedad Protectora de la Infancia, to the director of the Junta Central de Asistencia Pública, Quito, 21 September 1931, LCR 1931-II, AAP/MNM.

106. Pedro P. Garaicoa, minister of previsión social of the Junta de Gobierno Provisional, to the director de sanidad del Distrito Norte, Quito, 30 December 1925, LCR-1925-II, ASS/MNM.

107. While medical professionals provided significant unpaid services to institutions, such activities were taken into account when the state began to make paid appointments on a more competitive, less ad hoc, basis following the Juliana. Thus, for instance, on 21 December 1926 a special commission of the Junta Central de Asistencia Pública met to appoint the médico del Dispensario de Niños and of the San Vicente de Paul orphanage and the ayudante del médico de la Maternidad. Evaluating the candidates' records of theoretical training within and outside the country and practical experience in pediatrics and obstetrics, respectively, Dr. Araujo received the appointment at the dispensario and orphanage, while medical student Antonio Román demonstrated equal theoretical and practical training in obstetrics as his main competitor, but more "appointments in various positions [*nombramientos para diversos servicios*]" that were the deciding factor in giving him the ayudante position. Concurso, Quito, 21 December 1926, AAP/MNM.

108. M. Diaz B. and L. Calderón Paz to the director of the Junta Central de Asistencia Pública, Quito, 1 December 1926, AAP/MNM.

109. Señora Victoria de Cueva García, secretary of the Sociedad de La Gota de Leche, to the director of the Junta Central de Asistencia Pública, Quito, 4 September 1931, LCR 1931-II, AAP/MNM.

110. Sor Josefina to the president of the Junta de Beneficencia, Quito, 5 October 1916, LCR AAP/MNM.

111. "Informes sobre protección maternal y puericultura en el Ecuador, para la Asociación Internacional de Higiene Infantil de Washington," appendix to the subdirector of sanidad to the minister of sanidad, Quito, 18 October 1922, ASS/MNM.

112. Sor Josefina, superiora de San Carlos, Quito, 31 March 1924, AAP/MNM.

113. Draft budget, Casa Cuna, first half of 1924 (undated), AAP/MNM.

114. "Reglamento Interno de la Casa Cuna," second half of 1924, LCE 1924-II, AAP/MNM.

115. Dr. Luis G. Dávila to the director of the Junta Central de Beneficencia, Quito, 30 September 1924, AAP/MNM.

116. A more substantial reorganization occurred in February the next year, when among other things, the main office of the Servicio de Sanidad was moved to Quito from Guayaquil.

117. Dr. Luis G. Dávila, director of the Distrito Norte del Servicio de Sanidad Pública, to the director of the Junta Central de Beneficencia, Quito, 1 October 1925, AAP/MNM.

118. Luis G. Dávila to the director of the Junta Central de Beneficencia, Quito, 12 December 1925, AAP/MNM.

119. The quotations in this and the following paragraph are from Memorandum by Dr. Luis de la Torre to the director of the Junta Central de Asistencia Pública, Quito, 6 September 1927, LCR 1927-II, AAP/MNM.

120. Ibid.

121. Dr. Luis de la Torre, physician of the Casa Cuna, to the director general of Asistencia Pública, Quito, 24 December 1927, LCR 1927-II, AAP/MNM.

122. Dr. Luis de la Torre to the president of the Junta Central de Asistencia Pública, Quito, 20 December 1928, LCR 1928-II, AAP/MNM.

123. See Ann Blum's interesting analysis in her chapter "Dying of Sadness: Hospitalism and Child Welfare in Mexico City," in *Disease in the History of Modern Latin America*, edited by Diego Armus (Durham: Duke University Press, 2003), 209–36.

124. Dr. Cesar Jácome, secretary of the Sociedad Ecuatoriana de la Cruz Roja, to the director general of the Junta Central de Asistencia Pública, Quito, 18 March 1937 and 4 May 1937, both LCR 1937-I, AAP/MNM.

125. Director general of sanidad to the director of asistencia pública, Quito, 3 June 1929, LCR 1929, AAP/MNM.

126. Dr. Braulio Pozo i Diaz to the director of the Junta Central de Asistencia Pública, Quito, 30 July 1928, AAP/MNM.

127. Director general of sanidad to the director of the Junta Central de Asistencia Pública, Quito, 9 January 1930, LCE 1930-I, ASS/MNM.

128. Dr. Eduardo Batallas to the director of the Junta Central de Asistencia Pública, Quito, 6 February 1931, LCR 1931-I, AAP/MNM.

129. Dr. Carlos R. Sánchez, director of the Dispensario de Niños, to the director of the Junta de Asistencia Pública, Quito, 19 April 1932, LCR 1932-II, AAP/MNM.

130. In 1931 Señorita Carrera was twenty-four years old and unmarried. She was probably a paternal orphan (her mother was named in the university records as legally responsible for her). This is the first reference found in the AAP to the employment status of a nursing graduate.

131. There is a more modern feel to the facilities of the children's ward at the Hospital Eugenio Espejo, such as the establishment of a playground beside it to be used for convalescing children, staffed by a primary schoolteacher from the provincial department of education (provincial director of education for Pichincha to the director of the Junta Central de Asistencia Pública, Quito, 7 July 1934, LCR 1934-II, AAP/MNM).

132. Director general of sanidad to the director of the Junta Central de Asistencia Pública, Quito, 4 April 1933, LCR 1933-I, AAP/MNM.

133. Director of sanidad to the minister of previsión social y sanidad, Quito, 4 January 1938, LCE 1938-I, ASS/MNM.

134. In 1938 the first School of Social Workers was established, which functioned for two years and graduated approximately twenty-five women. In 1944 the minister of social welfare sought assistance from the Children's Bureau in Washington, D.C., to establish a professional social work school in Ecuador, which was created in Quito in 1945 as the Escuela Nacional de Trabajadores Sociales. That year also saw the establishment of the Catholic Mariana de Jesús Social Work School in Quito. See Leifsen, "Moralities and Politics of Belonging," chapter 7, for information on the interventions of social workers in child protection in the 1940s. While social workers undoubtedly advanced new forms of social control in some ways, they may also have promoted alternative visions of social responsibility. See Karin Rosemblatt's interesting discussion of Chilean social workers in her *Gendered Compromises: Political*

*Cultures and the State in Chile, 1920–1950* (Chapel Hill: University of North Carolina Press, 2000).

135. Report on child welfare presented to the Junta Central de Asistencia Pública by Pablo Arturo Suárez and Gregorio Ormaza, Quito, 12 May 1938, LCR 1938-I, AAP/MNM.

136. Sor María Josefa, visitadora of the Hijas de la Caridad, to the president of the Junta Central de Asistencia Pública, Quito, 9 December 1940, LCR 1940-II, AAP/MNM.

137. Abelardo Moncayo, *Informe del ministro de lo interior y policía, beneficencia, etc. al congreso ordinario de 1900* (Quito: Imprenta Nacional, 1900), xvi.

138. Modesto A. Peñaherrera, minister of the interior, to the president of the Junta de Beneficencia de Quito, Quito, 8 May 1914, AAP/MNM.

139. Sor Cecilia, superiora of the hospicio and manicomio de San Lázaro, to the president of the Junta de Beneficencia, Quito, 4 May 1914, AAP/MNM.

140. Modesto A. Peñaherrera, minister of the interior, to the president of the Junta de Beneficencia, Quito, 6 July 1915, APP/MNM.

141. Leopoldo Seminario to the president of the Junta de Beneficencia, Quito, undated 1915, AAP/MNM.

142. See, for instance, the appointments specified in subsecretary of the ministry of previsión social y trabajo to the director of the Junta Central de Asistencia Pública, Quito, 30 March 1939, LCR 1939-I, AAP/MNM.

143. César Mantilla to the president of the Beneficencia, Quito, 11 December 1915, AAP/MNM. Mantilla was also the founder and owner of Quito's most important daily newspaper, *El comercio*, which was founded in 1906 and continues to be published today.

144. President of the Escuela Militar's Comité "Pro Infancia" to the president of the Junta de Beneficencia, Quito, 9 August 1918, AAP/MNM.

145. President of the Rotary Club of Quito to the director of asistencia pública, Quito, 16 November 1935, LCR 1935-II, AAP/MNM.

146. Letter transcribed in provincial director of education for Pichincha to the director of the Junta Central de Asistencia Pública, Quito, 14 October 1932, LCR 1932-II, AAP/MNM.

147. Petition transcribed in minister of education to the director of asistencia pública, Quito, 4 December 1934, LCR 1934-II, AAP/MNM.

148. Petition transcribed in minister of gobierno y previsión social to the director of the Junta Central de Asistencia Pública, Quito, 8 February 1933, LCR 1933-I, AAP/MNM.

149. Director of the Hermandad Ferroviaria to the director of asistencia pública, Quito, 4 June 1933, LCR 1933-I, AAP/MNM.

150. Señora Agripina de Suárez, president of the Comité Pro-habilitamiento del Pabellón de Niños del Hospital Eugenio Espejo, to the president of the Junta de Asistencia Pública, Quito, 14 June 1933, LCR 1933-I, AAP/MNM.

151. Secretary of the Sindicato de Madera to the director of asistencia pública,

Quito, 6 September 1935, and president of the Sociedad de Carpinteros Unión y Trabajo to the director of asistencia pública, Quito, 30 August 1935, both LCR 1935-II, AAP/MNM.

152. General secretary of the Asociación Sindical de Trabajadores del Fósforo, to the director of the Junta de Beneficencia, Quito, 27 May 1937, 26 August 1937, and 21 September 1937, LCR 1937-I and 1937-II, AAP/MNM. Less frequently, factory owners also solicited spots for the children of their female workers (see, for instance, general director of the Compañía Anónima La Industrial to the director of asistencia pública, Quito, 1 June 1936, LCR 1936-I, AAP/MNM).

153. Octavio Díaz, *Informe que a la nación presenta el ministro de lo interior, policía, beneficencia, obras públicas, etc., en el año 1910* (Quito: Imprenta y Encuadernación Nacionales, 1910), xxii–xxiii. For an earlier period, see Cynthia Milton, *The Many Meanings of Poverty: Colonialism, Social Compacts, and Assistance in Eighteenth-Century Ecuador* (Stanford: Stanford University Press, 2007).

154. Transcribed in subsecretary of the ministry of previsión social, trabajo, agricultura e industrias to the director of sanidad for the central zone, Quito, 14 February 1938, LCR-Ministerio 1938, ASS/MNM.

155. Alfredo Espinosa Tamayo, *Consejos a las madres: Cartilla higiénica de puericultura* (Guayaquil: Imprenta La Reforma, 1914), 10.

156. Emiliano J. Crespo, "Conferencia sobre puericultura," *Revista de la Universidad de Cuenca* 7 (1926): 10.

157. R. P. Fr. Ricardo Delgado Capeáns, *Deberes de la madre cristiana* (Quito: Tipografía y Encuadernación de la "Prensa Católica," 1923).

158. Andrade Marín, *La protección a la infancia*, 89.

159. Dávila, "Gota de Leche," 202.

160. Bastidas, *La ilegitimidad*, 8.

161. María Cuvi Sánchez, ed., *Quito casa adentro: Narrado por mujeres* (Quito: FONSAL, 2009), 20.

## Chapter 3. Governing Sexuality and Disease

1. The minister of finance, acting for the minister of the interior, to the subdirector of sanidad, Quito, 23 June 1911, LC 1911–12, ASS/MNM.

2. For other activities of the Oficina de Higiene Municipal before 1908, see Eduardo Kingman Garcés, *La ciudad y los otros, Quito 1860–1940: Higienismo, ornato y policía* (Quito: FLACSO and Universidad Rovira e Virgili, 2006), chapter 6.

3. The jefe político, acting governor of Pichincha province, to the subdirector of sanidad, Quito, 5 September 1913, LC 1913, ASS/MNM.

4. Report of the chief of the servicio de profilaxis venérea to the director of sanidad for the central zone, Quito, 19 April 1943, Informes y Conferencias 1937–1946, ASS/ MNM. For a pioneering study of the concept of racial poisons in Latin America, see Nancy Leys Stepan, *"The Hour of Eugenics": Race, Gender, and Nation in Latin America* (Ithaca: Cornell University Press, 1991); for Ecuador, see A. Kim Clark, "Género, raza y nación: La protección a la infancia en el Ecuador, 1910–1945," in *Palabras*

*del silencio: Las mujeres latinoamericanas y su historia*, edited by Martha Moscoso (Quito: Abya-Yala, DGIS, and UNICEF, 1995), 219–56; and Clark, "Race, 'Culture' and Mestizaje: The Statistical Construction of the Ecuadorian Nation, 1930–1950," *Journal of Historical Sociology* 11, no. 2 (1998): 185–211.

5. The subdirector of sanidad to the acting governor of the province, Quito, 8 September 1913, LCE (Libro de Comunicaciones Enviadas) 1913, ASS/MNM.

6. The provincial chief of security and statistics to the subdirector of sanidad, Quito, 30 November 1920, LCR 1920, ASS/MNM. The chief was probably not suggesting that minor boys were prostituted, but rather that they had been exposed to venereal diseases via early sexual experiences.

7. The subdirector of sanidad to the provincial chief of security and statistics, Quito, 1 December 1920; and the subdirector of sanidad to the director of sanidad, Quito, 29 December 1920; both LCE 1920, ASS/MNM.

8. The arguments presented in this and the following paragraph were developed in support of a different analysis in A. Kim Clark, "El sexo y la responsabilidad en Quito: Prostitución, género y el estado, c. 1920–1950," *Procesos* 16 (2001): 35–59.

9. Donna J. Guy, *Sex and Danger in Buenos Aires: Prostitution, Family, and Nation in Argentina* (Lincoln: University of Nebraska Press, 1991); and Donna Guy, "Medical Imperialism Gone Awry: The Campaign against Legalized Prostitution in Latin America," in *Science, Medicine, and Cultural Imperialism*, edited by Teresa Meade and Mark Walker (New York: St. Martin's Press, 1991), 75–94.

10. Sueann Caulfield, "The Birth of Mangue: Race, Nation, and the Politics of Prostitution in Rio de Janeiro, 1850–1942," in *Sex and Sexuality in Latin America*, edited by Daniel Balderston and Donna J. Guy (New York: New York University Press, 1997), 86–100; and Sueann Caulfield, "Getting into Trouble: Dishonest Women, Modern Girls, and Women-Men in the Conceptual Language of *Vida Policial*, 1925–1927," *Signs* 19, no. 1 (1993): 146–76. See also Sandra Graham Lauderdale, "Slavery's Impasse: Slave Prostitutes, Small-Time Mistresses, and the Brazilian Law of 1871," *Comparative Studies in Society and History* 33–34 (1991): 669–94.

11. Katherine Elaine Bliss, *Compromised Positions: Prostitution, Public Health, and Gender Politics in Revolutionary Mexico City* (University Park: Pennsylvania State University Press, 2001). For an earlier period in Mexico, see William E. French, "Prostitutes and Guardian Angels: Women, Work, and the Family in Porfirian Mexico," *Hispanic American Historical Review* 72, no. 4 (1992): 529–53.

12. David McCreery, "'This Life of Misery and Shame': Female Prostitution in Guatemala City, 1880–1920," *Journal of Latin American Studies* 18, no. 2 (1986): 333–53.

13. "Breve noticia sobre protección maternal, puericultura y lucha antivenérea en el Ecuador," Quito, 15 February 1921, LCE 1921, ASS/MNM.

14. In subdirector of sanidad to the president of the Cruz Roja Ecuatoriana, Quito, undated (mid-January) 1925, LCE 1925-I, ASS/MNM.

15. Judith R. Walkowitz, *Prostitution and Victorian Society: Women, Class, and the State* (Cambridge: Cambridge University Press, 1980), 254.

16. When Salvarsan was discovered by Paul Ehrlich in 1909, it was more than a breakthrough for syphilis treatment; it was the first time a specific chemical compound was demonstrated to kill a specific microorganism. A modified version, Neosalvarsan, was the main treatment for syphilis until penicillin was shown to be effective in treating the disease in 1943, ushering in the era of antibiotics. Allan Brandt, "Sexually Transmitted Diseases," in *Companion Encyclopedia of the History of Medicine*, vol. 1, edited by W. F. Bynum and Roy Porter (London: Routledge, 1993), 572–73.

17. Pedro J. Zambrano, "Historia del reglamento de la prostitución," *Boletín sanitario* (Quito) 1, no. 1 (1926): 43.

18. Médico bacteriólogo of the servicio de profilaxis venérea to the subdirector of sanidad, Quito, 11 October 1921, LCR (Libro de Comunicaciones Recibidas) 1921, ASS/MNM.

19. The subdirector of sanidad to the director of sanidad, Quito, 8 July 1922, LCE 1922-II, ASS/MNM.

20. The subdirector of sanidad to the minister of sanidad, Quito, 8 February 1922, LCE 1922-I, ASS /MNM.

21. The subdirector of sanidad to the general jefe de estado mayor, Quito, 8 May 1922, LCE 1922-I, ASS/MNM.

22. The director of sanidad of the Distrito Norte to the corps of military surgeons, Quito, 5 December 1925, LCE 1925-II, ASS/MNM.

23. The presidential decree is dated 23 April 1927 and the regulation is dated 30 April 1927, ASS/MNM.

24. The inspector general of sanidad to the director general of sanidad, Quito, 14 September 1927, ASS HM 1927, ASS/MNM.

25. The director of sanidad of the Distrito Norte to the minister of sanidad, Quito, 12 December 1925, LCE 1925-II, ASS/MNM.

26. The director general of sanidad to the director of the Instituto Juan Montalvo, Quito, 2 June 1932, LCE-I 1932, ASS/MNM.

27. The acting director of sanidad to the director general of cárceles, Quito, 23 October 1926, LCE 1926-II, ASS/MNM.

28. The chief of the servicio de profilaxis venérea to the director general of sanidad, Quito, 10 June 1930, LCR-SI 1930, ASS/MNM. While the Sanidad could offer doses of mercury for the treatment of gonorrhea by the prison physician, the warden would have to send the prisoners under guard to the SPV for the administration of Neosalvarsan for syphilis, both because the injection technique was more complicated and because Zambrano carefully monitored the results of those treatments. The director general of sanidad to the director general of cárceles, Quito, 24 June 1930, LCE 1930-I, ASS/MNM.

29. In director of sanidad of the Distrito Norte to the director of the penitenciaria, Quito, 5 September 1925, LCE 1925-II, ASS/MNM, it is clear that prostitutes were freely entering and leaving the prison to offer their services. The director de sanidad

asked that the director of the prison suspend this practice for a few weeks during the reorganization of the Sanidad's services, since in the interim the SPV would be unable to monitor the health status of the prostitutes.

30. Zambrano, "Historia del reglamento," 44.

31. Circular of the director general of sanidad to the leaders of workers' organizations, Quito, 17 March 1927; and circular of the director general of sanidad to military and police surgeons, Quito, 19 March 1927; both LCE 1927, ASS/MNM.

32. Schedule of venereal prophylaxis classes offered in the dispensaries, 12 August 1927, DSTyOEC 1927, ASS/MNM.

33. The ayudante of the oficina de identificación dactiloscópica to the subdirector of sanidad, Quito, 15 June 1925, LCR 1925-I, ASS/MNM; and the subdirector of sanidad to the director of the oficina de identificación dactiloscópica, Quito, 14 August 1925, LCE 1925-II, ASS/MNM.

34. The director de sanidad for Pichincha to the intendente general of policía for Pichincha, Quito, 17 November 1925, LCE 1925-II, ASS/MNM.

35. The chief of identification of the intendencia de policía nacional to the director general of sanidad, Quito, 17 September 1928, LCR-G 1928, ASS/MNM.

36. Pedro Zambrano, *Estudio de la prostitución en Quito* (Quito: Imprenta Nacional, 1924), 21–28.

37. Zambrano, *Estudio de la prostitución*, 20.

38. Zambrano, *Estudio de la prostitución*, 26.

39. Enrique Garcés, *Por, para y del niño (tomo II)* (Quito: Talleres Gráficos de Educación, 1937), 116–24.

40. The subdirector of sanidad to the minister of sanidad, Quito, 8 February 1922, LCE 1922-I, ASS/MNM.

41. The subdirector of sanidad to the comisario tercero nacional, Quito, 15 March 1923, LCE 1923-I, ASS/MNM.

42. The director de sanidad to the juez primero cantonal, Quito, 10 December 1927, LCE 1927-II, ASS/MNM.

43. The director general of sanidad to the intendente general de policía de la provincia, Quito, 15 October 1934, LCE-II 1934, ASS/MNM.

44. The director general of sanidad to the comisario tercero nacional, Quito, 4 June 1935, and the director general of sanidad to the director of sanidad for the coastal zone, Quito, 18 June 1935, both LCE-I 1935, ASS/MNM; see also the director of sanidad to Señor Octavio Villafuerte, Quito, 11 March 1936, LCE-I 1936, ASS/MNM.

45. The inspector técnico of sanidad for the central zone to the director general of sanidad, Quito, 4 October 1945, LCE-JP 1945, ASS/MNM.

46. Report of Eustorgio Salgado, director of the servicio de profilaxis venérea, to the subdirector of sanidad, Quito, 30 June 1923, LCR 1923-I, ASS/MNM.

47. The director of sanidad to the minister of sanidad, Quito, 25 August 1927, LCE 1927-II, ASS/MNM.

48. The secretary of sanidad for the coastal zone to the director general of sanidad, Guayaquil, 27 December 1928, LCR-Sanidad del Litoral 1928, ASS/MNM.

49. The general director of sanidad to the director of sanidad of the Distrito Norte, Guayaquil, 29 October 1925, LCR 1925-II, ASS/MNM.

50. The director of sanidad of the Distrito Norte to the general director of sanidad, Quito, undated (end of October 1925), LCR 1925-II, ASS/MNM.

51. Both regulations were approved by the minister of previsión social y trabajo on 27 December 1926, on file in LDSSeH 1926–27, ASS/MNM.

52. Data from 1932 are from the chief of the servicio de profilaxis venérea to the director general of sanidad, Quito, 27 May 1932, LCR-SI 1932, ASS/MNM

53. The chief of the servicio de profilaxis venérea to the director general of sanidad, Quito, 27 May 1932, LCR-SI 1932, ASS/MNM.

54. The chief of the servicio de profilaxis venérea to the director of sanidad for the central zone, Quito, 12 June 1937, PDeInt 1937, ASS/MNM.

55. The chief of the servicio de profilaxis venérea to the director of sanidad for the central zone, Quito, 27 April 1942, Libro de Informes y Conferencias 1937–1946, ASS/MNM.

56. The inspector técnico of sanidad for the central zone to the director of the medical services of the Caja del Seguro, Quito, 18 March 1946, LCE-JP 1946, ASS/MNM.

57. The minister of sanidad to the inspector técnico of sanidad for the central zone, Quito, 30 December 1946, LCR-Presidencia y Ministerio 1946, ASS/MNM.

58. Reproduced in the secretary of congress's report on legislative project no. 17-D-1950, Quito, 21 August 1957, AFL [Archivo de la Función Legislativa], Cámara de Diputados, caja no. 58 [484], expedientes, serie DD-III-B, no. 1-23, 1957.

59. The subdirector of sanidad to the minister of gobierno, Quito, 29 October 1921, and the subdirector of sanidad to the intendente general of policía de la provincia, Quito, 10 November 1921, both LCE 1921-II, ASS/MNM; the minister of gobierno to the subdirector of sanidad, Quito, 21 October 1921, LCR 1921-II, ASS/MNM.

60. Dr. Pedro Zambrano to the director of sanidad, Quito, 17 January 1927, DSTyOEC 1927, ASS/MNM.

61. The subdirector of sanidad to the minister of gobierno, Quito, 29 October 1921, LCE 1921 ASS/MNM.

62. Communication from the chief of the servicio de profilaxis venérea transcribed in provincial director of sanidad for Pichincha to the primer jefe of the Regimento Quito No. 1, Quito, 19 July 1945, LCE (JPP) 1945(July–September), ASS/MNM.

63. Report on prostitution by Dr. Pedro Zambrano, transcribed in the director of sanidad to the minister of previsión social y sanidad, Quito, 19 August 1939, LCE 1939-II ASS/MNM. This report was written in response to a questionnaire from Dr. Enrique Garcés to assist him in writing a study of the issues that he had been asked to send to colleagues in England.

64. Alberto Correa, *Conferencias sustentadas en el Teatro Variedades el 14 y 15 de enero de 1930* (Quito: Imprenta Luis E. Giacometti, 1930).

65. The director of the dispensario de sifilografía y enfermedades venéreas of the

Hospital Civil to the director of the Junta de Beneficencia, Quito, 15 October 1925, LCR 1925-II, AAP/MNM.

66. The provincial director of sanidad for Pichincha to the chief of the servicio de venereología, Quito, 4 June 1945, LCE (JPP) 1945-I; and the chief of profilaxis venérea to the provincial director of sanidad for Pichincha, Quito, 9 June 1945, LCR-IV 1945 (L-U), both in ASS/MNM.

67. The director of sanidad for the Distrito Norte to the encargado de negocios de España, Quito, 5 December, 12 December, and 23 December 1925, LCE 1925-II, ASS/MNM.

68. The subdirector of sanidad to Eduardo Borja Pérez, Quito, 31 March 1922, LCE ASS/MNM.

69. Petition from R. C. to the director general of sanidad, Quito, undated (January 1927), Documentos sobre tifoidea y otras enfermedades contagiosas 1927, ASS/MNM.

70. Certificates regarding A. S.'s conduct, Quito, 20 June 1922, LCR 1922, ASS/MNM.

71. Certificates regarding M. P.'s conduct, Quito, undated (late July) 1923, LCR 1923-II, ASS /MNM.

72. Petition from A. T. to the subdirector of sanidad, Quito, 20 October 1921, LCR 1921-II, ASS/MNM.

73. Petition from M. D. to the subdirector of sanidad, Quito, undated (December 1921), LCR 1921-II, ASS/MNM.

74. Petition to the director general of sanidad, Quito, 22 May 1928, LCR-G 1928, ASS/MNM.

75. The chief of the servicio de profilaxis venérea to the director general of sanidad, Quito, 10 July 1928, LCR-G 1928, ASS/MNM.

76. Petition (signature illegible) to the director of sanidad for the central zone, with report, Quito, 9 March 1937, Solicitudes 1937, ASS/MNM.

77. Petition from E. N. to the director of sanidad, Quito, 27 February 1941, Solicitudes 1941, ASS/MNM.

78. Another way to leave prostitution was to seek shelter in the convent of the Buen Pastor. The Hermanas del Buen Pastor, specialists in the rehabilitation of "fallen" women, arrived from Montreal in 1871, contracted by President Gabriel García Moreno. See Francisco Miranda Ribadeneira, *Las religiosas del Buen Pastor en el Ecuador: Rasgos históricos* (Quito: Imprenta del Colegio Técnico Don Bosco, 1970); and Ana María Goetschel, "Educación e imágenes de mujer," in *Y el amor no era todo . . . Mujeres, imágenes y conflictos*, edited by Martha Moscoso (Quito: Abya Yala and DGIS, 1996), 59–83. However, one registered prostitute in Guayaquil in 1951 tried this but found that she was treated so badly by the nuns that she preferred to return to prostitution (included in Report from the medical director of the Oficina de Profilaxis Venérea in Guayaquil to the president of congress, Guayaquil, 11 April 1951, AFL, Cámara de Diputados, caja no. 11 (374), expedientes, serie DD-51-III-B, no. 1-35, 1951).

79. I. C. de C. to the minister of sanidad, Quito, 11 December 1923, LCR 1923-II, ASS/MNM. She was only eliminated in July 1926; perhaps the Sanidad was waiting

until she could demonstrate a clean bill of health. The secretary of sanidad to Señora I. C. de C., Quito, 30 July 1926, LCE 1926-II, ASS/MNM.

80. Petition from M. A. to the subdirector of sanidad, Quito, 11 October 1924, LCR 1924, ASS/MNM.

81. Petition from A. P. to the director of sanidad for Pichincha, Quito, undated (November 1925), LCR 1925-II, ASS/MNM.

82. Petition from O. B., with report from the servicio de profilaxis venérea, Quito, 11 February 1938, Solicitudes 1938, ASS/MNM.

83. Petition from L. J. to the director of sanidad, Quito, 1 November 1926, DSTyOEC 1926, ASS/MNM.

84. Petition from M. E. G. M. and A. R. to the director of sanidad, Quito, 14 June 1927, DSTyOEC 1927, ASS/MNM.

85. Petition from C. S. to the director general of sanidad, Quito, 1 July 1927, DSTyOEC 1927, ASS/MNM.

86. Petition from M. V. and her conviviente P. V., Quito, 19 December 1938, Solicitudes 1938, ASS/MNM.

87. Petition of R. J. and H. R. to the director of sanidad, Quito, 30 April 1942, Solicitudes 1942, ASS/MNM.

88. The historian Karin Rosemblatt also found that marriage was apparently not as appealing to some single mothers as dominant representations suggested it should be; see her *Gendered Compromises: Political Cultures and the State in Chile, 1920–1950* (Chapel Hill: University of North Carolina Press, 2000).

89. The 1933 figure is the only one taken from a list with all of the women's names and addresses. The figure of 704 was not the actual figure of prostitutes active in Quito but rather the number who had registered since the SPV had begun the registry; no doubt the totals given for other years also took this form. Some of the women had in fact been eliminated in the meantime (113), others had died (18), and others were absent from the city (247), supposedly on a temporary basis. "Meretrices inscritas en la Oficina de Profilaxis Venérea de la Dirección General de Sanidad," Quito, 10 May 1933, LCE 1933, ASS/MNM.

90. Report by Pedro Zambrano, director of the servicio de profilaxis venérea, transcribed in the director of sanidad to the minister of gobierno y sanidad, Quito, 9 March 1933, LCE 1933 ASS/MNM.

91. Garcés, *Por, para y del niño*, 118.

92. Report on prostitution by Pedro Zambrano, transcribed in the director of sanidad to the minister of previsión social y sanidad, Quito, 19 August 1939, LCE 1939-II ASS/MNM.

93. Linda Alexander Rodríguez, *The Search for Public Policy: Regional Politics and Government Finances in Ecuador, 1830–1940* (Berkeley: University of California Press, 1985).

94. Pablo Arturo Suárez, A. López, and Cornelio Donoso, "Estudio numérico y económico-social de la población de Quito," *Boletín del departamento médico social* 1, no. 1 (1937): 7–11.

95. For the mínimum wage, see Guillermo Bustos, "La politización del 'problema obrero': Los trabajadores quiteños entre la identidad 'pueblo' y la identidad 'clase' (1931–1934)," in *Las crises en el Ecuador: Los treinta y los ochenta* (Quito: Corporación Editora Nacional, 1991), 125. For workers' needs, see Pablo Arturo Suárez, *Contribución al estudio de las realidades entre las clases obreras y campesinas* (Quito: Imprenta de la Universidad Central, 1934), 80.

96. Report on prostitution by Pedro Zambrano, transcribed in the director of sanidad to the minister of previsión social y sanidad, Quito, 19 August 1939, LCE 1939-II ASS/MNM.

97. Report from the medical director of the Oficina de Profilaxis Venérea in Guayaquil to the president of congress, Guayaquil, 11 April 1951, AFL, Cámara de Diputados, caja no. 11 (374), expedientes, serie DD-51-III-B, no. 1-35, 1951.

98. Katherine Elaine Bliss, "The Right to Live as *Gente Decente*: Sex Work, Family Life, and Collective Identity in Early-Twentieth-Century Mexico," *Journal of Women's History* 15, no. 4 (2004): 165.

99. See, for instance, Zambrano, "Historia del reglamento," 55–56; and in a similar vein, Jaime Barrera B., "La mujer y el delito," *Archivos de criminología, neurosiquiatría y disciplinas conexas* (Quito), 6–7 (1942–43): 69.

100. "Problemas de las enfermedades venéreas en el Ecuador, plan de control de las mismas," undated (1945) in Informes y Conferencias 1937–1946, ASS/MNM. The report is unsigned but appears to be a commentary on (or perhaps the prologue to) the comprehensive plan of action developed in 1945 by the Sanidad in Quito.

101. Report from the medical director of the Oficina de Profilaxis Venérea in Guayaquil to the president of congress, Guayaquil, 11 April 1951, AFL, Cámara de Diputados, caja no. 11 (374), expedientes, serie DD-51-III-B, no. 1-35, 1951.

## Chapter 4. Midwifery, Morality, and the State

1. Consuelo Rueda to the director general of sanidad, Quito, 27 September 1929, Libro de Comunicaciones Recibidas (hereafter LCR) 1929, Archivo del Servicio de Sanidad/Museo Nacional de Medicina (ASS/MNM).

2. See Mariana Landázuri Camacho, *Juana Miranda: Fundadora de la Maternidad de Quito* (Quito: Banco Central, 2004), which is an essential source for the politics of the establishment of the Maternidad.

3. The data discussed here, and compiled in tables in this chapter, are drawn from the enrollment registries at the Universidad Central, in the Archivo General de la Universidad Central (hereafter AGUC), Quito: "Matrículas de Medicina—Obstetricia—Farmacia—Dentistas desde el Año de 1888 a 1912"; "Matrículas de la Facultad de Medicina, Farmacia, Odontología, Obstetricia, 15 Octubre de 1912—18 de Junio de 1930"; and "Matrículas de Medicina—Odontología—Enfermería—Obstetricia de los Años 5 Septiembre de 1930 al 27 de Noviembre de 1950." Supplementary data are drawn from individual student files ("Expedientes . . . ") and from the graduation records ("Grados . . . ") at the AGUC. In the tables presented, the women included are those who registered in their first year of obstetrical studies during the period speci-

fied; not all of these women completed their studies. Also, a few women transferred to the Universidad Central after their first year (for most of the period studied, women could only complete their studies in obstetrics in Quito, although they could begin them in the universities in Cuenca and Guayaquil). Several kinds of information are included in the university records only upon registration in the first year, so it is more difficult to draw conclusions about some of these other women.

4. There were also nineteen Hermanas de la Caridad who wrote exams at the university in 1905 and 1906 to verify their pharmaceutical knowledge, although they apparently did not actually engage in pharmacy coursework. Hermanas had traditionally served as apothecaries in hospitals administered by the order. "Matrículas de Medicina—Obstetricia—Farmacia—Dentistas desde el Año de 1888 a 1912," AGUC.

5. "Matrículas de Medicina—Odontología—Enfermería—Obstetricia de los Años 5 de Septiembre de 1930 al 27 de Noviembre de 1950," AGUC.

6. Formal records of nursing graduation only begin to appear in the archives of the Universidad Central in 1929, with forty-three graduates between that date and the fall of 1936. However, there were an additional twenty-three students who undertook two years of nursing study from 1917 through 1928 who may well have completed the curriculum, although apparently they were not considered university graduates.

7. This interim regulation was meant to be in effect only until a school of obstetrics or a maternity hospital was established. See the 13 February 1890 decree of the General Council of Public Education recorded in "Grados de Matronas y Obstetrices Mayo 31 de 1890 a Mayo 27 de 1934 . . . Enfermeras Marzo 8 de 1935 a 1944," AGUC.

8. Dirección General de Sanidad, *Nómina de médicos y cirujanos, dentistas, farmacéuticos y obstetrices, inscritos en Quito y Guayaquil* (Quito: Imprenta Nacional, 1932), updated with handwritten annotations in 1937, LCR-Solicitudes, ASS/MNM).

9. Discussion of the first three women in this paragraph is based on documents in a file located in the Museo Nacional de Medicina, "Documentaciones de Exámenes de Obstetricia, 1827–1899," which contains photocopied material from the AGUC.

10. An Executive Decree of 1 November 1904 authorized the national government to enter into contracts with women who wanted to study midwifery. Such contracts required women to present certificates verifying both their progress and conduct three times a year, complete the three-year program of studies or repay the monies received from the government, and upon graduation accept employment for three years "in a city of the government's choosing at a salary that the government designates," in exchange for a monthly stipend of twelve sucres during their studies. These contracts included waivers of examination fees (*derechos de exámenes*), and these women could also apply for a waiver of graduating fees (*derechos de grado*) if their grades were sufficiently high. See, for example, "Expedientes de Obstetrices 'Matronas' A-B Desde 11 de Enero de 1907 a . . . , " AGUC; file of Señora Rosario Almeida de Gabela.

11. Certificate from Federico González Suárez, archbishop of Quito, Quito, 26 July 1906, in file of Zoila M. Larrea contained in "Expedientes de Obstetrices 'Matronas' I-J-K-L 27 de Julio de 1906 hasta . . . , " AGUC.

12. For instance, at the time that the Sanidad was preparing to establish its

outreach program of maternal-infant care in 1935, the province of Imbabura had three licensed midwives: two were employed by the municipality of Otavalo (the Larrea sisters) and one was employed by the Asistencia Pública of Ibarra, practicing out of the provincial hospital and in the homes of the poor. The municipality of Cotacachi was at the time also trying to hire a midwife but had not met with success despite offering an unusually high salary. The provincial delegate of sanidad for Imbabura to the director general of sanidad, Ibarra, 25 April 1935, LCR-Delegaciones Provinciales 1935, ASS/MNM.

13. "Expedientes de Obstetrices 'Matronas' LL-M Desde el 19 de Julio de 1902 hasta . . . ," AGUC; file of Señora Alejandrina Miranda viuda de Yépez.

14. Parental concern about finding appropriate lodgings for female students from the provinces persisted beyond the period when this information was recorded in the university's records. For instance, in 1939 Elías Castillo, the owner of a textile factory in Riobamba, contacted the Junta Central de Asistencia Pública to request accommodations for his daughter within the Maternidad during her obstetrics studies in Quito, citing both her desire to study and his desire to find a place where she would be safe (Elías Castillo to the director of the Junta Central de Asistencia Pública, Riobamba, 18 December 1939, LCR 1939, AAP/MNM).

15. The 1950 census indicated that in that year (with a half century for their numbers to have accumulated in the population) only 4,635 of 692,543 people of marriageable age living in urban areas were divorced (that is, 0.67 percent); in rural areas the numbers were much smaller (1,515 of 1,096,878 people of marriageable age, or 0.14 percent). J. V. D. Saunders, *The People of Ecuador: A Demographic Analysis* (Gainesville: University of Florida Press, 1961), 38.

16. For instance, the state-funded midwife in the county seat of Machachi, south of Quito, explained to the regional director of sanidad in Quito that in September 1937 she had not attended a single delivery, because the women of the area had instead sought out empirics, a very shameful situation in her view. She asked that the director use his influence to ensure that empirics were investigated and punished for exercising a profession illegally, so that she could carry out her duties. Rosa M. Verdesoto to the director of sanidad for the North-Central Zone, Machachi, 5 October 1937, LCR (Comunicaciones Varias) 1937, ASS/MNM.

17. Although the physicians who worked at the Maternidad seem to have been generally well qualified, it is not so clear that the medical students—who included two students cycling through on one-month "voluntary internships" as well as the generally more capable intern who won his one-year position in a competitive process—lived up to Ayora's claims. For instance, in 1934 a workers' delegation registered a complaint with the director of the Junta Central de Asistencia Pública about how their mothers, sisters, and wives were treated by these students. As they characterized it, "The roughness and rudeness of the physician is beyond the pale. Many poor patients, timid and ignorant patients who turn to this hospital to be examined and to seek good advice from the physician, are examined brutally, and some of them have told us that they have been physically abused and affronted." They conclude with a request

that the Junta Central de Asistencia Pública "put an immediate end to such criminal abuses by people who are unqualified, immoral, and without conscience" (Segundino Aviles and Rafael Narváez to the director of the Junta Central de Asistencia Pública, Quito, 14 June 1934, LCR-1934, AAP/MNM). Ayora was consistently critical of midwives' competence, but apparently not all physicians themselves treated women with the professionalism and delicacy that Ayora himself suggested was important.

18. Isidro Ayora, director of the maternidad, to the director of the Junta Central de Asistencia Pública, Quito, 9 June 1916, LCR 1916-I, AAP/MNM.

19. This also marked an interruption in women's participation in training midwives, until Cecilia de Arrellano and her colleagues were formally appointed as profesoras at the school in the early 1970s (after having worked for several years there supervising midwifery students in their practical training). Interview with Cecilia de Arrellano, Quito, 7 July 2005.

20. "Proyecto de Plan General de Estudios de Medicina: Obstetricia," *Anales de la Universidad Central* (1916), reproduced in Landázuri Camacho, *Juana Miranda,* 189–90.

21. Responses from the directors of these institutions to this survey by the Sanidad are collected in the Libro de Comunicaciones Recibidas (LCR) by the Jefatura de Farmacias y Profesiones Médicas (JFyPM), November 1947, in the ASS/MNM.

22. Caja de Pensiones, *Segundo censo de afiliados, realizado el 30 de Abril de 1935* (Quito, 1936).

23. In 1932, for instance, the guide published by the Dirección General de Sanidad, *Nómina de médicos y cirujanos, dentistas, farmacéuticos y obstetrices, inscritos en Quito y Guayaquil* (Quito: Imprenta Nacional, 1932), lists fifty-four women who had registered their midwifery titles with the Sanidad office in Quito; another twenty-nine had done so in Guayaquil.

24. "Nómina del Cuerpo Médico Ecuatoriano en el año 1938," *Anales de la Sociedad Médico-Quirúrgica del Guayaquil* 18, no. 1 (1938): 27–42. The compilers of this list admitted that they might have inadvertently omitted some names, and they appealed to readers to send them any updates or corrections.

25. By 2005 the subdirector of the Escuela de Obstetricia in Quito estimated that in the capital city only two percent of births were attended by midwives, although in the provinces she calculated that midwives probably attended some forty percent of births. Although midwives are authorized to attend low-risk deliveries, at the Maternidad Isidro Ayora they are currently tasked with prenatal care and sexual health issues rather than delivering babies. Although midwifery students must assist at some thirty to forty births before graduating, the graduated midwives employed at the Maternidad do not deliver babies there. Interview with Ximena Cevallos (subdirectora de la Escuela de Obstetricia), Quito, 7 July 2005. While Ecuadorian women have the right to free maternity services at the Maternidad, midwives have encountered obstacles in their attempts to increase the number of positions earmarked for midwives within that and other state institutions. Interview with Rosa Santamaría (directora de la Escuela de Enfermería), Quito, 7 July 2005.

26. In this era there does not appear to have been any regulation of the amount of fees charged to private patients; indeed, physicians, for instance, set fees at their own discretion, based in part on their assessment of what clients could pay (interview with María Martínez de Suárez [Quito, 3 July 2006] regarding the medical practices of both her father-in-law, Dr. Pablo Arturo Suárez, and her father, Dr. Luis J. Martínez). The remuneration that state midwives received from the Sanidad for their provision of free services to the poor population was initially a monthly salary of 120 sucres.

27. "Al Público," Ambato, June 1935, LCR (Delegaciones Provinciales) 1935, ASS/ MNM.

28. "Protección Infantil," Ibarra, February 1936, LCR (Delegaciones Provinciales) 1936, ASS/MNM.

29. The director general of sanidad to the comisario of sanidad, Quito, 14 August 1936, LCE-II 1936, AAS/MNM.

30. The director of sanidad for the central zone to the president of the municipal council of Pelileo, Quito, 19 November 1946, LCE (Municipalidades) 1946, AAS/ MNM.

31. Hortensia Cevallos to the director general of sanidad, Pujilí, no date (second half of 1935), LCR 1934-5 ASS/MNM.

32. The technical inspector of sanidad of the central zone to the director general of sanidad, Quito, 20 September 1946, LCE-DG/R/T/L 1946, ASS/MNM.

33. "Memorandum para las obstetrices de la Dirección de Sanidad de la Zona Central," Quito, 18 January 1939, LCR-Dirección 1939, ASS/MNM.

34. Consuelo Rueda to the director of sanidad for the central zone, 12 February 1938, LCR (Delegaciones Provinciales-I) 1938, ASS/MNM.

35. For instance, in February 1930, 24 of 73 births were attended by professionals; in March, 31 of 108; in April, 37 of 105 (provincial delegate of sanidad for Tungurahua to the director general of sanidad [trimestral report], Ambato, May 1930, LCR-IAD 1928-1930, ASS/MNM). Some six months earlier, the delegate had reported (in a request to the Asistencia Pública that they outfit a small maternity ward at the provincial hospital) that the number of both stillbirths and maternal deaths in Ambato was perhaps the highest in the country on a per capita basis, largely due to the fact that 90 percent of births were attended by empirics (delegate of sanidad for Tungurahua to the director general of asistencia pública, Ambato, 19 September 1929, LCR 1929-II, AAP/MNM).

36. The delegate of sanidad for Tungurahua to the director general of sanidad, Ambato, 26 June 1936, LCR (Delegaciones Provinciales) 1936, ASS/MNM.

37. The delegate of sanidad for Tungurahua to the director of sanidad for the central zone, Ambato, 21 April 1939, LCR (Delegaciones Provinciales-I) 1939, ASS/ MNM.

38. Consuelo Rueda to the Tungurahua provincial sanidad delegate, Ambato, 5 September 1940, LCR-Delegaciones Provinciales-II 1940, ASS/MNM.

39. "Expedientes Obstetrices 'Matronas' R desde 14 de Julio de 1903 a . . . ," AGUC; file of Consolación Rueda Saénz.

40. Consuelo Rueda to the director of sanidad for the central zone, Ambato, 1 August 1940, LCR (Delegaciones Provinciales-II) 1940, ASS/MNM.

41. The Carchi provincial sanidad delegate to the director of sanidad of the Central Zone, Tulcán, 4 July 1940, LCR-Delegaciones Provinciales-II 1940, ASS/MNM.

42. Dolores Ayabaca de Lippke to the regional director of sanidad in Quito, Guaranda, 29 January 1938, LCR (Comunicaciones Varias) 1938, ASS/MNM.

43. Juana Miranda to the rector of the Universidad Central, Quito, 31 October 1892, *Anales de la Universidad Central* (1892), reproduced in Landázuri Camacho, *Juana Miranda*, 248.

44. In 1934 the Colegio 24 de Mayo became Quito's principal state secondary school for girls, when the Instituto Nacional Mejía was converted from a coeducational institution to a young men's school that year. Interestingly, none of the Quiteñas who studied midwifery had graduated from another prominent institution in the capital: the Liceo Fernández Madrid, established in 1930 as a technical school for young women of a somewhat lower social class. The academic program of the Colegio 24 de Mayo was apparently more in keeping with the preparation necessary for the study of midwifery. All of this contrasted with the background of the young women who studied nursing in the same era, where in some cases we find women who had studied in the Liceo Fernández Madrid as well as some women who had attended Catholic girls' schools.

45. Consuelo Rueda to the director of sanidad, Ambato, 22 January 1937, LCR (Comunicaciones Varias) 1937, ASS/MNM.

46. The provincial sanidad delegate for Tungurahua to the director of sanidad, Ambato, 11 January 1937, LCR (Delegaciones Provinciales) 1937, ASS/MNM.

47. The director of sanidad to the minister of gobierno y sanidad, Quito, 29 April 1936, LCE 1936-I, ASS/MNM.

48. Ann Zulawski, *Unequal Cures: Public Health and Political Change in Bolivia, 1900-1950* (Durham: Duke University Press, 2007), chapter 4.

49. Kristin Ruggiero, "Honor, Maternity, and the Disciplining of Women: Infanticide in Late Nineteenth-Century Buenos Aires," *Hispanic American Historical Review* 72, no. 3 (1992): 368-70.

50. Steven Palmer, *From Popular Medicine to Medical Populism: Doctors, Healers, and Public Power in Costa Rica, 1800-1940* (Durham: Duke University Press, 2003), chapter 6.

51. The notion that professionals participate in a larger system of practitioners who struggle for jurisdiction over areas of expertise and practice was developed by Andrew Abbott in *The System of Professions: An Essay on the Division of Expert Labor* (Chicago: University of Chicago Press, 1988).

52. In rector of the Universidad Central to the governor of Pichincha province, Quito, 15 November 1895, *Anales de la Universidad Central* (1898), reproduced in Landázuri Camacho, *Juana Miranda*, 255.

53. Following a presentation of some of these ideas at a history conference in Quito in July 2009, Luis González Palacios commented that during an oral history project

in a working-class neighborhood in Quito, La Libertad, residents said that from the 1950s to about 1970, Carmela Granja was associated with a brothel frequented by wealthy Quiteños called El Rincón Chileno, where she continued to offer her controversial obstetrical services up to the time of her death. None of the archival documents encountered through the 1940s suggested an association with prostitution, but popular memory in the neighborhood casts her as the owner of a brothel in subsequent decades. This might reflect a change in her circumstances over time or perhaps simply profound ambiguity around the association between her means of livelihood and issues of sexuality. Thanks to Luis González for sharing these stories.

54. The director of sanidad to the chief of investigations, Quito, 11 May 1929; LCE 1929-I, ASS/MNM.

55. He also characterized the level of noise made by both the employees and the radio that the Maternidad's administrator played at all hours as a martyrdom for the laboring women. Gabriel Moreno y Rosales to the director of the Junta Central de Asistencia Pública, Quito, 28 August 1942, LCE-1942 AAP/MNM.

56. "Circular del ayudante encargado del despacho del servicio de sanidad to the propietarios y representantes legales de las boticas de Quito," Quito, 11 September 1926, LCE-1926 ASS/MNM. Thanks to Ecuadorian botanist Patricio Mena for his assistance in identifying the herbs mentioned in this communication.

57. This may help to explain why the minister of previsión social himself sent a handwritten note to the director of the Sanidad in 1929 asking him to seek a "conciliatory arrangement" in an incident involving Granja, assuring him that in the future she would respect the dispositions of the public health authorities (minister of previsión social, trabajo, agricultura, etc. to the director general of sanidad, Quito, 22 March 1929, LCR-PL/PR/M/PJ 1929, ASS/MNM). A month later, the city's pharmacists were informed that midwives, whether licensed or not, did not have the right to prescribe medication of any kind (circular from the director of sanidad to the representantes de las boticas de Quito, Quito, 23 April 1929, LCR-EP/SI 1929, ASS/ MNM). It was a few weeks later, in early May, that Granja's clinic was raided.

58. The earlier conviction is referred to in the director of sanidad to the chief of investigations, Quito, 23 November 1935, LCE-1935-II, ASS/MNM. For a published reference to her later incarceration, see criminologist Jaime Barrera B.'s article "La mujer y el delito" in *Archivos de criminología, neurosiquiatría y disciplinas conexas* (Quito) 6–7 (1942–43): 118.

59. Interview with Dr. Eduardo Luna Yépez, Quito, July 2006.

60. The director of the Hospital Civil San Juan de Dios to the minister of gobierno y municipalidades, Quito, 24 October 1941, Libro de Comunicaciones Recibidas y Enviadas (LCRyE), Archivo del Hospital Civil San Juan de Dios (AHCSJD)/MNM.

61. The chief of farmacias y profesiones médicas to the comisario of sanidad, Quito, 4 April 1946, LCE-JFyPM 1946, ASS/MNM.

62. Conversations in Quito with Rocío Bedón have been useful in considering this question.

63. In Ecuador during the second quarter of the twentieth century, there was no

parallel to the extensive political and medical debates over abortion that occurred in Chile and Uruguay (see Jadwiga Pieper Mooney, *The Politics of Motherhood: Maternity and Women's Rights in Twentieth-Century Chile* [Pittsburgh: University of Pittsburgh Press, 2009], chapter 2; and Asunción Lavrin, *Women, Feminism, and Social Change in Argentina, Chile, and Uruguay, 1890–1940* [Lincoln: University of Nebraska Press, 1995], chapter 5). The scattered archival evidence about Carmela Granja's practice thus provides us with rare although partial insight into these issues.

64. The director general of sanidad to the intendente general de policía, Quito, 4 June 1929, LCE-1929-I, ASS/MNM.

65. Like Granja, the second midwife referred to here was fully trained in the biomedical model, although unlike Granja she had graduated (in 1907).

66. Anne-Claire Defossez, "Un hospital testigo del siglo: Historia social y reproductiva de mujeres enfermas en Quito (1925–1965)," in *Mujeres de los Andes: Condiciones de vida y salud*, edited by Anne-Claire Defossez, Didier Fassin, and Mara Viveros (Colombia: Instituto Francés de Estudios Andinos and Universidad Externado de Colombia, 1992), 59.

67. Luis F. Domínguez, "Reforma al Código Penal: Aborto Criminal," in *Memoria del II Congreso Médico Ecuatoriano* (Guayaquil: Imprenta y Literatura La Reforma, 1931), 228.

68. When these research results were presented to students and faculty at the Escuela de Obstetricia at the Universidad Central in May 2010, the identification of midwives with abortion in the historical record struck a strong chord with the audience, provoking a heated discussion about the continuing weight of this presumed association in determining the professional position and general status of midwives in Ecuador into the present.

69. These calculations are based on Caja de Pensiones, *Segundo censo*.

## Chapter 5. The Transformation of Ecuadorian Nursing

1. Research for this chapter was greatly enhanced by several provocative oral history interviews: thanks to Adrila Aguirre (student at the ENE 1949–52), Iralda Benítez de Núñez (student 1956–59, directora of the ENE 1978–80), Clemencia Gía (student 1964–67), Georgina Morales de Carrillo (student 1953–56, directora 1971–78), Rosa Santamaría (student 1961–64, directora 2002–07), and Margarita Velasco (student 1973–76) for their willingness to share their memories and insightful analyses. While interviews are only cited here where direct quotations are used, those conversations were enormously helpful in interpreting the archival materials throughout this chapter. The feedback offered by an interested audience of students and professional nurses when some of these research results were presented at the Escuela Nacional de Enfermería in May 2010 is also greatly appreciated.

2. Considerable information about the agreement and the negotiations around it can be found in United States Department of State, *Foreign Relations of the United States Diplomatic Papers, 1942: The American Republics*, volume 6 (Washington, D.C.: U.S. Government Printing Office, 1942), which can be accessed via the University

of Wisconsin Digital Collection (http://digicoll.library.wisc.edu/FRUS/). There is also useful information about the larger agreement in Ronn Pineo, *Ecuador and the United States: Useful Strangers* (Athens: University of Georgia Press, 2007), chapter 4, although Pineo does not analyze the health and sanitation dimensions of the agreement.

3. Patricia de la Torre and Margarita Velasco, "La educación de enfermería en el estado liberal ecuatoriano," *Boletín de informaciones científicas nacionales* 117 (1985): 92–93.

4. "Empleados que necesitan nuevo nombramiento por cambio de denominación en el nuevo presupuesto desde April 1 de este año," director of the Hospital Civil San Juan de Dios, Quito, 12 April 1938, LCRyE 1938, AHCSJD/MNM.

5. The director of the Hospital Civil San Juan de Dios to the director of the Junta Central de Asistencia Pública, Quito, undated (September) 1938, LCRyE 1938, AHCSJD/MNM.

6. The director of the Junta Central de Asistencia Pública to the director of the Hospital Civil San Juan de Dios, Quito, 10 January 1946, LCR-1946, AHCSJD/MNM.

7. For 368 years the Hospital San Juan de Dios was the only civil hospital in Quito, until the Hospital Eugenio Espejo was inaugurated in 1933. With the opening of the Espejo, a new division of labor was instituted such that the Hospital San Juan de Dios provided medical care to patients with cancer, skin and venereal infections, tuberculosis, and contagious diseases, and the Espejo offered services in other areas. After 409 years of continuous operation, the Hospital San Juan de Dios was closed at its original site in 1974 and its operations were transferred to the newly inaugurated Hospital Pablo Arturo Suárez.

8. Compañía de las Hijas de la Caridad, *Trescientos cincuenta aniversario de la fundación (1633–1983): Aporte de las Hijas de la Caridad para el desarrollo de enfermería en el Ecuador* (Quito, 1982), i.

9. Sioban Nelson, *Say Little, Do Much: Nursing, Nuns, and Hospitals in the Nineteenth Century* (Philadelphia: University of Pennsylvania Press, 2001), 22–23.

10. Compañía de las Hijas de la Caridad, *Trescientos Cincuenta Aniversario*, 6.

11. Nelson, *Say Little, Do Much*. In contrast to the Ecuadorian case, Nelson has characterized Sisters in the United States and Australia as being immigrants in immigrant societies (often dealing precisely with the immigrant poor). The records of enrollment at the Universidad Central of those Hermanas who studied either pharmacy or nursing there, indicate that in Ecuador the Hermanas de la Caridad quickly became an Ecuadorian institution, primarily made up of women born locally. Interestingly, many of them came from relatively small population centers, a fact that raises some intriguing questions for future research about the process of recruitment into the religious community. Other than a very small number of foreign-born women, Hermanas who studied nursing before the 1942 establishment of the ENE were about evenly split among three groups: women born in Ecuador's largest cities (Quito and Guayaquil), those born in provincial capitals, and those born in county seats or even smaller towns. Their secular counterparts were much more likely to be

born in Quito or neighboring provincial capitals until 1942, when a new system of scholarships aimed to bring women from across the national territory to Quito for nursing training (although they were still more likely to be born in provincial capitals than in smaller towns).

12. Established by Acuerdo no. 8 of 28 February 1917.

13. Universidad Central records show that five students did indeed undertake three years of study (two began in 1921 and were in their third year in 1923–24; three began in 1923 and were in their third year in 1925–26), although subsequently the program continued to be for two years.

14. Information about the material covered in each year of study is offered in the *Acuerdo del Consejo General de Instrucción Pública reorganizando la Escuela de Enfermeras anexa a la Facultad de Medicina de la Universidad Central* (Quito: Imprenta de la Universidad Central, 1921).

15. *Reglamento interno de la Escuela de Enfermeras anexa a la Facultad de Medicina de la Universidad Central del Ecuador* (Quito: Imprenta Nacional, 1921), 6.

16. Leopoldo Brauer to Isidro Ayora, Hamburg, 16 May 1922, LCR-1922, AAP/ MNM.

17. Isidro Ayora, "Crónicas Médicas de la Capital: Escuela de Enfermeras de Quito," *Anales de la Sociedad Médico-Quirúrgico del Guayas*, no. 22 (December 1922): 516–17.

18. Information about enrollments comes from the university registration records held at the Archivo General de la Universidad Central (AGUC).

19. The earliest employment reference found in the documentation of the Archivo de la Asistencia Pública for a trained nurse mentioned that by 1931 a nurse was working in the children's free medical dispensary at the Hospital San Juan de Dios.

20. There is some slippage in the university enrollment registries due to inconsistent use of the birth names of Hermanas versus their religious names, which makes it difficult to affirm the religious or secular identity of one or two of the 1933 graduates.

21. By the 1950s the process had changed: sponsoring institutions undertook their own process of selection locally, then their candidates underwent a final interview with the directora (interview with Georgina Morales de Carrillo, Quito, 11 July 2005).

22. Actas del Concejo Ejecutivo, 1942–1946, meeting minutes for 9 January 1943, Archivo de la Escuela Nacional de Enfermeras (AENE).

23. Actas del Concejo Ejecutivo, 1947–1952, meeting minutes for 2 June 1949, AENE.

24. This information is culled from the university registration records, AGUC.

25. When Margarita Velasco did the interviews with nursing leaders that underlay the publication *La historia contada desde las líderes: Precursoras 1940–1980* (coauthored with Soledad Alvarez [Quito: Federación Ecuatoriana de Enfermeras/ os, 2002]), she found that several such leaders were maternal orphans and eldest sisters, accustomed to managing a household from a young age (interview, Quito, 6 July 2005). This differs from the situation among midwives, where not only were there proportionately more orphans but also the majority had lost their fathers rather than their mothers.

26. Fanny de Mora's elder sister, Mercedes, began in medical school with her but then transferred to dentistry. In 1939, Mercedes de Mora became the second woman to graduate from the Universidad Central as a *doctora de odontología*, twelve years after her only predecessor (according to registration and graduation records at the AGUC).

27. Actas del Concejo Ejecutivo, 1942–1946, meeting minutes for 8 November 1943, AENE.

28. Actas del Concejo Ejecutivo, 1942–1946, meeting minutes for 10 January 1944, AENE.

29. Some of the difficulties with physicians were alluded to when Doctora Fanny de Mora resigned to leave for Panama in mid-1944 and the council discussed who should replace her for the remaining few months of her contract. The physicians on the council thought it should be a physician because the nursing students "study better with a man than with a woman; a male professor inspires more respect and therefore confidence." Middlemiss pointed out, however, that "the male professors have not proven to be very reliable, unlike Dra. de Mora" (Actas del Concejo Ejecutivo, 1942–1946, meeting minutes for 18 September 1944, AENE). Judith Egas, a licentiate in medicine who needed only to complete her thesis to graduate as doctora, was accepted following the dean's positive recommendation of her. Egas went on to become the eighth woman to graduate as doctora de medicina from the Universidad Central (AGUC).

30. Actas del Concejo Ejecutivo, 1947–1952, meeting minutes for 16 March 1950 (discussion of the 1950 budget), AENE. This reflected the curriculum established from the beginning by las Americanas, with the addition in the mid-1940s of English classes.

31. Actas del Concejo Ejecutivo, 1947–1952, meeting minutes for 10 July 1947, AENE.

32. Actas del Concejo Ejecutivo, 1947–1952, meeting minutes for 10 October 1947, AENE.

33. This had begun in early 1944 as a per-class payment only to those who were not already employed by the university; in 1948 hourly payments were finally extended to all members of the teaching staff who did not work full-time at the school (by 1950, paid at the rate of thirty sucres per hour).

34. Interview with Judith Armas's niece, Iralda Benítez de Núñez, Quito, 5 July 2005.

35. Actas del Concejo Ejecutivo, 1947–1952, meeting minutes for 23 March 1950, AENE.

36. Actas del Concejo Ejecutivo, 1947–1952, meeting minutes for 3 May 1951, AENE. In 1958 the Asociación de Enfermeras del Ecuador was founded to meet this need (de la Torre and Velasco, "La educación de enfermería en el estado liberal . . . ," 92).

37. Actas del Concejo Ejecutivo, 1942–1946, meeting minutes for 17 May 1943, AENE.

38. Actas del Concejo Ejecutivo, 1947–1952, meeting minutes for 11 October 1952,

AENE. Eventually the ENE itself took on a leadership role in providing training to the *auxiliares*, following the departure of the Servicio Cooperativo.

39. Actas del Concejo Ejecutivo, 1942–1946, meeting minutes for 19 April 1943, AENE.

40. They established the Escuela de Enfermeras San Vicente de Paul in 1946 for the purposes of training nursing nuns. Later, following the establishment of the private Pontificia Universidad Católica del Ecuador, in 1965 a faculty of nursing was opened there, which recruited secular students. Before that, Ligia Gomezjurado during her directorship of the Escuela successfully built bridges with the Hermanas de la Caridad, some of whom did undertake some coursework at the school (interview with Iralda Benítez de Núñez, Quito, 5 July 2005).

41. Actas del Concejo Ejecutivo, 1942–1946, meeting minutes for 9 January 1943, AENE.

42. Actas del Concejo Ejecutivo, 1942–1946, meeting minutes for 31 May 1943, AENE.

43. Actas del Concejo Ejecutivo, 1942–1946, meeting minutes for 27 August 1945, AENE. Documents housed at the Rockefeller Archive Center reveal that the Rockefeller Foundation determined after her arrival in the United States that Colombia Galvis was suffering from equine encephalitis rather than polio. The foundation's decision that they therefore were not responsible for her treatment may explain why she returned so quickly to Quito to complete her training at the ENE (Nicola Foote, personal communication, June 2011). For analysis of some of the Rockefeller documentation about the Ecuadorian nursing school, see Nicola Foote, "International Discourses of Domesticity in Ecuador: Race, Gender, and the Home in Missionary Work and Modernization Projects, 1900–1960," paper presented at the American Historical Association conference, Boston, January 2011.

44. Actas del Concejo Ejecutivo, 1942–1946, meeting minutes for 3 June 1946, AENE.

45. Actas del Concejo Ejecutivo, 1947–1952, meeting minutes for 5 February 1948, AENE.

46. Actas del Concejo Ejecutivo, 1942–1946, meeting minutes for 9 April 1945, AENE.

47. Actas del Concejo Ejecutivo, 1942–1946, meeting minutes for 26 November 1946, AENE.

48. Actas del Concejo Ejecutivo, 1947–1952, meeting minutes for 11 October 1952, AENE.

49. Actas del Concejo Ejecutivo, 1947–1952, meeting minutes for 29 January 1948, AENE.

50. Actas del Concejo Ejecutivo, 1942–1946, meeting minutes for 29 November 1943, AENE.

51. The following discussion and quotations are drawn from Actas del Concejo Ejecutivo, 1942–1946, meeting minutes for 6 December 1943, AENE.

52. Actas del Concejo Ejecutivo, 1942–1946, meeting minutes for 10 January 1944, AENE.

53. Actas del Concejo Ejecutivo, 1942–1946, meeting minutes for 8 March 1943, AENE.

54. Actas del Concejo Ejecutivo, 1947–1952, meeting minutes for 8 December 1949, AENE.

55. Actas del Concejo Ejecutivo, 1947–1952, meeting minutes for 5 October 1950, AENE.

56. Actas del Concejo Ejecutivo, 1942–1946, meeting minutes for 19 March 1945, AENE. In an interview Margarita Velasco, an acute observer of Ecuadorian society, commented that in the early twenty-first century still the central figure around which all hospital work turned was not the patient but the physician (Quito, 6 July 2005).

57. The director of the nursing school to the director of the Hospital Eugenio Espejo, Quito, 2 April 1945, LCR 1945-I, AAP/MNM; director of the nursing school to the director of the Junta Central de Asistencia Pública, Quito, 6 April 1945, LCR 1945-I, AAP/MNM.

58. Actas del Concejo Ejecutivo, 1942–1946, meeting minutes for 9 April 1945, AENE.

59. The dean of medicine to Dr. Estupiñán, Quito, 10 April 1945, LCR 1945-I, AAP/MNM.

60. Actas del Concejo Ejecutivo, 1942–1946, meeting minutes for 11 March 1946, AENE.

61. Actas del Concejo Ejecutivo, 1942–1946, meeting minutes for 3 June 1946, AENE.

62. Actas del Concejo Ejecutivo, 1947–1952, meeting minutes for 21 April 1947, AENE.

63. Adrila Aguirre (who was a student from 1949 through 1952) recounted an experience she had as a nursing student in the operating room that mirrored this case very closely (interview, 13 July 2005).

64. Actas del Concejo Ejecutivo, 1942–1946, meeting minutes for 1 July 1944, AENE.

65. Written submission by Tula Espinosa, 28 July 1948, discussed at the council meeting on 29 July. Actas del Concejo Ejecutivo, 1947–1952, meeting minutes for 29 July 1948, AENE. Some of the spirit she shows here led Espinosa to become a leader of Ecuadorian nursing in the 1970s, both of the nurses' professional association and then of the first union that included nurses (Velasco and Alvarez, *La historia contada desde las líderes*).

66. Actas del Concejo Ejecutivo, 1947–1952, meeting minutes for 29 July 1948, AENE.

67. When this anecdote was recounted to the nurses interviewed, they reflected on the direct transfer into the space of the hospital of the male-female relation existing in society. They also commented on their experiences and observations that nurses were expected to serve physicians coffee, and on their training that as subordinates

they should greet physicians on passing them in the hallway (rather than physicians, as men, having the courtesy to greet them first, as women). In other words, nurses' identity as women might lead to contradictory expectations—that they be subordinate to men but also that men should observe gendered courtesies with them. These were difficult waters to navigate.

68. The "problem of orthopedics" was discussed at meetings between August and October 1949; Actas del Concejo Ejecutivo, 1947–1952, AENE.

69. Nelson, *Say Little, Do Much.*

70. Actas del Concejo Ejecutivo, 1947–1952, meeting minutes for 22 November 1952, AENE.

71. Reproduced in "El décimo aniversario de la Fundación de la Escuela Nacional de Enfermeras de la Universidad Central," *Boletín de informaciones científicas nacionales* 5, no. 50 (1952): 352–53.

72. "El décimo aniversario," 356.

73. Interview with Rosa Santamaría, Quito, 7 July 2005. Following a guest lecture to the students and staff of the school in May 2010, Rosa Santamaría further commented that despite receiving a scholarship to attend the nursing school in the Universidad Católica, she fought instead to study at the Escuela Nacional, since she was from a liberal family. However, once she enrolled, she discovered that the atmosphere at the latter was even more Catholic than at the former. Indeed, at the Universidad Católica, nursing students were permitted to entertain their boyfriends in the public reception areas of the school's residence—something that was never allowed in her student days at the Escuela Nacional.

74. Interview with Iralda Benítez de Núñez, Quito, 5 July 2005.

75. Actas del Concejo Ejecutivo, 1942–1946, meeting minutes for 14 October 1946, AENE.

76. Actas del Concejo Ejecutivo, 1947–1952, meeting minutes for 4 August 1949, AENE.

77. Actas del Concejo Ejecutivo, 1947–1952, meeting minutes for 3 May 1952, AENE.

78. Actas del Concejo Ejecutivo, 1942–1946, meeting minutes for 19 June 1944, AENE.

79. This was not the only case where a student enrolled against the wishes of her parents. Adrila Aguirre, who began her studies in 1949, also chose nursing over her father's objections. He still saw nursing in its former terms: as a servile job, as a servant to physicians. Adrila enrolled anyway, and because her father would not provide the necessary financial guarantee, she asked her sister's fiancé to do so. Interview in Quito, 13 July 2005.

80. Actas del Concejo Ejecutivo, 1942–1946, meeting minutes for 6 November 1945, AENE.

81. "Reunión de todas las alumnas del plantel convocada por el Dr. Ricaurte, el 10 de Noviembre de 1945"; Actas del Concejo Ejecutivo, 1942–1946, AENE.

82. Actas del Concejo Ejecutivo, 1942–1946, meeting minutes for 1 July 1944, AENE.

83. Indeed, several nurses were interviewed who upon graduating in the 1950s, 1960s, and even 1970s were placed in charge of new medical facilities or were asked to thoroughly reorganize the structures of work at existing ones, as the only professional nurses onsite.

84. There was some early ambiguity over marital status of students (and teachers), but a clear model emerged by the end of the school's first decade that required both to be single. It was only in the early 1960s that Georgina Morales de Carrillo became the first member of the school's teaching staff who married without resigning her position. However, to achieve this right, she had to go over Directora Gomezjurado's head, requesting successfully that the dean and the executive council overrule the directora's decision (interview with Georgina Morales de Carrillo, 11 July 2005).

85. Actas del Concejo Ejecutivo, 1947–1952, meeting minutes for 4 March 1948, AENE.

86. Actas del Concejo Ejecutivo, 1947–1952, meeting minutes for 9 September 1948, AENE.

87. Actas del Concejo Ejecutivo, 1947–1952, meeting minutes for 3 August 1950, AENE.

88. Actas del Concejo Ejecutivo, 1947–1952, meeting minutes for 3 May 1952, AENE.

89. Actas del Concejo Ejecutivo, 1947–1952, meeting minutes for 16 June 1947, AENE.

90. Actas del Concejo Ejecutivo, 1947–1952, meeting minutes for 16 June 1947, AENE.

91. Actas del Concejo Ejecutivo, 1947–1952, meeting minutes for 26 June 1947, AENE.

92. Actas del Concejo Ejecutivo, 1947–1952, meeting minutes for 24 July 1947, AENE.

93. Actas del Concejo Ejecutivo, 1947–1952, meeting minutes for 18 January 1948, AENE.

94. This was emphasized especially in the interview with Clemencia Gía, Quito, 11 July 2005; however, many interviewees commented on this dimension of their training.

95. Interview with Adrila Aguirre, Quito, 13 July 2005.

96. Interview with Georgina Morales de Carrillo, Quito, 11 July 2005.

97. Interview with Adrila Aguirre, Quito, 13 July 2005.

98. Interview with Georgina Morales de Carrillo, Quito, 11 July 2005.

99. Interview with Iralda Benítez de Núñez, Quito, 5 July 2005.

100. Interview with Georgina Morales de Carrillo, Quito, 11 July 2005.

101. Interview with Georgina Morales de Carrillo, Quito, 11 July 2005.

102. Interview with Iralda Benítez de Núñez, Quito, 5 July 2005.

103. Interview with Margarita Velasco, Quito, 6 July 2005.

104. These norms of conduct are in Actas del Concejo Ejecutivo, 1947–1952, AENE.

105. In Ana María Goetschel, *Educación de las mujeres, maestras y esferas públicas: Quito en la primera mitad del siglo XX* (Quito: FLACSO/Abya Yala, 2007), 185.

106. Fernando Jurado Noboa, *Las Quiteñas* (Quito: Dinediciones, 1995), 298.

107. Interview with Adrila Aguirre, Quito, 13 July 2005.

108. Information on this period can be found in Patricia de la Torre and Margarita Velasco, "La educación de la enfermería en el estado capitalista ecuatoriano, 1960–1983," *Boletín de informaciones científicas nacionales* 119 (1986): 71–103.

109. Caroline Moser, "Adjustment from Below: Low Income Women, Time, and the Triple Role in Guayaquil, Ecuador," in *"Viva": Women and Popular Protest in Latin America*, edited by Sarah Radcliffe and Sallie Westwood (London: Routledge, 1993), 177.

## Conclusion

1. Philip Corrigan, *State Forms/Human Capacities: Essays in Authority and Difference* (London: Routledge, 1990), 265.

2. Report from the medical director of the Oficina de Profilaxis Venérea in Guayaquil to the president of congress, Guayaquil, 11 April 1951, AFL, Cámara de Diputados, caja no. 11 (374), expedientes, serie DD-51-III-B, no. 1-35, 1951.

3. Interview with Rosa Santamaría, Quito, 7 July 2005.

4. Interviews with Ximena Cevallos, Quito, 7 July 2005, and Margarita Velasco, Quito, 6 July 2005.

5. Elizabeth F. S. Roberts, *God's Laboratory: Assisted Reproduction in the Andes* (Berkeley: University of California Press, 2012).

6. Esben Leifsen, "Moralities and Politics of Belonging: Governing Female Reproduction in Twentieth-Century Quito" (PhD diss., University of Oslo, 2006), 246–47.

7. Eric R. Wolf, *Peasant Wars of the Twentieth Century* (New York: Harper and Row, 1969), chapter 7.

8. I was inspired in this by Adriana Premat's unpublished manuscript "Popular Culture, Politics, and Gender Imaginaries in the Argentina of the 1960s and 1970s."

9. Guillermo Bustos, "Notas sobre economía y sociedad en Quito y la Sierra centro norte durante las primeras décadas del siglo XX," *Quitumbe* 7 (1990): 101–17.

10. Philip Abrams, "Notes on the Difficulty of Studying the State," *Journal of Historical Sociology* 1, no. 1 (1988): 58–89.

# BIBLIOGRAPHY

## Archives

AAP/MNM   Archivo de la Asistencia Pública, Museo Nacional de Medicina, Quito

AENE   Archivo de la Escuela Nacional de Enfermeras, Quito

AFL   Archivo de la Función Legislativa, Quito

AGUC   Archivo General de la Universidad Central, Quito

AHCSJD/MNM   Archivo del Hospital Civil San Juan de Dios, Museo Nacional de Medicina, Quito

ASS/MNM   Archivo del Servicio de Sanidad, Museo Nacional de Medicina, Quito

## Books and Articles

Abbott, Andrew. *The System of Professions: An Essay on the Division of Expert Labor.* Chicago: University of Chicago Press, 1988.

Abrams, Philip. *Historical Sociology.* Ithaca: Cornell University Press, 1982.

———. "Notes on the Difficulty of Studying the State." *Journal of Historical Sociology* 1, no. 1 (1988): 58–89.

*Acuerdo del Consejo General de Instrucción Pública reorganizando la Escuela de Enfermeras anexa a la Facultad de Medicina de la Universidad Central.* Quito: Imprenta de la Universidad Central, 1921.

Alfaro, Eloy. "Mensaje de Eloy Alfaro a los diputados, sesión ordinario de 13 de Junio de 1897." *Diario de debates* (1897): 1734–35.

Allende, Salvador. *La realidad médico-social Chilena.* 1939; reprint, Santiago: Editorial Cuarto Propio, 1999.

Andrade Marín, Carlos. *La protección a la infancia en el Ecuador.* Quito, 1929.

Arcos, Carlos. "El espíritu de progreso: Los hacendados en el Ecuador del 900." *Cultura* 19 (1984): 107–34.

Ayala Mora, Enrique. *Historia de la revolución liberal ecuatoriana.* Quito: Corporación Editora Nacional, 1994.

———, ed. *Federico González Suárez y la polémica sobre el estado laico.* Quito: Banco Central and Corporación Editora Nacional, 1978.

Ayora, Isidro. "Crónicas médicas de la capital: Escuela de Enfermeras de Quito." *Anales de la Sociedad Médico-Quirúrgica del Guayas* 22, no. 1 (1922): 516–17.

Barrera B., Jaime. "La mujer y el delito." *Archivos de criminología, neuropsiquiatría y disciplinas conexas* (Quito) nos. 6–7 (1943): 50–119.

Bastidas, Antonio J. *Contribución al estudio de la protección infantil en el Ecuador y demografía nacional.* Quito: Imprenta Municipal, 1924.

———. *La ilegitimidad, factor de letalidad infantil.* Quito: Imprenta de la Universidad Central, 1932.

Becerra, León. "Informe de la Dirección del Servicio de Sanidad Pública del Ecuador." Appendix to *Informe que Modesto A. Peñaherrera, ministro de lo interior, municipalidades, policía, obras públicas, etc., presenta a la nación en 1914.* By Modesto A. Peñaherrera. 429–38. Quito: Imprenta y Encuadernación Nacionales, 1914.

Becker, Marc. *Indians and Leftists in the Making of Ecuador's Indian Movements.* Durham: Duke University Press, 2007.

Besse, Susan K. *Restructuring Patriarchy: The Modernization of Gender Inequality in Brazil, 1914–1940.* Chapel Hill: University of North Carolina Press, 1996.

Black, Chad Thomas. *The Limits of Gender Domination: Women, the Law, and Political Crisis in Quito, 1765–1830.* Albuquerque: University of New Mexico Press, 2010.

Bliss, Katherine Elaine. *Compromised Positions: Prostitution, Public Health, and Gender Politics in Revolutionary Mexico City.* University Park: Pennsylvania State University Press, 2001.

———. "The Right to Live as *Gente Decente*: Sex Work, Family Life, and Collective Identity in Early Twentieth-Century Mexico." *Journal of Women's History* 15, no. 4 (2004): 164–69.

Blum, Ann S. "Cleaning the Revolutionary Household: Domestic Servants and Public Welfare in Mexico City, 1900–1935." *Journal of Women's History* 15, no. 4 (2004): 67–90.

———. *Domestic Economies: Family, Work, and Welfare in Mexico City, 1884–1943.* Lincoln: University of Nebraska Press, 2010.

———. "Dying of Sadness: Hospitalism and Child Welfare in Mexico City, 1920–1940." In *Disease in the History of Modern Latin America.* Edited by Diego Armus. 209–36. Durham: Duke University Press, 2003.

Bourdieu, Pierre. "The Forms of the Capital." In *The Handbook of Theory and Research for the Sociology of Education.* Edited by John Richardson. 241–58. New York: Greenwood Press, 1986.

Brandt, Allan. "Sexually Transmitted Diseases." In *Companion Encyclopedia of the History of Medicine.* Volume 1. Edited by W. F. Bynum and Roy Porter. 562–84. London: Routledge, 1993.

Bustos, Guillermo. "La politización del 'problema obrero': Los trabajadores quiteños entre la identidad 'pueblo' y la identidad 'clase' (1931–1934)." In *Las crises en el Ecuador: Los treinta y los ochenta*. Quito: Corporación Editora Nacional, 1991.

———. "Notas sobre economía y sociedad en Quito y la sierra centro norte durante las primeras décadas del siglo XX." *Quitumbe* 7 (1990): 101–17.

———. "Quito en la transición: Actores colectivos e identidades culturales urbanas (1920–1950)." In *Quito a través de la historia*. 163–88. Quito: Municipio de Quito, 1992.

Caja de Pensiones. *Segundo censo de afiliados realizado el 30 de Abril de 1935*. Quito, 1936.

Carranza, María. "'In the Name of Forests': Highlights of the History of Family Planning in Costa Rica." *Canadian Journal of Latin American and Caribbean Studies* 35, no. 69 (2010): 119–54.

Caulfield, Sueann. "The Birth of Mangue: Race, Nation, and the Politics of Prostitution in Rio de Janeiro, 1850–1942." In *Sex and Sexuality in Latin America*. Edited by Daniel Balderston and Donna J. Guy. 86–100. New York: New York University Press, 1997.

———. "Getting into Trouble: Dishonest Women, Modern Girls, and Women-Men in the Conceptual Language of *Vida Policial*, 1925–1927." *Signs* 19, no. 1 (1993): 146–76.

———, Sarah C. Chambers, and Lara Putnam, eds. *Honor, Status, and Law in Modern Latin America*. Durham: Duke University Press, 2005.

Christiansen, Tanja. *Disobedience, Slander, Seduction, and Assault: Women and Men in Cajamarca, Peru, 1862–1900*. Austin: University of Texas Press, 2004.

Clark, A. Kim. "El sexo y la responsabilidad en Quito: Prostitución, género y el estado, c. 1920–1950." *Procesos* 16 (2001): 35–59.

———. "Feminismos estéticos y antiestéticos en el Ecuador de principios del siglo XX: Un análisis de género y generaciones." *Procesos* 22 (2005): 85–105.

———. "Género, raza y nación: La protección a la infancia en el Ecuador, 1910–1945." In *Palabras del silencio: Las mujeres latinoamericanas y su historia*. Edited by Martha Moscoso. 219–56. Quito: Abya-Yala, Netherlands' Directorate-General for International Cooperation (DGIS), and UNICEF, 1995.

———. "Race, 'Culture' and Mestizaje: The Statistical Construction of the Ecuadorian Nation, 1930–1950." *Journal of Historical Sociology* 11, no. 2 (1998): 185–211.

———. *The Redemptive Work: Railway and Nation in Ecuador, 1895–1930*. Wilmington: Scholarly Resources, 1998.

———, and Marc Becker, eds. *Highland Indians and the State in Modern Ecuador*. Pittsburgh: University of Pittsburgh Press, 2007.

Compañía de las Hijas de la Caridad. *Trescientos cincuenta aniversario de la fundación (1633– 1983): Aporte de las hijas de la caridad para el desarrollo de enfermería en el Ecuador*. Quito, 1982.

Compañía Guía del Ecuador. *El Ecuador: Guía comercial, agrícola e industrial de la república*. Guayaquil: Talleres de Artes Gráficos de E. Rodenas, 1909.

Córdova, Gonzalo. *Informe del ministro de lo interior y policía, obras públicas, etc. al congreso ordinario de 1903*. Quito: Imprenta Nacional, 1903.

Coronel, Adriana Valeria. "A Revolution in Stages: Subaltern Politics, Nation-State Formation, and the Origins of Social Rights in Ecuador, 1834–1943." PhD diss., New York University, 2011.

Correa, Alberto. *Conferencias sustentadas en el Teatro Variedades el 14 y 15 de enero de 1930*. Quito: Imprenta Luis E. Giacometti, 1930.

Corrigan, Philip. *State Forms/Human Capacities: Essays in Authority and Difference*. London: Routledge, 1990.

——, and Derek Sayer. *The Great Arch: English State Formation as Cultural Revolution*. New York: Basil Blackwell, 1985.

Crespo de Ortíz Bilbao, Lola. *Mi vida tal como la conté a uno de mis hijos*. Quito: Corporación Editora Nacional, 2003.

Crespo, Emiliano J. "Conferencia sobre puericultura." *Revista de la Universidad de Cuenca* 7 (1926): 1–34.

Curtis, Bruce. *The Politics of Population: State Formation, Statistics, and the Census of Canada, 1840–1875*. Toronto: University of Toronto Press, 2001.

Cuvi Sánchez, María, ed. *Quito casa adentro: Narrado por mujeres*. Quito: Fondo de Salvamento del Patrimonio Cultural (FONSAL), 2009.

Dávila, Luis G. "La Gota de Leche: Lo que se puede aguardar en Quito de esta obra de protección infantil." *Anales de la Universidad Central* 31, no. 247 (1923): 199–254.

Dean, Mitchell. "'Demonic Societies': Liberalism, Biopolitics, and Sovereignty." In *States of Imagination: Ethnographic Explorations of the Postcolonial State*. Edited by Thomas Blom Hansen and Finn Stepputat. 41–64. Durham: Duke University Press, 2001.

Defossez, Anne-Claire. "Un hospital testigo del siglo: Historia social y reproductiva de mujeres enfermas en Quito (1925–1965)." In *Mujeres de los Andes: Condiciones de vida y salud*. Edited by Anne-Claire Defossez, Didier Fassin, and Mara Viveros. 39–60. Colombia: Instituto Francés de Estudios Andinos and Universidad Externado de Colombia, 1992.

de la Cadena, Marisol. "'Women Are More Indian': Ethnicity and Gender in a Community near Cuzco." In *Ethnicity, Markets, and Migration in the Andes*. Edited by Brooke Larson and Olivia Harris. 329–48. Durham: Duke University Press, 1995.

de la Torre, Carlos. *La seducción velasquista*. Quito: Libri Mundi, 1993.

de la Torre, Patricia. *Lo privado y local en el Estado ecuatoriano: La Junta de Beneficencia de Guayaquil*. Quito: Abya Yala, 1999.

——, and Margarita Velasco. "La educación de enfermería en el estado liberal ecuatoriano." *Boletín de informaciones científicas nacionales* 117 (1985): 85–97.

——. "La educación de la enfermería en el estado capitalista ecuatoriano, 1960–1983." *Boletín de informaciones científicas nacionales* 119 (1986): 71–103.

Delgado Capeáns, R.P.Fr. Ricardo. *Deberes de la madre cristiana*. Quito: Tipografía y Encuadernación de la "Prensa Católica," 1923.

Demélas, Marie-Danielle, and Yves Saint-Geours. *Jerusalén y Babilonia: Religión y política en el Ecuador, 1780–1880.* Quito: Corporación Editora Nacional y Instituto Francés de Estudios Andinos, 1988.

Díaz, Octavio. *Informe que a la nación presenta el ministro de lo interior, policía, beneficencia, obras públicas, etc. en el año 1910.* Quito: Imprenta y Encuadernación Nacionales, 1910.

Dirección General de Sanidad. *Nómina de médicos y cirujanos, dentistas, farmacéuticos y obstetrices, inscritos en Quito y Guayaquil.* Quito: Imprenta Nacional, 1932.

Domínguez, Luis F. "Reforma al Código Penal: Aborto criminal." In *Memoria del II Congreso Médico Ecuatoriano.* 225–33. Guayaquil: Imprenta y Literatura La Reforma, 1931.

Drinot, Paulo. *The Allure of Labor: Workers, Race, and the Making of the Peruvian State.* Durham: Duke University Press, 2011.

Durán, Cecilia. *Irrupción del sector burócrata en el estado ecuatoriano, 1925–1944.* Quito: Abya Yala and Pontificia Universidad Católica del Ecuador, 2000.

"El décimo aniversario de la fundación de la Escuela Nacional de Enfermeras de la Universidad Central." *Boletín de informaciones científicas nacionales* 5, no. 50 (1952): 350–56.

Espinosa Tamayo, Alfredo. *Consejos a las madres: Cartilla higiénica de puericultura.* Guayaquil: Imprenta La Reforma, 1914.

Estrada, Jenny. *Mujeres de Guayaquil.* Guayaquil: Banco Central and Archivo Histórico del Guayas, 1984.

———. *Una mujer total: Matilde Hidalgo de Prócel (biografía).* Guayaquil: Imprenta de la Universidad de Guayaquil, 1980.

Ferguson, James, and Akhil Gupta. "Spatializing States: Toward an Ethnography of Neoliberal Governmentality." *American Ethnologist* 29, no. 4 (2002): 981–1002.

Foote, Nicola. "International Discourses of Domesticity in Ecuador: Race, Gender, and the Home in Missionary Work and Modernization Projects, 1900–1960." Paper presented at the American Historical Association conference. Boston. January 2011.

Foucault, Michel. "Governmentality." In *The Foucault Effect: Studies in Governmentality.* Edited by Graham Burchell, Colin Gordon, and Peter Miller. 87–104. Chicago: University of Chicago Press, 1991.

———. *The History of Sexuality.* Volume 1, *An Introduction.* New York: Vintage Books, 1980.

French, William E. "Prostitutes and Guardian Angels: Women, Work, and the Family in Porfirian Mexico." *Hispanic American Historical Review* 72, no. 4 (1992): 529–53.

Garcés, Enrique. *Por, para y del niño (tomo II).* Quito: Talleres Gráficos de Educación, 1937.

Goetschel, Ana María. *Educación de las mujeres, maestras y esferas públicas: Quito en la primera mitad del siglo XX.* Quito: Facultad Latinoamericana de Ciencias Sociales and Abya Yala, 2007.

———. "Educación e imágenes de mujer." In *Y el amor no era todo . . . Mujeres, imágenes y conflictos.* Edited by Martha Moscoso. 59–83. Quito: Abya Yala and DGIS, 1996.

———. "Las paradojas del liberalismo y las mujeres: Coyuntura 1907–1909." In *Celebraciones centenarias y negociaciones por al nación ecuatoriana.* Edited by Valeria Coronel and Mercedes Prieto. 209–40. Quito: FLACSO and Ministerio de Cultura, 2010.

Goetschel, Ana María, Andrea Pequeño, Mercedes Prieto, and Gioconda Herrera. *De memorias: Imágenes públicas de las mujeres ecuatorianas de comienzos y fines del siglo veinte.* Quito: FONSAL and FLACSO, 2007.

Gómez, Jorge. *Las misiones pedagógicas alemanas y la educación en el Ecuador.* Quito: Abya Yala, Proyecto EBI-MEC-GTZ, 1993.

Gómez de la Torre, Rafael. *Informe concerniente a las secciones de instrucción pública, justicia y beneficencia que presenta el ministro de gobierno a la convención nacional de 1896–1897.* Quito: Imprenta Nacional, 1897.

Graham Lauderdale, Sandra. "Slavery's Impasse: Slave Prostitutes, Small-Time Mistresses, and the Brazilian Law of 1871." *Comparative Studies in Society and History* 33–34 (1991): 669–94.

Gupta, Akhil. "Blurred Boundaries: The Discourse of Corruption, the Culture of Politics, and the Imagined State." *American Ethnologist* 22, no. 2 (1995): 375–402.

———. "Governing Population: The Integrated Child Development Services Program in India." In *States of Imagination: Ethnographic Explorations of the Postcolonial State.* Edited by Thomas Blom Hansen and Finn Stepputat. 65–96. Durham: Duke University Press, 2001.

Guy, Donna J. "Medical Imperialism Gone Awry: The Campaign against Legalized Prostitution in Latin America." In *Science, Medicine, and Cultural Imperialism.* Edited by Teresa Meade and Mark Walker. 75–94. New York: St. Martin's Press, 1991.

———. *Sex and Danger in Buenos Aires: Prostitution, Family, and Nation in Argentina.* Lincoln: University of Nebraska Press, 1991.

———. *Women Build the Welfare State: Performing Charity and Creating Rights in Argentina, 1880–1955.* Durham: Duke University Press, 2009.

Hansen, Thomas Blom, and Finn Stepputat, eds. *States of Imagination: Ethnographic Explorations of the Postcolonial State.* Durham: Duke University Press, 2001.

Hecht, Tobias, ed. *Minor Omissions: Children in Latin American History.* Madison: University of Wisconsin Press, 2002.

Herrera, Gioconda. "El congreso católico de mujeres en 1909 y la regeneración de la nación." In *Celebraciones centenarias y negociaciones por la nación ecuatoriana.* Edited by Valeria Coronel and Mercedes Prieto, 241–63. Quito: FLACSO and Ministerio de Cultura, 2010.

Joseph, Gilbert, and Daniel Nugent, eds. *Everyday Forms of State Formation: Revolution and the Negotiation of Rule in Mexico.* Durham: Duke University Press, 1994.

Jurado Noboa, Fernando. *Las Quiteñas.* Quito: Dinediciones, 1995.

Kingman Garcés, Eduardo. *La ciudad y los otros, Quito 1860–1940: Higienismo, ornato y policía.* Quito: FLACSO and Universidad Rovira e Virgili, 2006.

Koven, Seth, and Sonya Michel, eds. *Mothers of a New World: Maternalist Politics and the Origins of Welfare States.* New York: Routledge, 1993.

Krupa, Christopher. "State by Proxy: Privatized Government in the Andes." *Comparative Studies in Society and History* 52, no. 2 (2010): 319–50.

Landázuri Camacho, Mariana. *Juana Miranda: Fundadora de la Maternidad de Quito.* Quito: Banco Central, 2004.

Larrea Borja, Piedad. "Biografía de la mujer en el Ecuador: Romanticismo y siglo XX." *El espectador* (Quito) 1 (1943): 3.

Lavrin, Asunción. *Women, Feminism, and Social Change in Argentina, Chile, and Uruguay, 1890–1940.* Lincoln: University of Nebraska Press, 1995.

Leifsen, Esben. "Moralities and Politics of Belonging: Governing Female Reproduction in Twentieth Century Quito." PhD diss., University of Oslo, 2006.

Leinaweaver, Jessaca. *The Circulation of Children: Kinship, Adoption, and Morality in Andean Peru.* Durham: Duke University Press, 2008.

Linke, Lilo. *Ecuador: Country of Contrasts.* London: Royal Institute of International Affairs, 1954.

Lucero, José Antonio. *Struggles of Voice: The Politics of Indigenous Representation in the Andes.* Pittsburgh: University of Pittsburgh Press, 2008.

Maiguashca, Juan. "Los sectores subalternos en los años 30 y el aparecimiento del velasquismo." In *Las crises en el Ecuador: Los treinta y ochenta.* Edited by Rosemary Thorp. 79–94. Quito: Corporación Editora Nacional, 1991.

———, and Liisa North. "Orígenes y significado del velasquismo: Lucha de clases y participación política en el Ecuador, 1920–1972." In *La cuestión regional y el poder.* Edited by Rafael Quintero. 89–159. Quito: Corporación Editora Nacional, 1991.

Marchán Romero, Carlos. "La crisis de los años treinta: Diferenciación social de sus efectos económicos." In *Las crises en el Ecuador: Los treinta y ochenta.* Edited by Rosemary Thorp. 31–60. Quito: Corporación Editora Nacional, 1991.

Martínez, Luis A. *Memoria del secretario de instrucción pública, correos y telégrafos, etc. al congreso ordinario de 1905.* Quito: Tipografía de la Escuela de Artes y Oficios, 1905.

Martínez-Alier, Verena. *Marriage, Class, and Color in Nineteenth-Century Cuba.* Cambridge: Cambridge University Press, 1974.

McCreery, David. "'This Life of Misery and Shame': Female Prostitution in Guatemala City, 1880–1920." *Journal of Latin American Studies* 18, no. 2 (1986): 333–53.

Milton, Cynthia. *The Many Meanings of Poverty: Colonialism, Social Compacts, and Assistance in Eighteenth-Century Ecuador.* Stanford: Stanford University Press, 2007.

Miño, Carlos. "Informe de la Subdirección de Sanidad de la provincia de Pichincha al ministro de Sanidad y al director del Servicio de Sanidad Pública." Appendix to *Informe que Modesto A. Peñaherrera, ministro de lo interior, municipalidades,*

*policía, obras públicas, etc., presenta a la nación en 1914*. By Modesto A. Peñaherrera. 439–46. Quito: Imprenta y Encuadernación Nacionales, 1914.

Miño Grijalva, Wilson. *Eduardo Larrea Stacey: Visionario y precursor de un nuevo
Ecuador*. Quito: Banco Central, 2006.

Miranda Ribadeneira, Francisco. *Las religiosas del buen pastor en el Ecuador: Rasgos
históricos*. Quito: Imprenta del Colegio Técnico Don Bosco, 1970.

Moncayo, Abelardo. *Informe del ministro de lo interior y policía, beneficencia, etc. al
congreso ordinario de 1898*. Quito: Imprenta Nacional, 1898.

———. *Informe del ministro de lo interior y policía, beneficencia, etc. al congreso de
1899*. Quito: Imprenta Nacional, 1899.

———. *Informe del ministro de lo interior y policía, beneficencia, etc. al congreso
ordinario de 1900*. Quito: Imprenta Nacional, 1900.

Morgan, Lynn, and Elizabeth Roberts. "Rights and Reproduction in Latin America."
*Anthropology News* (March 2009): 12–13.

Moscoso, Martha. "Discurso religioso y discurso estatal: La mujer sumisa." In *Y el
amor no era todo . . . Mujeres, imágenes y conflictos*. Edited by Martha Moscoso.
21–57. Quito: Abya Yala and DGIS, 1996.

———. "Imagen de la mujer y la familia a inicios del siglo XX." *Procesos* 8 (1996):
67–82.

Moser, Caroline. "Adjustment from Below: Low Income Women, Time, and the
Triple Role in Guayaquil, Ecuador." In *"Viva!": Women and Popular Protest in
Latin America*. Edited by Sarah Radcliffe and Sallie Westwood. 173–96. London:
Routledge, 1993.

Muñoz, Leonardo J. *Testimonio de lucha: Memorias sobre la historia del socialismo en
el Ecuador*. Quito: Corporación Editora Nacional, 1988.

Nelson, Sioban. *Say Little, Do Much: Nursing, Nuns, and Hospitals in the Nineteenth
Century*. Philadelphia: University of Pennsylvania Press, 2001.

"Nómina del cuerpo médico ecuatoriano en el año 1938." *Anales de la Sociedad
Médico-Quirúrgica del Guayaquil* 18, no. 1 (1938): 27–42.

Nugent, David. "State and Shadow State in Northern Peru circa 1900: Illegal Political
Networks and the Problem of State Boundaries." In *States and Illegal Practices*.
Edited by Josiah McC. Heyman. 63–98. New York: Berg, 1999.

Núñez, Jorge, Cecilia Mantilla, Enrique Abad, Lenin Miño, Mónica León, Matilde
Wolter, Hugo Vaca, Juan Carrera, and Selma Merino. *Historia del Seguro Social
Ecuatoriano*. Quito: Instituto Ecuatoriano de Seguridad Social, 1984.

O'Connor, Erin. *Gender, Indian, Nation: The Contradictions of Making Ecuador,
1830–1925*. Tucson: University of Arizona Press, 2007.

Painter, Joe. "Prosaic Geographies of Stateness." *Political Geography* 25 (2006): 752–74.

Palleres, Amalia. *From Peasant Struggles to Indian Resistance: The Ecuadorian Andes
in the Late Twentieth Century*. Norman: University of Oklahoma Press, 2002.

Palmer, Steven. *From Popular Medicine to Medical Populism: Doctors, Healers, and
Public Power in Costa Rica, 1800–1940*. Durham: Duke University Press, 2003.

Paz y Miño Cepeda, Juan. *Revolución Juliana: Nación, ejército y bancocracia.* Second edition. Quito: Abya Yala, 2000.

Peñaherrera, Modesto A. *Informe que Modesto A. Peñaherrera, ministro de lo interior, municipalidades, policía, obras públicas, etc., presenta a la nación en 1913.* Quito: Imprenta y Encuadernación Nacionales, 1913.

———. *Informe que Modesto A. Peñaherrera, ministro de lo interior, municipalidades, policía, obras públicas, etc., presenta a la nación en 1914.* Quito: Imprenta y Encuadernación Nacionales, 1914.

———. *Informe que Modesto A. Peñaherrera, ministro de lo interior, municipalidades, policía, obras públicas, etc., presenta a la nación en 1916.* Quito: Imprenta y Encuadernación Nacionales, 1916.

Peralta, José. *Informe del ministro de instrucción pública al congreso ordinario de 1900.* Quito: Imprenta de la Universidad Central, 1900.

Pieper Mooney, Jadwiga. *The Politics of Motherhood: Maternity and Women's Rights in Twentieth-Century Chile.* Pittsburgh: University of Pittsburgh Press, 2009.

Pineo, Ronn. *Ecuador and the United States: Useful Strangers.* Athens: University of Georgia Press, 2007.

Prado, L. Estuardo. "La protección de la infancia en el Ecuador." *Revista del Centro de Estudiantes de Medicina* 13–14 (third series, 1930): 14–66.

Premat, Adriana. "Popular Culture, Politics, and Alternative Gender Imaginaries in the Argentina of the 1960s and 1970s." Unpublished manuscript.

Prieto, Mercedes. "Las trampas del silencio: Estado y mujeres indígenas en Ecuador, 1925–1975." Paper presented at the conference Off-Centered States: State Formation and Deformation in the Andes. Quito. May 2010.

———. *Liberalismo y temor: Imaginando los sujetos indígenas en el Ecuador postcolonial, 1895–1950.* Quito: FLACSO, 2004.

———. "Rosa Lema y la misión cultural ecuatoriana indígena a Estados Unidos: turismo, artesanías y desarrollo." In *Galo Plaza y su época.* Edited by Carlos de la Torre and Mireya Salgado. 157–91. Quito: FLACSO and Fundación Galo Plaza Lasso, 2008.

Quintero, Rafael, and Erika Silva. *Ecuador: Una nación en ciernes.* Volume 1. Quito: FLACSO and Abya Yala, 1991.

*Reglamento interno de la Escuela de Enfermeras anexa a la Facultad de Medicina de la Universidad Central del Ecuador.* Quito: Imprenta Nacional, 1921.

Roberts, Elizabeth F. S. *God's Laboratory: Assisted Reproduction in the Andes.* Berkeley: University of California Press, 2012.

Rodas, Raquel. *Crónica de un sueño: Las escuelas indígenas de Dolores Cacuango.* Quito: Proyecto EBI-MEC-GTZ, 1989.

———. "De los inicios de la República a la Revolución Juliana." In *Historia del voto femenino en el Ecuador.* Edited by Raquel Rodas Morales. 19–134. Quito: Consejo Nacional de las Mujeres, 2009.

———. *Nosotras que del amor hicimos . . . .* Quito: Fraga, 1992.

Rodríguez, Linda Alexander. *The Search for Public Policy: Regional Politics and Government Finances in Ecuador, 1830–1940*. Berkeley: University of California Press, 1985.

Roseberry, William. *Anthropologies and Histories: Essays in Culture, History, and Political Economy*. New Brunswick: Rutgers University Press, 1989.

Rosemblatt, Karin. *Gendered Compromises: Political Cultures and the State in Chile, 1920–1950*. Chapel Hill: University of North Carolina Press, 2000.

Ruggiero, Kristin. "Honor, Maternity, and the Disciplining of Women: Infanticide in Late Nineteenth-Century Buenos Aires." *Hispanic American Historical Review* 72, no. 3 (1992): 353–73.

———. "Wives on 'Deposit': Internment and the Preservation of Husbands' Honor in Late Nineteenth-Century Buenos Aires." *Journal of Family History* 17, no. 3 (1992): 253–70.

Sánchez, Carlos R. "La importancia del estudio de puericultura en la enseñanza escolar." *Anales de la Universidad Central* 41, no. 265 (1928): 16–19.

———. "Protección a la infancia." *Anales de la Universidad Central* 31, no. 246 (1923): 57–64.

Saunders, J. V. D. *The People of Ecuador: A Demographic Analysis*. Gainesville: University of Florida Press, 1961.

Schild, Verónica. "Empowering Consumer Citizens or Governing Poor Female Subjects? The Institutionalization of 'Self-Development' in the Chilean Social Policy Field." *Journal of Consumer Culture* 7, no. 2 (2007): 179–203.

———. "Neoliberalism's New Gendered Market Citizens: The 'Civilizing' Dimension of Social Programs in Chile." *Citizenship Studies* 4, no. 3 (2000): 275–305.

Smith, Carol A. "Race-Class-Gender Ideology in Guatemala: Modern and Anti-Modern Forms." *Comparative Studies in Society and History* 37, no. 4 (1995): 723–49.

Stepan, Nancy Leys. *"The Hour of Eugenics": Race, Gender, and Nation in Latin America*. Ithaca: Cornell University Press, 1991.

Stoler, Ann. *Along the Archival Grain: Epistemic Anxieties and Colonial Common Sense*. Princeton: Princeton University Press, 2009.

Suárez, Pablo Arturo. *Contribución al estudio de las realidades entre las clases obreras y campesinas*. Quito: Imprenta de la Universidad Central, 1934.

———, A. López, and Cornelio Donoso. "Estudio numérico y económico-social de la población de Quito." *Boletín del departamento médico social* 1, no. 1 (1937): 7–11.

Velasco, Margarita, and Soledad Alvarez. *La historia contada desde las líderes: Precursoras 1940–1980*. Quito: Federación Ecuatoriana de Enfermeras/os, 2002.

Walkowitz, Judith R. *Prostitution and Victorian Society: Women, Class, and the State*. Cambridge: Cambridge University Press, 1980.

Williams, Derek. "Assembling the 'Empire of Morality': State Building Strategies in Catholic Ecuador, 1861–1875." *Journal of Historical Sociology* 14, no. 2 (2001): 149–74.

Wolf, Eric R. *Peasant Wars of the Twentieth Century.* New York: Harper and Row, 1969.

Zambrano, Pedro J. *Estudio de la prostitución en Quito.* Quito: Imprenta Nacional, 1924.

———. "Historia del reglamento de la prostitución." *Boletín sanitario* (Quito) 1, no. 1 (1926): 41–58.

Zulawski, Ann. *Unequal Cures: Public Health and Political Change in Bolivia, 1900–1950.* Durham: Duke University Press, 2007.

# INDEX

*Note:* page numbers in italic type indicate tables and a map

Abbott, Andrew, 223n51

abortion, 137–41, 185, 187, 224n63, 225n68

Abrams, Philip, 3

Acijuela, Manuela, 43

Afro-Ecuadorians, 175

A.G. (orphan), 43

agency, 3, 9, 193n3

agrarian reform (1960s), 32

Aguirre, Adrila, x, 225n1, 231n79

alcoholism, 92

Alfaro, Colón E., 150

Alfaro, Eloy, 10, 13–14, 23

Allende, Salvador (physician), 57

Americanas, las, 143, 154, 156–58, 176–77, 228n30

anatomo-politics (Foucault), 24

Andrade Marín, Carlos, 57, 76, 96, 144, 177

Andrade Stacey, Alicia and Ximena, x, 194n17

Araujo, Angel F. and Obdulia Chiriboga de, 40–41

Araujo, Gabriel, 63, 208n107

Arauz (Doctor), 162–63

Armas, Judith, 157

Arrellano, Cecilia de, x, 221n19

Arroyo del Río, Carlos, 7, 12

Asilo Antonio Gil, 48–50, 61

Asistencia Pública. *See* Beneficencia/ Asistencia Pública, Junta de

Asociación de Empleados, 87

Asociación de Trabajadores del Fósforo Libertad y Justicia, 74

Ayabaca, Dolores, 134

Ayora, Isidro, 4–5, 62, 92, 206n92, 207n101; nurses and midwives, 115, 125–26, 142, 145, 148–49; venereal disease prophylaxis, 84

Baca, Héctor, 73–74

Baker, Charles, 54

banana production, 12–13

Barberis, Luis, 62, 65

barchilonas, 145–46, 182

Barrera, Jaime, 10

Bastidas, Antonio, 61, 76–77, 187, 207n100

Batallas, Eduardo, 68

Becker, Marc, x, 31

Beneficencia/Asistencia Pública, Junta de, xi, 30, 34–36, 70, 200n4; and children's hospital ward, 54–55, 61; daycare, 49, 64–67; and Escuela Nacional de Enfermeras, 151–52; home medical visits, 68–69; infant care, 64; and Maternidad de Quito, 115; and orphanages, 36, 38–39

Besse, Susan, 22

biopolitics (Foucault), 24–25

Black, Chad, 26

Bliss, Katherine, 107

Blum, Ann, 203n54

Bourdieu, Pierre, 29

bronchitis, 54, 57, 68–69

bubonic plague, 35, 80

Buen Pastor convent, 34, 38–39, 42, 44, 72, 216n78

Bustamante, Carlos, 151, 163–64, 173–74, 176–77

Byron, George Gordon (Lord), 9

cacao production, 12, 106

Cacciopo de Cevallos, Anne, 153–55, 161

Cacuango, Dolores, 7, 31

Cadena, Reina, 116

Caesarean section, 187

Caja del Seguro, 20, 152

Caja de Pensiones, 20

Camarote de Santa Marta (Hospital San Juan de Dios), 139

Carrera, Inés, 68, 209n130

Casares Rivera, Manuel María, 59

Catholic Church: and education, 6, 11, 194nn10–11; and nursing, 147, 190, 231n73; and rehabilitation of prostitutes, 216n78; and sexuality, 108; and social welfare, 11, 34–36, 60; and state, 6, 11, 13, 15–16, 34–35, 51–52. See also specific institutions and religious orders

census, 28, 53

Central Bank, 12

Centro de Re-educación Femenina, 72

Cevallos, Hortensia, 129

charity, 36, 58–60, 70–72, 74–75, 200n3, 207n95

child protection and welfare: abandoned children, 37–48, 64–66, 203n52; child labor, 37–42; daycare, 42, 48–51, 63–64, 66–67; digestive problems, 54–57, 64, 66, 75–77; and eugenics and genetic constitution, 72, 76–77, 82; as gendered social policy, 33, 36–40, 46–48, 75–77; infant mortality, 53–69, 57, 113–14, 183, 203n52, 222n35; mothers as responsible for, 55–56, 66, 75–77; mothers receiving state support and education, 52, 58, 62, 64, 112–13, 127–29; orphans and orphanages, 34, 36–51, 66–67, 71, 203n52; and population expansion for economic growth, 50–53, 114; provision of sterilized milk, 54–56, 58, 63–64, 66, 73, 184; state medical care, 50–69, 184; use by poor of state facilities for temporary care, 44–48, 73–74; venereal disease, 81, 92, 100–101, 104, 212n6. See also illegitimacy

Children's Bureau (U.S.), 176, 209n134

chulla quiteña, la, 182

Civil Code (1967), 187

Civil Guard, 97–98

Civil Marriage and Divorce Law (1902), 15

civil registry, 15, 52–54

Civil Registry Law (1900), 52

Clínica de la Caja del Seguro (CCS), 126, 161, 165

Clínica Endara, 126

Clínica Moderna, 126

Clínica Narváez, 126
Clínica Pasteur, 126, 153
Clínica Quito, 126
Clínica Román, 126
Club de Profesores del Instituto Nacional Mejía, 7
Código de Menores (Child Code, 1938), 2, 33, 41, 69–70
Colegio 24 de Mayo, 135, 223n44
Colegio de La Providencia, 38
Colegio Normal Juan Montalvo, 85
Colegio Normal Manuela Cañizares, 6
colonias infantiles sanitarias, 69
Comedor de la Madre, 64
Comité Pro-habilitamiento del Pabellón de Niños del Hospital Eugenio Espejo, 74
Comité "Pro Infancia" (Quito military academy), 72
Concordat with Vatican (1862), 6, 16
Confederación de Nacionalidades Indígenas del Ecuador (CONAIE), 7
Conferencia de San Vicente de Paul, 59
Consejo General de Instrucción Pública, 116
Consejo Nacional de Menores, 72
Constitution (1897), 16
Constitution (1929), 5
contraception, 109
Coronel, Valeria, x, 11
Correa, Alberto, 98
Corrigan, Philip, 184
Coyan, Ambrocia, 40
Crespo, Emiliano, 76
Crespo de Ortiz Bilbao, Lola, 42
Customs Service, 17–18
Cuvi Sánchez, María, 10

Dávila, Luis G., 65–66, 76, 92
Defenses Services Corporation (U.S.), 144

de la Cruz, Francisca, 116–17
de la Torre, Luis, 66
del Pino, Blanca Rosa, 123
de Mora, Fanny, 156
de Mora, Mercedes, 228n26
dentistry, 18, 116
Depression (1930s), 12, 93–95, 106
Diaz, Marina, 157
Díaz, Octavio, 74
Di Capua, Alberto, 160
divorce, 15–16, 124, 220n15
Drinot, Paulo, x, 25

Ecuador Peru War (1941), 144
education: and church and state, 6, 8, 13, 16–17, 117, 190, 194nn10–11; and women, 4–6, 10, 16–17, 117, 186, 196n38, 197n47, 199n78. See also specific schools and professions
Egas, Judith, 228n29
Ehrlich, Paul, 213n16
El Labrador, 37
enfermeras, 145–46, 148
Escobar de Ruiz, Emperatriz, 45–46
Escuela de Enfermeras San Vicente de Paul, 229n40
Escuela Nacional de Enfermeras (ENE, National Nurses School), 2, 30, 71, 143–45, 151–58, 155, 172, 189
Escuela Nacional de Trabajadores Sociales, 209n134
Escuela-Taller de Mujeres, 8
Espinosa, Tula, 157, 167–68, 230n65
Espinosa Tamayo, Alfredo, 75
estado terrateniente, 15
Estupiñán, Augusto, 162, 166–67, 170
Estupiñan, Dolores de, 42
expósitos, 36

Faculty of Law (Universidad Central), 18, 116, 159

Faculty of Medicine (Universidad Central), 18, 30, 114, 116

Federación Ecuatoriana de Indios, 7

feminism. *See* women's rights movement and reforms

Ferguson, Ruth, 154

Flores, Diana, 153

Foley, Dorothy, 154–55, 176

Foucault, Michel, 24–25, 50

Franco, Emma, 117

French Revolution (1789), 147

Gallegos Anda, Enrique, 19–20, 58

Galvis, Colombia, 157, 160–61, 229n43

Garcés, Enrique, 89, 91

García Drouet, Carlos, 55–56

García Moreno, Gabriel, 13, 35, 114–15, 146, 216n78

gender ideologies and attitudes, ix; and child protection policies, 33, 36–40, 46–48, 75–77; in combating venereal disease, 79, 81, 84–85, 87, 99, 110; and concepts of honor, 26–27; and elite charity work, 60; and indigenous women, 31–32; and midwifery, 26, 120; and nursing, 164, 169–70, 182, 230n65; protection policies, 33, 36–40, 46–48, 75–77; and sexuality, 79–80, 170, 182, 185; and state formation and reform, 1–2, 16, 23–24

gender relations, 16, 164, 169–70, 182, 186, 196n38, 230n65, 230n67. *See also* male protector

gender studies, ix, 26–27, 198n65

Geneva Declaration of the Rights of the Child (1923), 60

Gil, Antonio, 48

Goetschel, Ana María, x, 9–10

Gómez de la Torre, Joaquín, 5

Gómez de la Torre, Jóse, 177

Gómez de la Torre, María Luisa, 5–9, 187

Gomezjurado Narváez, Ligia, 154–55, 157–58, 161, 165, 168, 170–72, 176–83, 229n40

gonorrhea, 84, 213n28. *See also* venereal disease

González Delgado, Julia, 123

González Palacios, Luis, 223n53

González Suárez, Federico, 119

Gota de Leche, Sociedad de La, 58–64, 69–70, 189–90, 206n89

governmentality (Foucault), 24–25

Granja, Carmela, 137–40, 223n53

Granja, Olga, 157

Grijalva, Victoria, 157

Grijalva Polanco, Rafael, 54, 79–80

Groves, Ruth, 154

Guayas province, *xiv*, 18

*Guía comercial, agrícola e industrial* (1909), 17

Guy, Donna, 81

haciendas de asistencia pública, 34, 69

Hermanas de la Caridad (Sisters of Charity), 21, 189–90, 226n11; and healthcare administration, 35–36, 66, 70–71, 139, 145–47, 153, 165; and midwifery, 115; and nursing, 145–46, 149–50, 159–65, 168, 170, 172, 182, 229n40; and pharmacy, 219n4

Hermanas del Buen Pastor, 216n78

Hermanas Dominicanas, 63–64

Hermandad Ferroviaria, 74

Hidalgo de Prócel, Matilde, 3–5, 7–9, 18, 22, 122–23

Hierro, Luis and Maria H. del, 46–47

highland Ecuador, *xiv*, 15, 23, 26–32, 58, 207n95

Higiene Escolar (Department of Education), 70, 150, 152

Hogares de Protección Social, 72, 152

honor, 45–46, 48, 140, 179; concept in gender studies, 26–27, 198n65; male protector as guarantor, 27–30, 45, 99–104, 110; work as establishing, 13–15, 111, 114, 190

Hospicio y Manicomio, 34, 46

Hospital Civil San Juan de Dios, xi, 21, 30, 34, 54, 146, 165, 226n7; and children, 55–58, 61, 68

Hospital de la Misericordia de Nuestro Señor Jesucristo, 146

Hospital de Niños Baca-Ortiz, 61

Hospital Eugenio Espejo, 68, 73–74, 150, 160–61, 226n7

hospitalism (Mexico), 67

Hospital Militar, 54, 126

Hospital Pablo Arturo Suárez, 226n7

hospital servants (barchilonas), 145–46, 182

huérfanos, 36

illegitimacy, ix, xii, 29, 42, 187–88; and economic vulnerability, 120, 120–24, 122, 141; as health risk, 76–77, 101, 108–9

indigenous people, 7, 31–32, 88, 120

inheritance tax, 63

Institute for Inter-American Affairs (U.S. State Department), 143, 154, 176

Instituto Nacional Mejía, 6, 8, 17, 85, 117, 223n44

Instituto Normal Manuela Cañizares, 117

International Handbook of Child Health, 57

J.A.O. (expósito), 43

J.G.L. (expósito), 42

Jijón Larrea, Manuel, 37–38

Josefina (superiora of San Vicente), 38

Juan López, Pedro, 45

Junta Central de Asistencia Pública. See Beneficencia/Asistencia Pública, Junta de

Junta de Beneficencia. See Beneficencia/Asistencia Pública, Junta de

J.V.M. (adopted child), 43

La Providencia convent, 34, 44

Larrea, Zoila and Rosa, 119

Larrea Borja, Piedad, 23–24

Larrea Stacey, Eduardo, ix, xi

Lasso, Sergio, 62

Lasso de Eastman, María, 62, 207n101

Latorre, Delfina, 119

Law of Civil Registry (1900), 15

Lazareto de Pifo (lepers' colony), 34

Leifson, Esben, x, 31, 41, 200n2, 206n93

Ley de Beneficencia (1908), 34

Ley de Boticas (1920), 120

Ley de Cultos (1904), 34

Ley de Educación Sexual (1951), 109

Ley de Fomento Agrícola (1918), 58

Ley de Sanidad (1908), 78–79

Liberal Revolution (1895) and social policies, 3, 6, 8, 11, 15, 17, 115, 190

Liceo Fernández Madrid, 223n44

life expectancy, 24, 28, 183, 190

literacy, 7, 88, 109, 194–95n7, 199n78

Lituma, Filomena, 157, 171

L.J.M. (expósito), 47

L.L (expósita), 40

Logan, Kathleen, 154–55, 162–64

male protector, 10–11, 27–30, 45, 99–107, 110, 122–24, 123–24

Mantilla, César, 72

María de San José (Superiora Sor), 38–39
Mariana de Jesús Social Work School, 209n134
marriage, 28–29, 53–54, 93–94, 102–4
Martínez, Luis A., 18–19
Martínez, Nela, 5
Martínez, Rosa, 134
Martínez Serrano, Francisco, 78
Maternidad de Quito, 2, 34, 68, 115, 125, 138, 220n17
Maternidad Isidro Ayora, 126, 158, 165
M.D. (expósita), 40
Mena de Barrera, Rosario, 10, 18
mental illness, 34, 37, 46, 48–50, 61
methodology and sources, ix–xi, 1, 24–32
Mexican Revolution (1910), 22
Middlemiss, Anne, 154–55, 166, 176, 228n29
midwifery, 9, 131–32, 221n25, 222n26; background and economic status, 113, 117–24, 118, 120, 123–24, 134, 137, 189; as both independent and marginalized, 41, 141–42, 186–87; as morally suspect, 134–41, 185–86, 225n68; profession open to women, 4, 113, 186; relations with physicians and unlicensed midwives, 26, 124–40, 131, 220n16; training and licensing, 2, 112–18, 120–21
Ministerio de Previsión Social, Trabajo y Agricultura, 52
Ministry of Health, 141. See also Sanidad, Servicio de (Public Health Service)
Miño, Carlos, 35–36, 48–50, 53–55, 60–61, 79–81, 83, 85
Miranda, Alejandrina, 120
Miranda, Juana, 63, 125, 135, 137
M.L.L. (child given up by widowed father), 45
modernization and industrialization, 1, 12–15, 17, 22, 38, 58–59

Morales de Carrillo, Georgina, x, 179, 183, 225n1
Morgan, Lynn, 25
Mosquera, Lucelina, 157
Mosquera Narváez, Alfonso, 61–62, 68, 140, 155
Mosquera Narváez, Aurelio, 155
mujer, La (magazine), 18, 24
Muñoz, Leonardo, 7
Muñoz v. de Vega, Carmen, 49, 59
Murillo, Guillermina, 157
Murphy, Pansy Virginia, 154–55, 157, 162, 177–78

National Library, 18
Navarro, Juan Francisco, 40
Needham, Isabel, 154–55
Nelson, Siobhan, 170, 226n11
Neosalvarsan, 82, 213n16, 213n28
Nicklin, Olive, 154–55, 176–77
nodrizas, 62
notificadores, 89
nursing, 9, 186–87, 189; background of students, 146, 153, 171–75, 186, 189, 227n25; establishment as profession, 162–83, 185; and gender relations, 164, 169–70, 182, 230n65; and morality, 144–45, 147, 176–83, 185–86, 190, 231n73; precursors, 145–50; profession open to women, 18, 116; relations with physicians and midwives, 142, 165–70, 230n65, 231n79; training, 2–3, 118, 144, 158–61, 164–67, 171–72

obstetricia, 114
Ochoa, Carlos, 43
Ochoa, Piedad, 153, 157
O'Connor, Erin, x, 31
Oficina de Higiene Municipal, 78–79
oil production, 183

Ormaza, Gregorio, 69–70
Ortega, Genoveva, 43
Ortega, Manuela, 118
Ortiz, Dolores, 61, 73–74
Ortiz, Miguel, 45

Páez, Francisca, 5
Palmer, Steven, x, 137
Palmieri, Aurelia, 16, 196n38
Panagra airline (U.S.), 144
Pareja, Wenceslao, 91–92
partera, 114
Partido Socialista Ecuatoriano, 7
patria potestad, 46–48
peasant revolutions, 188
Peñaherrera, Modesto, 11
penicillin, 80, 96, 213n16
Peralta, José, 14–15
pharmacy, 4, 18, 113, 116
physicians, 228n26, 228n29
Pichincha province, xiv, 18
Plaza, Leonidas, 11, 13, 62
Plaza Lasso, Galo, 12–13
police, 84–85, 92–93, 96–98
Policía de Higiene y Salubridad, 79
poliomyelitis, 160, 170
Pólit, Carlos, 168
Polytechnic School, 114
Pontificia Universidad Católica del
    Ecuador, 229n40
Population Council (New York), 51
populism, 12, 183
postal system, 17–18
Pozo i Diaz, Braulio, 68
Prieto, Mercedes, x, 31
prisons, 86, 213n29
Prócel, Fernando, 4–5
prostitution, 1–2, 9, 72, 184–85, 213n29,
    216n78, 217n89; causes and ethnic and

social makeup, 88–89, *88–89*, 105–10;
    combating and regulation, 14, 78–83,
    87–93, 101–3

Quevedo Coronel, Rafael, 69

Racines, Isabel María, 119
R.C. (juvenile delinquent), 46
Red Cross, 60, 67, 158, 189, 206n89,
    206n92
Reglamento de Profilaxis de la Prosti-
    tución (1926), 81, 83
Reglamento de Vigilancia de la Prosti-
    tución (1926), 81
reproductive governance, 25
Reverendas Madres de los Sagrados
    Corazones, 35
Revolución Gloriosa (1944), 7, 12
Revolución Juliana (1925), 5, 12, 52, 84
Robalino, Isabel, 116
Robalino Dávila, Luis, 206n92
Roberts, Elizabeth, x, 25, 187
Rockefeller, John D., 51
Rockefeller, Nelson A., 143
Rockefeller Foundation, 143–44, 151, 177,
    189, 229n43
Rodas, Raquel, 23
Román, Antonio, 208n107
Rosalino Cruz, Luis, 42–43
Rosemblatt, Karin, 217n88
Rotary Club of Quito, 72–73
Rueda Sáenz, Consuelo, 112–13, 122, 125,
    128, 132–36
Ruggiero, Kristin, 137

Sagrados Corazones convent, 34–35, 44,
    117
Salazar, María Luisa, 10
Salgado, Mireya, 10–11, 18, 77

Salgado Vivanco, Eustorgio, 10, 83, 162

San Carlos orphanage, 34, 36–39, 44

Sánchez, Carlos R., 44, 51, 56, 156, 162–63, 166–67, 205n79

San Gabriel orphanage, 37

Sanidad, Servicio de (Public Health Service), xi, 30–31, 61, 70, 208n116; antivenereal campaign and regulation of prostitution, 84–104; and infants and children, 2, 35–36, 61–63, 68–69; and nurses and midwives, 120, 151

Sanidad Militar, 84

San Juan orphanage, 39

Santamaría, Rosa, x, 225n1, 231n73

Santo Domingo de Conocoto, 69

San Vicente orphanage, 34, 36–39

Sares, Adelina, 157

Saunders, John, 28, 188

School of Obstetrics (Universidad Central), 115, 121

Schwarz, Frida, 148–49

secularization and separation of church and state, 15–16, 52; and child protection, 35–36, 71; and education, 17, 117, 190; and nursing, 147, 149–50

Sedta airline (German), 144

Señoras de la Caridad. See Sociedad de las Señoras de la Caridad

Servicio Cooperativo Interamericano, 95, 143, 151, 172, 177, 189

Servicio de Profilaxis Venérea (SPV, Veneral Prophylaxis Service), 2, 81–104, 184–85, 213n28. See also venereal disease

sexuality, 24–25, 77, 79–80, 106–10, 170, 182, 185, 223–24n53

Sindicato de la Madera, 74

Sindicato de Profesores, 7

socialism and communism, 5, 7

social mobility and transformation, 12, 85, 188–89

social workers, 69, 209n134

Sociedad Artística e Industrial de Pichincha, 73–74, 87

Sociedad Bar de Pichincha, 87

Sociedad de Carpinteros Union y Progreso, 74

Sociedad de La Gota de Leche. See Gota de Leche, Sociedad de La

Sociedad de las Señoras de la Caridad, 59, 190, 206n90

Sociedad de Puericultura, 63

Sociedad de San Vicenta de Paul, 59, 206n90

Sociedad Funeraria Nacional, 54

Sociedad Nacional de Agricultura (SNA), 58–59

Sociedad Protectora de la Infancia, 48–50, 62–63

Spanish influenza, 56, 60

Stacey, Diego (James), 9

Stacey, Rosa, 8–9, 18, 187

Stacey Sanz, Manuel, 9, 18

state formation and institutions, 3, 5, 7, 11–12, 25–26, 52, 84, 184; and women, 1–2, 142, 190. See also Liberal Revolution (1895) and social policies; modernization and industrialization; secularization and separation of church and state

Sternberg, Alicia, 70–71

Stoler, Ann, 30–31

Suárez, Pablo Arturo, 62–63, 69–70, 106, 207n101

Surette, Genoveva, 154–55

syphilis, 79–80, 84, 90, 93–94, 213n16, 213n28. See also venereal disease

Tamayo, José Luis, 81
telegraph system, 18
Tolóntag (hacienda de asistencia pública), 69
Torres, Angela, 123
Tribunales de Menores, 41

Ugarte de Landívar, Zoila, 18, 23
Unión Internacional Contra el Peligro Venéreo (France), 82
United States, 2, 95, 143–45, 153–54, 158, 176–77
Universidad Central, xi, 18, 116; female students, 30, 32; nurse and midwife training, 114, 152, 158–59
urbanization, 28

Vaca v. de Aguirre, Rosario, 47
Valencia de Valencia, Margarita, 44–45
Vallejo, Juliana, 115
Velasco Ibarra, José María, 7, 12
Velásquez, María, 43
venereal disease, 1, 24–25, 78–80, 107–10, 212n6, 213n16; Servicio de Profilaxis Venérea (SPV), 2, 81–104, 184–85, 189, 213n28
Vera, José María, 45
Verduga, Teresa, 158
Villavicencio, Salomón and Jacinta Andrade de, 40

Vivero, Lusitania, 18
voting rights, 5, 12, 22–23, 193–94nn6–8
V. v. de Pinto, Virginia, 41

Walkowitz, Judith, 82
Wandemberg, Benjamin, 83, 158
wet nurses, 43–44, 62–67, 76
white slavery, 82
whooping cough, 60, 68
Wolf, Eric, 188
women's rights movement and reforms, 5, 8, 12–17, 22–24, 193–94nn6–8
work open to women, 9, 12–15, 17, 22; domestic service, 199n72; education, 24, 125, 221n19; factory labor, 199n69; government employment, 16–22; medical professions, 4, 18–20, 113, 116, 186, 228n26, 228n29
World War I, 12, 35, 106
World War II, 144

yellow fever, 80
Yépez, Ligia, 157

Zambrano, Pedro, 83, 86, 88–89, 94–95, 101–3, 105, 213n28
Zulawski, Ann, 137
Zumba v. de Latorre, Rosa, 44